The Promise of Sleep

A Pioneer in Sleep Medicine
Explores the Vital Connection
Between Health, Happiness,
and a Good Night's Sleep

WILLIAM C. DEMENT, M.D., PH.D.
and Christopher Vaughan

A Living Planet Press Book

Delacorte Press

IMPORTANT NOTE:

This book is not intended to take the place of medical advice from your medical professional. Readers are advised to consult a physician or other qualified health professional regarding treatment of all of their health problems. Neither the publisher nor the authors take any responsibility for any possible consequences from any treatment, action, or application of medicine or preparation by any person reading or following the information in this book.

Published by
Delacorte Press
Random House, Inc.
1540 Broadway
New York, New York 10036

Copyright © 1999 by William C. Dement

Library of Congress Cataloging in Publication Data

Dement, William C., 1928–
    The promise of sleep : a pioneer in sleep medicine
  explores the vital connection between health, happiness,
  and a good night's sleep / by William C. Dement and
  Christopher Vaughan.
        p.   cm.
    ISBN 0-385-32008-6
    1. Sleep—Popular works.   2. Sleep disorders—
  Popular works.   I. Vaughan, Christopher C., 1961–   .
  II. Title.
  RA786.D43   1999
  612.8′21—dc21   98-23527
                                                                  CIP

Manufactured in the United States of America
Published simultaneously in Canada

March 1999

10 9 8 7 6 5 4 3 2 1

First and foremost, to my wife, Pat, who was the first to show me that women also have rapid eye movements during sleep. She has put up with the life of a sleep researcher for more than four decades, and set a world record for "putting up with" during the writing of this book. In order to avoid chaos and minimize confusion over the past year, each room of our house has been the work site for one or two chapters. Insomnia was in the guest bedroom and sleep debt in the kitchen.

And to my children: Cathy, Elizabeth, and Nick, and my son-in-law, Gary Roos. And to my grandsons, David, Matthew, and Christopher, and my mother, who gave me a pretty good start and drew me ever back to Walla Walla.

Acknowledgments

IT IS a real challenge to get one's arms around nearly half a century of work and have the description of it remain meaningful and interesting to the people for whom it is intended. Successful or not, this book could not have been written without lots of help and for this I first acknowledge Chris Vaughan.

Excellent hands-on help is very hard to come by, but I have been lucky enough to be blessed with an amazing assistant, Adam Strom, who has put in an incredible amount of work. For their invaluable assistance I would like to thank Sonia Barragan, Kathy Ho, Natasha Belanger, and Pam Hyde.

Also, I thank the staff at Living Planet Press and Delacorte Press, with a special thanks to Tom Spain and Mitch Hoffman. And from the perspective of what it's all about, I thank the more than 15,000 Stanford students who have made three decades of "Sleep and Dreams" much more fun than work.

Before mentioning more individuals, I would like to acknowledge a very special organization, the National Sleep Foundation. Its mission statement reads: "The National Sleep Foundation promotes public understanding of sleep and sleep disorders and supports sleep-related education, research, and advocacy to improve public health and safety." It is my great privilege to be a member of the board of directors and chairman of its standing committee on government affairs. A number of my most distinguished and public-spirited colleagues are also on the Board or are participating with the Foundation in many ways to advance its great mission. Among many outstanding activities, the Foundation conducts polls that have created an expanding database of knowledge about sleep, and there will now be an omnibus poll every year as part of National Sleep Awareness Week, which will give us a longitudinal database. I have referred to the results of these polls many times throughout this book, and I am grateful to the Foundation and its truly outstanding and dedicated staff for acquiring this information and look forward to exciting new findings in the future. The work of the National Sleep Foundation deserves everyone's support, financial and otherwise. Information about the Foundation, as well as other professional and patient organizations, may be found in the Appendix.

I would now like to thank the numerous people who have helped and/or inspired me throughout my career and life. So as to overlook as few as possible, I have arranged them by the stage in my life in which they first appeared.

From the University of Chicago, I begin with Nathaniel Kleitman who, at over 100 years of age, lives in Santa Monica, and in my heart as well, now and forever. Next is Eugene Aserinsky—if he hadn't temporarily lost interest in sleep I might have become a rich surgeon. I also acknowledge Kao Liang Chow and John Perkins, each an epitome of pure science; Elliot Weitzman, classmate and then colleague; and finally, Chris Athas then and now— "Ere the end some work of noble note may yet be done."

From the years in New York City, I must first mention Howie Roffwarg, who became a lifelong colleague and friend. I would also like to thank Charles Fisher at Mount Sinai, Allan Rechtschaffen, who has stayed in the field to make great contributions, and Fred Snyder whose herculean efforts are not fully appreciated.

From the years of the Quonset hut at Stanford I would like to acknowledge Jim Ferguson, Kathy McGarr, Peter Henry, Stuart Rawlings, Vince Zarcone, Greg Belenky, George Mitchell, Jon Glick, Bill Gonda, Terry Pivik, Steve Henriksen, Vicki Varner, and Barbara Scavullo.

Later at Stanford, in the years of the museum basement, I had the privilege of working with Merrill Mitler, Christian Guilleminault, John Orem, Barry Jacobs, and Gary Richardson.

The period of expansion and the Association of Sleep Disorders Centers brought me in contact with innumerable good people, including Tom Roth, David Kupfer, John Karacan, Bill Orr, Charles Pollack, Chip Reynolds, Mitchell Balter, Bob Purpura, and Mark Rosekind.

During the past two decades Wes Seidel, Dale Edgar, Tom Kilduff, Craig Heller, Nelson Powell, Jed Black, Bob Riley, Clete Kushida, Raphael Pelayo, Joe Miller, Emmanuel Mignot, Seiji Nishino, Meir Kryger, Phil and Carol Westbrook, Carolyn Hiller, Lynn Lamberg, and Andy Monjan have made my job both enjoyable and rewarding.

Senator Mark Hatfield—I wish our paths had crossed much earlier. All of the members of the National Commission on Sleep Disorders Research and Mollly Haselhorst deserve high praise and boundless gratitude.

A very special thanks to Jim Walsh, Dale Dirks, Senator Ted Kennedy, Congresswoman Anna Eshoo, John Lauber, Barbara Shoup, Michael Thorpy, and Don Bliwise. And in Walla Walla and Moscow, Dick Simon, Eric Ball, Jennings Falcon, John Grauke, and Debee Nichols.

Mary O'Brien, Neil Feldman, Sue Cohen, Laurose Richter, Elisabeth Chowning, Kathleen Chittenden, and Frankie Roman have been the most outstanding members of the tiny group of "do-gooders" to whom the world owes much. Additionally, I would like to acknowledge all of the Chairs of the standing committees of what has evolved into the American Academy of Sleep Medicine, and had started as the Association of Sleep Disorders Centers.

Thanks also go out to Helio Lemmi, Pierre Passouant, Michel Billiard, Jay Cinque, and Charles Krauthammer from Project Sleep; Chris Gillen, and Wally Mendelson.

A super special acknowledgment to Barbara Corneille, Peter Bing, Michel Jouvet, Elio Lugaresi, Mary Carskadon, Sharon Keenan, Tibby Simon, Jim Dewson, Darrell Drobnich, Peter Farrell, Pat Gonzales-Casey, and Lynn Hassler.

And spanning all these years, David and Betty Hamburg, ever my wise mentors and faithful friends.

To those (probably many) of you whom I have failed to mention and who certainly deserve acknowledgment, thank you and I must plead sleep loss amnesia.—WCD

I would like the thank the many people who pulled together, year-round, to make the publication of this book possible. First of all, I would like to thank our excellent and patient editor, Tom Spain, and his steadfast assistant, Mitch Hoffman, at Delacorte Press. Big thanks go to the many others at Delacorte who made the extra effort to push the book through, particularly Susan Schwartz, Mark Pensavalle, and Johanna Tani, for their professional oversight of the project, and to both Debra Manette and Tom Kleh for their heroic red-pencil work. In addition I would like to thank our agent, Gail Ross, and the persistent folks who worked on the book at Living Planet Press: Joshua Horwitz, Julie Kuzniski, and Diana Morgan. We owe a great deal to the hardship and sweat of those in the Dement office who worked on the book—Adam Strom, Kathy Ho, Natasha Belanger, Clarence Miao, Sonia Barragan, and many others. A big hug and thanks go to Pat Dement for her support and back-channel diplomacy. Lastly, and most of all, I would like to thank my family for their undying patience, support, and faith—particularly my wife, Laurie. I can truly say that without extraordinary efforts by everyone this book would never have been created.—CV

Contents

Part Four: The Principles of Healthy Sleep

The Promise of Sleep

Prescription for Sleep-Sick Society

JUST A FEW MONTHS ago a colleague of mine had the good fortune of being able to save her nephew's life. Adam was only 12 months old, but it was clear that something was terribly wrong with him. While other kids his age were beginning to walk and talk, Adam couldn't even crawl. His weight and height were far below the norm for his age. He was a tiny, sad, emaciated specter. Every single day of the year, Adam's parents held him and hovered over him, frustrated, heartbroken, frantic with worry. Did Adam have cancer? Some awful birth defect? No. After tens of thousands of dollars' worth of medical testing, their child had been categorized only as having a "failure to thrive." This is actually a nondiagnosis—a medical throwing up of the hands that meant his doctors had no idea what was wrong. The small army of pediatricians who saw Adam could only say that this baby might waste away and die, or might never be normal if he did survive.

During a visit to her sister's house, my colleague observed Adam while he slept. Being knowledgeable about sleep disorders, she realized right away that the boy could not breathe when he was asleep. His disorder, well known to sleep specialists, was, in this instance, caused mainly by large tonsils and adenoids. His tiny air passages, barely adequate while he was awake, were completely closed off during sleep. A moment after falling asleep he would stop breathing, and within a minute Adam's oxygen-starved brain would wake him up. After taking a few breaths he would fall asleep again and repeat the cycle.

The sleep specialist's diagnosis was passed on to Adam's pediatrician, who still could not be persuaded to have the boy's tonsils and adenoids taken out. When the procedure was finally performed by another, more enlightened doctor found by the family, the thin and weak little boy underwent a dramatic change. Within a few weeks he was clearly thriving physically and mentally.

Today, as I write, six months have passed, and this previously despairing family is living with a miracle. Their little boy is taking his first steps, he can crawl everywhere, he is beginning to talk, and he is gaining a pound a month. Sadly, the first terrible year of Adam's life may have lasting effects on his development, but at the moment there is too much relief and happiness to dwell on that.

This story is only one of hundreds I hear year after year that confirm something almost no one will acknowledge: We are a sleep-sick society. I understand this sad fact all too well. I have spent my entire career, more than 45 years of nights, studying sleep. When I first entered medical school in 1951, sleep was little more than a curiosity to the scientific world, and it was almost totally ignored in medical practice. Over the ensuing decades, we have learned an enormous amount about the nocturnal third of our lives. Today sleep science is exciting and diversified, utilizing all the tools of modern molecular biology and addressing great scientific questions. Sleep medicine, which I started at Stanford University, where several passionately committed colleagues and I struggled to nurture it through its first uncertain and difficult years, has grown into a mature clinical discipline with stunningly skilled practitioners able to diagnose and treat a huge array of disorders. We have accumulated an enormous reservoir of knowledge about how sleep works and how it affects our other bodily systems. Quite frankly, when I was the only person in the world grinding out all-night sleep recordings at the University of Chicago, and when I decided to extend the practice of medicine to the sleeping patient at Stanford University, I did not expect to achieve or participate in success on such a large scale.

Unfortunately, doctors and the general public know almost nothing of this vast store of knowledge. A diagnosis like Adam's, which could have been made by a six-year-old child with the right information, was completely missed by medical specialists for months. If even the basic facts about sleep had been known and understood by the general public and its doctors over the years, there's no way of knowing how many human beings now dead—possibly millions; perhaps even relatives of yours—might be alive today. Never before in human history has a disparity between the amount of scientific knowledge and the benefit of that knowledge to society been so tragically vast.

As a result of this alarming lack of awareness about sleep in the medical community, doctors simply miss or ignore a veritable flood of sleep disorders. Hundreds of thousands of people worldwide are dying each year in large part because of undiagnosed and untreated sleep problems—tens of thousands in the United States alone. For instance, if someone you know has had a heart attack, there is a good chance (especially if the victim is young) that an undiagnosed sleep disorder contributed to the problem. I have seen near-miraculous cases in which a patient's advanced heart disease was dramatically reversed after his sleep problem was diagnosed and treated—although cardiologists had overlooked the underlying sleep problem for years.

Ignorance about sleep results in far more than medical problems, however. Less dramatic than medical tragedy, but nearly as sad, are the people all around us who are fatigued and exhausted every day because they don't understand how to manage their sleep, betrayed by their ignorance about the mechanics of sleep debt and the intricate biological clock that ticks away inside us. Consider these statistics: Half of us mismanage our sleep to the point where it negatively affects our health and safety. On average, each of us sleeps one and a half fewer hours each night than our great-grandparents did a century ago. I have observed people stagger through their lives in a daze, misunderstanding the roots of their sleepiness, or not even recognizing that they are sleepy. It may seem impossible that people can be very sleepy and not know it, but this fact has been proven beyond the shadow of a doubt. Study after study has revealed that people who are chronically sleep deprived can be completely unaware of the root cause of their overwhelming fatigue. Many people conclude that being run down, apathetic, and glum must be the normal human condition, or can be attributed to boredom, warm rooms, or heavy meals.

All too often, lack of awareness leads to a tragedy like the one that befell Michael Doucette. In 1989 the New Hampshire teenager competed in a national driver safety competition and won the distinction of being dubbed America's Safest Teen Driver. He was awarded a Dodge Shadow automobile in recognition of his mastery of the principles of safe driving. Early the next year, while driving his new car 25 miles home from college, he fell asleep at the wheel. As the road curved to the right, his car continued straight into the oncoming lane and collided head-on with another car. Both Michael and the young woman in the other car were killed.

When I talked to Michael's father, he told me that "Safe driving was an obsession with Michael." The teenager's driving instructor later told me that the issue of sleep deprivation and drowsy driving was never discussed in his school or anywhere else, as far as he knew. Although Michael was fanatical about driving safety, he was never taught about one of the gravest threats to road safely. In a recent survey by the National Sleep Foundation, 23 percent of the people who were polled admitted falling asleep while driving in the past year. With this in mind, it should be no surprise that sleep deprivation plays a major role in most accidents labeled "cause unknown," or that an estimated 24,000 people die each year in accidents caused directly or in part by falling asleep at the wheel. Almost all of us, regardless of our formal education, are dangerously uninformed about drowsy driving and its causes.

For most of my career as scientist, sleep doctor, and clinic and laboratory administrator, I have worked unceasingly to change the way society deals with sleep. Why? Because the current way, or nonway, is so very bad. As a compassionate person, I have a deep concern about the millions of people whose suffering could be greatly reduced by implementing the knowledge we now possess. It greatly saddens me to think about the millions, possibly billions, of people whose lives could be improved if they understood only a few simple principles. Changing the way society and its institutions deal with sleep will do more good than almost anything else I can conceive, or certainly anything that was ever remotely within my grasp to accomplish.

For a number of years, I helped lobby the U.S. Congress at least to take a look at the problem. It responded in 1990 by creating the National Commission on Sleep Disorders Research, of which I was named chairman. When we fulfilled our mandate to study and make recommendations about sleep disorders in the United States, the commission estimated the financial cost of sleep disorders at tens of billions of dollars per year. The human costs, of course, are incalculable.

Although I had already been trying to promote change for many years, my work on this commission truly separated me from the so-called academic ivory tower. I had always believed that successful medical research—the research that leads to treatments and cures for disease—would quickly flow to those in need. The work of the National Commission clearly demonstrated that the flow of benefits to the general public is largely blocked where sleep deprivation and sleep disorders are concerned.

For me and the other 19 commissioners, the information-gathering public hearings we held in several American cities brought the statistics to life, connecting them to human faces, human dramas. We heard heartbreaking stories about people living through years of failure and fatigue, suffering terribly from the needless death of a spouse or child. We also learned how the medical establishment could allow this to go on with the shocking discovery that doctors-in-training often get only an hour or two of instruction in sleep problems in their four years of medical school—and frequently none at all.

These hearings revealed to me how very little of the wealth of information mined by sleep specialists has gotten out to the general population. The many millions who need help, whose lives can be changed or saved by a little knowledge about sleep, might just as well be living in 1950. For the majority of the population that could feel revitalized and renewed by understanding a few simple sleep principles, I might as well have been running a chain of beauty parlors for the last four decades.

The commission titled its final report to the Congress "Wake Up America! A National Sleep Alert," and recommended increased support for sleep research, and an effective national awareness campaign to be carried out by the federal government. We commissioners naively thought that our report was a "job well done" and that we could go back to our laboratories and clinics. Well, that was seven years ago, and America slumbers on. The Congress may ask for recommendations but that doesn't mean it acts upon them. My faith in government, the Congress, the Public Health Service, and the National Institutes of Health has been sorely challenged. We should all feel outrage and shame if even one child or one adult is allowed to sicken and die unnecessarily, or if even one life is blighted needlessly by fatigue or pernicious insomnia.

Very sadly for my personal life and family, I had learned far too much to return meekly to academia. I have since been sounding the alarm in every way I know. Almost every week of the year, I travel across the country to speak to civic and business groups, governmental bodies, and health professionals; I even continue to hound the Congress about the hidden epidemic of sleep disorders in our midst. But little that I report finds its way to the wider public, and the costs to us, both individually and as a society, continue to mount.

Another top priority of the National Commission was education and training of primary care physicians. Clearly, as the gatekeepers of medicine, knowledgeable primary care physicians could do an enormous amount. When I decided that I would do whatever I could to educate primary care physicians, it occurred to me that the very best place to launch the crusade to change the way society deals with sleep would be in my own hometown, Walla Walla, Washington.

When I left Walla Walla as a young man, I never imagined that my professional life would come full circle, back to the little town where I grew up. I have now lived all over the United States, and visited many of the world's great cities to attend scientific sleep meetings, but my return to Walla Walla has been the most rewarding and exciting phase of my professional career.

My professional involvement with my hometown began slowly. I often (but not often enough) returned to Walla Walla to visit my mother, Kathryn Dement, and on these trips I began to talk to doctors about sleep medicine. In 1988 I was invited to Walla Walla to give a public lecture on sleep in the big auditorium at Whitman College. Afraid that the auditorium would be nearly empty, I devoted my whole $500 honorarium to advertising the upcoming lecture. It turned out that $500 could buy a lot of advertising in Walla Walla. There were daily half-page advertisements in the city newspaper, and when I walked into the auditorium on the night of the lecture, I was delighted to find it absolutely packed. My mother may not have understood exactly how I earned my living, but as she looked around at the packed house it was obvious that people were interested in hearing me talk about it. People whose careers are mysterious to their parents in this rapidly changing world can understand what a magical moment it was. I will cherish it as long as I live.

In a flash of inspiration, I realized that the best way to start changing the way society deals with sleep was to start with my own hometown, which had already demonstrated its interest. In what has come to be known as the Walla Walla Project, I set out to educate and train Walla Walla doctors in the basics of sleep medicine and to see what impact that knowledge had on their practices and patients. An added benefit of the study was my new need to travel there relatively frequently, allowing me to visit my mother more often.

I was extremely fortunate to be joined by my friend and colleague in sleep medicine at Stanford, the late Dr. Gèrman Nino-Murcia. To establish a baseline, we first reviewed the records of approximately 750 patients; as expected, sleep disorder diagnoses were absent. After the baseline review, Dr. Nino-Murcia and I conducted training sessions for all interested health professionals. The Walla Walla primary care physicians then began diagnosing and treating sleep disorders patients. All the cases were discussed in detail in weekly telephone conferences held with Dr. Nino-Murcia and me. Then, as the Walla Walla physicians acquired more and more expertise, only complicated and difficult cases were discussed.

Since it was the first time anything like it had been attempted, the Walla Walla Project began slowly. However, from today's perspective, the results of this project have been astounding. The Walla Walla physicians were amazed by the large number of patients they found to have serious sleep disorders. All of these patients had been seen at the clinic on multiple occasions previously, yet their sleep disorders were not recognized until the Walla Walla Project was well under way. The physicians participating in the project have since acquired the skills and experience to manage any sleep disorder entirely on their own. Three Walla Walla physicians have learned to score and interpret sleep tests. Four Walla Walla primary care physician, Dr. Richard Simon, is now a diplomate of the American Board of Sleep Medicine, and with several colleagues, has founded a fully accredited sleep disorders center. In a most touching gesture, this excellent clinical resource was christened as the Kathryn Severyns Dement Sleep Disorders Center.

I am excited and gratified that sleep has now entered the mainstream of Walla Walla society as a fully qualified member of the basic triumvirate of health: good nutrition, physical fitness, healthy sleep. A sleep curriculum is being prepared for Walla Walla's two middle schools and high schools. Material covering the nature of sleep, sleep deprivation, biological rhythms, and the essentials of healthy sleep is being introduced in its three small colleges.

In addition to our work in Walla Walla, we are working nearby in Moscow, Idaho, where we have evaluated every patient in a single primary care practice, with startling results. No patient in the practice had received a specific sleep disorders diagnosis as of the end of 1996. But when we evaluated this patient population, we found that more than half of them presented obvious symptoms of one or more sleep disorders. Given these results, and assuming that the Moscow doctors are representative of those in the rest of the nation, it is clear that primary care physicians are missing important diagnoses and must fully integrate sleep medicine into the general practice of medicines.

There is one thing I must make absolutely sure that everyone understands. Primary care physicians are absolutely not responsible for the neglect of sleep disorders in America today. They are as much the victims of the lack of medical school teaching as everyone else. In my opinion, the tiny band of primary care physicians who have already tackled the sleep disorders problem head-on are heroes worthy of the highest accolades.

In Walla Walla as I write, about 2,000 seriously ill citizens have been diagnosed and treated, first at the Walla Walla clinic and in the past two years at the Kathryn Severyns Dement Sleep Disorders Center. The results of the Walla Walla project have been a mind-boggling revelation. In those suspected of having apnea, 80 percent of the sleep tests have revealed far-advanced illness. This means that these patients became ill decades ago, and as the years passed, they simply got sicker and sicker. The 80 percent figure is likely the same as would be found in other communities but such an effective sleep disorder and awareness program has not been done beyond Walla Walla.

Several thousand Walla Walla citizens have already received or will soon receive clinical salvation through treatment, and the potential for salvation elsewhere is awesome. An example: One of Dick Simon's many patients was an overweight 60-year-old who was overwhelmingly fatigued. The only thing he could do was sit around all day long, frequently dozing off in his chair. He was also in far advanced congestive heart failure. The slow failure of his heart muscle caused massive tissue swelling called edema. He could not walk one block without becoming very short of breath. When he lay down, the pressure of tissue and body fluids on the heart and lungs also made it hard to breathe. He had been hospitalized many times. The heart failure was assumed to be secondary to high blood pressure, which did not respond to treatment.

In less than a minute, Dick recognized his true condition, obstructive sleep apnea. The man's sleep test revealed a very high level of severity. He stopped breathing nearly 100 times every hour. After several weeks of treatment, this patient was reborn. He can breathe when lying down, he can walk many blocks without shortness of breath, his edema is gone, and he feels great. Of the eight medications he was taking for his heart, blood pressure, and fluid retention, he now takes only two. And each night his sleep is deep, healthy, and restorative.

After all the research I've done on sleep problems over the past four decades, my most significant finding is that ignorance is the worst sleep disorder of them all. People lack the most basic information about how to manage their sleep, leading to a huge amount of unnecessary suffering. My goal for this book is not to tell everyone about all the exciting discoveries in sleep science and sleep medicine—outstanding researchers and clinicians have filled volumes with that information. Rather, my goal is to give people the fundamental knowledge they need to change the way they sleep and live. What I am trying to do is akin to teaching the alphabet of sleep so that people can start learning to read. We are not healthy unless our sleep is healthy, and we cannot make our sleep healthy unless we become thoroughly aware of both its peril and its promise.

For nearly half a century, a huge reservoir of knowledge about sleep, sleep deprivation, and sleep disorders has been building up behind a dam of pervasive lack of awareness and unresponsive bureaucracies. We don't know how many preventable tragedies are occurring right now, today, this very instant. It is time to blow up the dam. The gentler approach of convincing authorities to lower the floodgates has not worked. Therefore, I hope and pray that this book will allow sleep knowledge to flow to the millions of people whose lives it can change—and save.

PART ONE

The Fundamentals of Sleep

Chapter 1

Long Night's Journey into Day

EVERY NIGHT nearly every person on the planet undergoes an astounding metamorphosis. As the sun sets, a delicate timing device at the base of our brain sends a chemical signal throughout our body, and the gradual slide toward sleep begins. Our body becomes inert, and our lidded eyes roll slowly from side to side. Later the eyes begin the rapid eye movements that accompany dreams, and our mind enters a highly active state where vivid dreams trace our deepest emotions. Throughout the night we traverse a broad landscape of dreaming and nondreaming realms, wholly unaware of the world outside. Hours later, as the sun rises, we are transported back to our bodies and to waking consciousness.

And we remember almost nothing.

Sleep is a miraculous journey made all the more extraordinary by this one simple fact: We never know we're sleeping while we're asleep. It is impossible to have conscious, experiential knowledge of nondreaming sleep; indeed, one of sleep's defining aspects is that we don't know that we are sleeping while we are doing it. Limited to an abstract knowledge of sleep, we are less able to identify any problems we have while sleeping. Sleep is a perceptual hole in time. I saw this firsthand in an experiment we conducted 25 years ago, one that helped me make a huge leap forward in my understanding of this essential difference between sleep and awake. Picture this:

A young man is lying on a bed, eyes wide open, staring straight up. As part of our experiment, he is allowed only four hours of sleep the previous night. Much of the time he is sleepy but unambiguously awake. We have positioned his head so that he is looking directly into a very bright strobe light—essentially like a camera flash, except his flash is only six inches away. We have asked him to stare at the light and to press a tiny switch taped to his index finger whenever he sees the flash. To make sure he cannot possibly miss the flash during a blink, we have taped his eyelids open. To some it looks uncomfortable, but it doesn't hurt.

The light goes off straight into his eyes—flash!—like a photographer ambushing a celebrity. Our volunteer presses the switch. A few seconds later another flash, another press of the response key. The strobe light is programmed to go off irregularly, on average every six seconds. For a few minutes the sleepy volunteer taps the switch after each flash. Then the bright flash surges through his pupils, and the switch is not pressed.

"Why didn't you press the switch just now?" we ask.

"Because there was no flash," the young man replies.

But there was a flash. I saw it. The three other people in the room saw it. And this unblinking volunteer didn't see it. Looking straight into the strobe light six inches away from his nose, he could not possibly have missed it. His retina was flooded with light many times brighter than the brightest bulb in his home, and yet he is absolutely sure that there was no flash. How is this possible?

The answer to the puzzle was revealed by the machines we use to monitor brain activity. They showed us that something had happened to his brain at the very moment the light flashed. The young man actually had fallen asleep for two seconds, so briefly that he wasn't even aware he had slept. And yet, in that moment of sleep, the door of perception between the brain and the outside world had slammed shut, barring entry to even a bright light.

Until that afternoon in the laboratory a quarter century ago, I had not been very concerned about the precise moment of sleep onset. Since we were customarily studying entire nights—eight or more hours, 400 to 500 minutes—we were happy to designate the beginning of sleep as the point where the brain-wave patterns were absolutely unambiguously different even to a casual observer. Like everyone else, I assumed that falling asleep was a relatively slow process coinciding with the reduction of activity and stimulation.

The strobe light result could be explained only if the switch from wakefulness to sleep is accomplished by a powerful, active process that abruptly blocks or alters sensory nerve impulses and shuts off sight. In other words, we are seeing, we are conscious of our environment, and a millisecond later we are totally blind. The moment of sleep is when the brain flips a switch and isolates itself from the outer world. Although at this point I had already been studying sleep for more than 20 years, until this experiment it hadn't been possible to see this truth.

Human beings have great difficulty monitoring their own exact "moment of sleep." It is not like a pinprick. Often I ask my students to describe the moment of falling asleep, and invariably they can't. They can recall lying in bed before sleep and then no more. Indeed, that flipping of neural switches and the leap from one reality into another is so complete that describing the experience of sleep itself is very difficult. What we have left when we wake is not so much a memory of sleeping as a residue of sleepiness, a vague feeling of having slept well or not, and vague fragments of dreams.

This experiment motivated me yet again to think about the question that has intrigued me nearly my whole adult life: What is sleep? For 46 years I've stalked the sleeping self to understand what happens when we sleep. Night after night I've watched people in our lab and our clinic undergo the commonplace and profound transformation called falling asleep. I've come to appreciate sleep as an inseparable part of our lives, the nightly yin to the yang of waking life, an essential part of the cycle of existence. I've also learned that when we fail to acknowledge sleep's sovereignty over our lives or fail to keep sleep healthy, it has the power to kill.

Mostly, people describe sleep by saying what it is not. We say that sleeping is not being awake. Or we say that sleeping is shutting down for the night. If asked to give a simile for sleep, you might say it is something like putting a car in the garage and turning off the ignition. Or turning off a computer. Or the ultimate switching off—death. It is common in many cultures to believe that sleep is a little death; some go so far to suggest that the soul leaves the body as we sleep and returns in the morning. Even without such elaborate explanations, most of us have the idea that sleep is a cessation of all activity, an oblivion we slip into where nothing happens.

The truth is completely the opposite. As the muscles relax, the mind shifts, and the brain starts behaving differently. During sleep the brain releases new combinations of the hormones and chemical messengers that stimulate cellular activity throughout the body. At some times the sleeping brain actually appears to be more active than it is while awake, burning large quantities of sugar and oxygen as neurons fire rapidly. When dreaming, the mind takes on a different consciousness, inhabits a new world that is as real as the world it experiences when awake.

I sometimes liken the study of sleep to oceanography. Like the ocean, sleep is little charted in its depths and is stunning in its vastness. The first trip I took on the high seas was a cruise to Japan, courtesy of Uncle Sam. In January 1946 I looked forward to a great adventure as my troop ship sailed under the Golden Gate Bridge. As soon as we cleared the harbor, though, the first real ocean swells started to slide under the ship, and a less happy feeling settled in my stomach. When I struggled onto deck after a few days of seasickness, I was overwhelmed by the watery mountains and troughs of midocean. I began to feel a sense of awe at the size of the Pacific. Day after day, night after night, we had surged steadily through the ocean at 20 miles an hour, and yet the scenery never changed: an expanse of water without end, stretching to the horizons. On that trip I came to understand in a very tangible way how much of Earth's real estate is buried under miles of water.

Just as a voyage across the ocean made me truly appreciate the ocean's size, staying up all night (especially if plagued by insomnia or a crying baby) will give you a better understanding of the length and breadth of those sleeping hours. And like the scientists who study the ocean, the scientists who study sleep historically have been limited to sampling the surface and hungering to uncover the great discoveries we know lie below. The history of sleep science is the story of what our nets have brought up from the deep and the unseen mysteries those catches hint at. With genetic probes and advances in neuroscience, we are now starting to dive deep into the ocean of sleep and illuminate much more of what lies below.

The Definition of Sleep

I am glad that I made the decision to develop an introductory course on sleep and dreams for undergraduates at Stanford. Teaching forced me to find the best and clearest answers to basic questions, including the most important question: What is sleep? Over the years humans have observed people sleeping and noted that the clearest changes are from activity to quiescence, eyes open to eyes closed. Sleep became defined as a state of rest as opposed to wakefulness, the state of activity. But these changes all can occur without the person being asleep. I asked the question: What is there about sleep that absolutely cannot be simulated? We can lie quietly with our eyes closed, we can even fake a snore. Also, as you will see later in the book, we can do all sorts of things when we are certainly not fully awake even outrageous activities like screaming, running, or even attacking someone. What is the absolute sign of sleep?

I define sleep in terms of only two essential features. The first, and by far the most important, is that sleep erects a perceptual wall between the conscious mind and the outside world. Closing our eyelids makes it easier to sleep, but even if our eyelids were shorn off, we would sleep just the same. Of course, if a sound is loud enough, it can leap over the sensory wall and wake the sleeper. The second defining feature of normal sleep is that it is immediately reversible. Even when someone is deeply asleep, intense and persistent stimulation will always awaken the sleeper. If not, the person is not asleep, but unconscious or dead.

These two essential features distinguish sleep from other apparently sleeplike states. For instance, we can't be immediately aroused from coma and anesthesia. Since sleep cuts people off from most outside sounds, hypnosis—which allows its subjects to respond to suggestion—can't be considered sleep in any sense of the word. Hibernation is not easily reversible, and so is also not sleep—although it may have evolved out of sleep. These nonsleep states point to two more important qualities of sleep: It occurs naturally, unlike coma, anesthesia, or hypnosis, which require injury, drugs, or some other outside influence; and it occurs periodically—daily in humans—unlike the annual hibernation pattern. In fact, animals just coming out of hibernation show signs of sleep deprivation, so hibernation actually may get in the way of the tasks sleep usually performs for the body.

Sleep also is characterized by electrical changes in the brain, which scientists can measure using machines called electroencephalographs (EEGs), which graphically show brain waves. The ability to chart the brain's activity with EEGs changed the essential nature of sleep research. This made it possible to go beyond the observations of philosophers and poets, to peek at the inner workings of the sleeping brain. In the sleep lab, we now attach electrodes to a person's scalp so that brain activity appears as squiggly lines on a moving sheet of paper produced by a machine called a polygraph. The squiggly lines the pens make resemble those of the polygraphs used as lie detector machines. Because the brain's electrical activity has a rhythmic rise and fall in strength, we call them brain waves. These brain waves change shape and oscillate slowly or quickly—depending on the brain's state.

Portrait of a Family Through a Night of Sleep

To get a better feeling for what happens when we sleep, and for the panorama of sleep styles and problems that people can have, let's look in on a fictional family of four. Imagine a mother in her early 40s, a husband pushing 50, their 16-year-old daughter, and a 10-year-old son. They live in a large house in a cozy suburb. We will follow them through one night and observe the differences among four sleepers spread around the house and across nearly four decades.

After dinner, the son is allowed to watch a little television, and around 8:30 P.M. he starts getting ready for bed. He puts on pajamas, brushes his teeth, dawdles a little, and then is off to his room. After good-night kisses, the Mickey Mouse night-light is turned on, and the room light goes out. Our 10-year-old closes his eyes and begins to relax.

The boy may think about his day, or tomorrow, or the television show. His breathing slows, his muscles grow limp, and his mind begins to wander. He is not asleep yet, but relaxing and preparing for sleep. His body temperature has been falling slightly over the last few hours, and his pineal gland has been releasing the hormone melatonin into the bloodstream, which indicates to his brain and body that it is dark and time to prepare for the transition to sleep.

If the boy were hooked up to one of the EEG machines in our sleep lab, we could observe the electrical activity of his brain. When the boy is fully awake, his brain waves are a rapid, low-voltage type called beta waves. (See Figure 1.1.) As he closes his eyes and falls into a state of calm wakefulness, his brain waves change to a slower, higher-strength type called alpha waves. Then the alpha waves quickly disappear, replaced by an even lower-frequency type called theta waves. His mind has been wandering toward the unmarked border that separates wakefulness from sleep, and in one quick step he is over it.

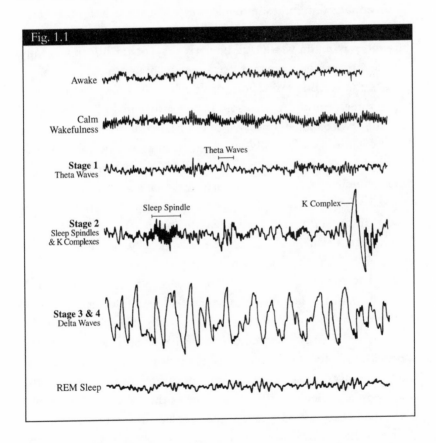

Fig. 1.1

Awake

Calm Wakefulness

Theta Waves

Stage 1
Theta Waves

Sleep Spindle

K Complex

Stage 2
Sleep Spindles
& K Complexes

Stage 3 & 4
Delta Waves

REM Sleep

At the moment when the alpha waves of drowsiness yield to the theta waves of stage 1 sleep, a sensory curtain drops and isolates his mind from the outside world. He no longer perceives the sounds of the household—his mother talking on the phone and the dishwasher humming. He no longer smells the soapy scent of the clean sheets or feels the crispness of the cotton he noticed when he climbed into bed. He briefly becomes conscious of his right leg when it makes a small jerk, but very quickly he is back into his own sleeping world. Stage 1 sleep is light sleep; a nudge or the sound of a cat screeching might rouse him. If the boy were to be awakened right now, he might say he had not been asleep at all. Yet during stage 1 sleep he will not respond to his whispered name—his mind is closed off. His eyes are engaged in slow back-and-forth movements (not the rapid movements of rapid-eye-movement, or REM, sleep).

After about five minutes in stage 1 sleep, the boy moves on to stage 2. If awakened now he is more likely to know he had been asleep, although waking up would still be fairly easy. Stage 2 sleep is readily identified by two new types of sleep-specific brain waves, called sleep spindles and K-complexes, both of which are episodic and last only two to three seconds. A sleep spindle is a short burst of waves with a frequency two to three times that of the background theta waves. On the EEG, it looks a little like the spindle on an old spinning wheel. K-complexes are large waves that usually seem to come out of no-where and disappear, like a little earthquake on a seismograph. These two wave forms are thought to reflect the massive changes in how sensory information is processed in the brain. Regardless of what they represent exactly, for me they are exquisite. They allow us to be absolutely certain that the brain is asleep and in non-REM, stage 2 sleep. I have stared at these beautiful waves on the EEG, and as each makes way for the next and the next I feel great pleasure.

After another five or 10 minutes, the boy falls into stage 3 sleep, the first stage of what is called deep sleep. This stage is heralded by the appearance of the final species of brain wave, the delta wave. If the theta waves of stage 2 sleep are comparable to the waves at the beach—small, uneven, of varying shapes—then delta waves are like the great ocean swells: larger, more regular, and with a lower frequency. Theta waves, sleep spindles, and K-complexes are still present in stage 3 sleep, but like the wind-blown waves running over ocean swells, they are harder to see.

The boy will spend relatively little time in stage 3 sleep as the oceanic delta waves start to swallow the smaller theta waves. When the theta waves are gone and the sleep spindles and K-complexes nearly impossible to detect, he has entered the deepest stage of sleep, stage 4, which is sometimes called slow-wave sleep. At last the boy is completely adrift on a sea of sleep, his brain waves rising and falling in a deep delta pattern, out of sight of the land we know as consciousness. He is deeply asleep, difficult to wake up, his heart and breathing are regular and relatively slow, his muscles are almost completely relaxed.

During this first deep sleep of the night, the boy's body secretes a pulse of growth hormone. This hormone helps cells divide and multiply, building new tissue for his growing body and rebuilding damaged tissue. In a few years, an increase in the amount of growth hormone secreted nightly will be one of the first indications that the boy has begun puberty. During this stage of sleep his body is also releasing the hormone prolactin. We know that prolactin is essential for milk production in nursing mothers, but we don't know what it does in children and nonnursing adults, or why its greatest release is during sleep.

It is now about 10:00 P.M., and the boy drifts along in stage 4 sleep for another 45 minutes, substantially more than adults spend in this stage. Around 10:45 P.M., signs of a lighter sleep begin to appear again. Like the certain birds at sea that warn mariners of the nearness of land, the theta waves, sleep spindles, and K-complexes of stage 3 sleep reemerge. The boy stirs, but he is not waking up, only preparing for a very different kind of sleep. After 10 minutes in stage 3, it comes. His eyes start jerking back and forth under closed eyelids. All voluntary muscles become completely paralyzed, and brain activity increases greatly. The boy is dreaming. He has made landfall and found consciousness once again, but like Gulliver he is now in a strange land far from the one he inhabits in waking life.

This period of sleep is called REM sleep, because of the rapid eye movements that always accompany it. (REM usually is pronounced to rhyme with "them.") The delta waves have disappeared and the choppy theta waves are back, but now there are also short bursts of the alpha and beta waves that on their own characterize wakefulness.

The first dreaming period will usually last no more than 10 minutes, and then the boy will descend once again into the deep sleep of stages 3 and 4. Throughout the night he will repeatedly travel up and down through deep and shallow sleep, and also wake many times for a few unremembered moments like a porpoise swimming up and down and occasionally skimming the surface for air. He will have four, or five, or even six more dream periods, alternating between two totally different kinds of sleep—REM and non-REM sleep.

By 2:00 A.M. the boy is in the middle of the sleep cycle, and his body temperature is reaching its lowest level, about two full degrees Fahrenheit below his peak daytime temperature. The next half of the night is more dream rich because each REM period tends to be longer. During these early-morning hours, levels of a hormone called cortisol start rising in the boy's bloodstream. Cortisol is released during times of stress, but its main job now is to mobilize energy stores, preparing the body for the demands of the coming day. It reaches its peak right before the boy awakes.

By 6:30 A.M. he is nearing the end of the final REM period. As first light appears at the window a few minutes later, he awakes, opens his eyes, and lies quietly thinking of the dream that just ended, about flying over a beach. For 10 minutes or so he will experience sleep inertia, the transitory sleepy feeling that hangs on after awaking. Any nighttime awakenings he experienced have been wiped from his memory; he feels as if he had just lain his head on the pillow at night, blinked his eyes, and it was morning. A few yawns and minutes later, the boy is energetic and ready to take on the day.

To me, the 10-year-old's journey through the night is a thing of beauty. So many of the things that disrupt adult sleep just aren't there. Even after 45 years of reading brain-wave recordings from the EEG machine, I am amazed to find myself still entranced by the perfect sleep spindles, the textbook theta waves, the absolutely perfect night of childhood sleep.

Given what we now know, the end of childhood may well be the end of the Golden Age of sleep for most of us. Certainly our initial casting or exploration of the ocean of sleep has netted an almost unbelievably large catch of sleep deprivation and sleep disorders. This same night, the boy's mother sleeps poorly. Instead of going to bed at the usual time, she puts in a couple of hours on an annual report due soon at work. She has been sleeping less and less the past few nights, staying up late, worrying over the impending deadline.

She labors past midnight, then has a nightcap to ease her mind into low gear. She checks her e-mail one last time and finds herself typing replies. She can't let go of the day. She turns on the television for a few minutes to watch the end of the *Tonight Show*. She slouches toward bed, dead tired.

Once in bed, the sleep debt built up from a day of hard work and the nightcap she drank combine to put her quickly into stage 1 sleep and then into the true sleep of stage 2. She has slept little the past few nights and is very sleep deprived.

Two hours later, though, the effect of the alcohol on the brain is wearing off and its effect on her bladder growing. At 3:00 A.M. her body forces her awake. The mother goes to the bathroom and shuffles back to bed but cannot fall asleep. Her mind churns through budget figures, and her adrenal glands pump her body full of stress hormones. She lies awake, staring at the ceiling, listening to her husband's snoring on the other side of a king-size bed, trying to turn off her brain. It's happening again: the sleepless night she's embarrassed to mention at the office and never even thinks about reporting to her doctor. For the next two hours she feels she checks the clock constantly, worrying that sleep will never come, but in fact she does sleep fitfully for a total of one and a half hours, even slipping briefly into deep sleep a couple of times. By 5:00 A.M., an hour before she knows she has to climb out of bed, she has just about given up on ever falling asleep. As she resigns herself to getting up shortly, she relaxes enough to fall into an unbroken sleep for another hour before the alarm goes off at 6:00 A.M.

The teenage daughter's alarm is also set for 6:00 A.M.—an hour before she has to be dressed and on the corner to catch her school bus. She spends the evening in her room, ostensibly doing homework. She's listening to her favorite band through earphones but manages to stay focused on a set of algebra problems. At 10:00 P.M., her father bangs on the door and says, "Time for bed." She acknowledges him but doesn't move. "I've got to finish these problems," she says. She doesn't feel at all like going to bed. At 11:00 P.M. her mother opens the door. "Get into bed right now," she says severely. Her husband has already gone to bed.

By 11:15 the daughter is in pajamas sitting on the edge of her bed doing her nails. This takes a fair amount of time. At 11:30, her mother is back in her room, turning out the ceiling light and saying, "If I have to come back one more time . . ." The daughter turns out the bedside lamp and gets in bed, but she is still wide awake and has many things on her mind. There is a fashion magazine she wants to look at, and she's learned to use the flashlight under the covers. A little after midnight, she knows she will be incredibly tired when the alarm goes off. She gets comfortable and tries to fall asleep but begins to worry about her algebra exam. Finally, at 12:30, after a bit of tossing and turning, she begins to settle down and falls asleep.

Her sleep is somewhat similar to her brother's. She very quickly gets into a deep sleep because she is sleep deprived from so many nights of staying up late. About an hour later she stirs as if the REM sleep were about to begin, but after a bit of restlessness, she is back in stage 4. As 4:00 A.M. approaches, her eyes begin to move, marking the onset of a long period of REM sleep. After another 90-minute cycle of all the sleep stages, the alarm goes off. It rings loudly and intrusively. She groggily reaches over and turns it off—an action she will not remember—and immediately falls asleep again. Her mother comes in shortly and gently shakes her shoulder until she really wakes up.

The father has also had a tough night, although he doesn't know it. After dinner, he does a little paperwork, then uses the treadmill in the basement and takes a shower. Afterward, he steps on the scale and notices that he is easily twenty pounds overweight. He is tired. After sitting in a trance and thinking of nothing, he remembers that he needs to fix the shelf in the laundry room. He finally gets up, forgetting where he left his tools. He finds them and methodically works on the shelf. He notices it is 9:30 and thinks, "Ha, I'll be able to go to bed soon." At 10:00 P.M. he knocks on his daughter's door and tells her it's bedtime, then goes off to bed himself. He puts on his pajamas, climbs into bed, and is asleep and snoring almost at once.

Soon after he falls asleep, he rolls over onto his back. In this position, the volume of his snoring begins to build. Anytime the family is on a camping trip, the rest of them complain about it. Sometimes his wife sleeps on the very comfortable couch in the recreation room, but mostly she sleeps with him. She wears earplugs to bed, and she thinks she's learned to ignore the sound. Every five or ten minutes he emits a restless snort and a series of deep breaths until he shifts position and settles back down. If we were measuring his heart-beat and the level of oxygen in his blood, we would see unquestion-able ups and downs. This goes on through the night, and he never gets the deep sleep his children achieve, because this snorting, gasp-ing breathing interrupts his sleep—not enough for him to remem-ber, but enough to deprive his brain and body of the uninterrupted sleep he needs. There is a period in which he rolls onto his stomach and the snoring subsides a bit. During this time he enters REM sleep. His alarm goes off at 6:30 A.M. It isn't easy to get up, but he gets into the shower immediately to help him get going.

In the morning father, mother, and daughter struggle to start their day in a fog of sleepiness. The mother showers groggily, then stum-bles toward the kitchen to grab a cup of coffee. The father has a light breakfast; his doctor has expressed concern about his elevated blood pressure and suggested he should think about taking medication for it. The daughter picks at her breakfast. Like most teenage girls, she wants to keep weight off for cosmetic reasons. All three of them will struggle against fatigue throughout the day, especially after lunch. The father is especially dazed, struggling to stay awake in a meeting and totally missing a stop sign on his drive home; he makes a mental note to mention his fatigue again to his doctor, who seemed more concerned with his weight and blood pressure the last time he brought up being tired all the time. The daughter drags a little through the school day, but by late afternoon she is starting to feel much more wide awake and energetic.

The 10-year-old son, meanwhile, is a bundle of energy all day. He tears around the kitchen during breakfast and can barely control himself enough to sit down to eat. The mother rubs her temples and glares at him as she makes his lunch. The noise irritates her, but deep down she also feels a vague envy of her son's energy, the energy she used to have, before time and the tide of responsibilities and worries stole it away.

Everyone spent the night in bed, but each had a very different journey through the night and arrived at the morning in very differ-ent shape—the son ready for the day ahead, everyone else feeling run over by the night train that delivered them to another fully scheduled day.

It doesn't have to be this way. With a little knowledge and a little effort, every member of this family could make their sleep healthy again and give themselves some of that magical sleep of childhood. You can too. We all have our own patterns of sleep and wakefulness, and it is up to you to understand your own sleep, to observe its unique patterns and anatomy. If you are like nearly every other adult in the industrial world, you will begin to see that you are handicapping yourself by sleeping poorly. You are not fully alert and awake during the day.

Sleep medicine is still young, but we now know enough about the dynamics and mechanics of sleep that we can help most people sleep better at night and feel more alive during the day. I feel that everyone can regain at least some of the energy and well-being of the 10-year-old, the kind of nighttime sleep and daytime alertness that we all used to have before childhood ended. We can be better parents, workers, and friends. We can learn to sleep.

Chapter 2

A Short and Personal History
of Sleep Research

IN EARLY SEPTEMBER 1951, with my University of Washington degree in my suitcase, my dad and I drove from Walla Walla to Pendleton, Oregon, where I caught the train for Chicago to begin medical school. Like everyone else, I had little curiosity about the nature of sleep and would never have dreamed that I would study it at all, let alone as a career. To whatever extent I thought about sleep, I am sure that I totally accepted the prevailing notion that except for the occasional occurrence of a dream, sleep is simply the brain "turned off." Like about half of my medical school classmates, I wanted to be a psychiatrist—in particular a Freudian psychoanalyst. I had been exposed to abnormal psychology and psychoanalytic theories as an undergraduate, and like Sigmund Freud, I had become fascinated by the "the problem of consciousness": What is it, and how does it work? By the 1950s, a fair amount had been learned about the brain and the question had become more pointed: How can nerve cells and nerve impulses in the brain give rise to consciousness?

But at the beginning of my second year of medical school in the fall of 1952, Nathaniel Kleitman gave a lecture on higher brain function in a required neurophysiology course. Although I didn't know it at the time, this was a turning point in my life. During that lecture it occurred to me that the way to understand consciousness is to understand what must be given up to enter unconsciousness. In other words, since we are conscious while awake and unconscious while asleep, if we determine what brain functions are lost when we move from wakefulness to sleep, then we can understand what is required for us to be conscious. It was a simple notion but very exciting to me at the time. When the lecture ended, I sat for a few minutes to gather my thoughts and decide what to do next. I had never done research, nor had I worked directly with a professor in any other capacity. I had nothing to offer but my enthusiasm. However, I knew that several of my classmates were working with professors. If they could do it, so could I.

I immediately went to Kleitman's office and tapped on the closed door. No response. Taking a deep breath, I knocked louder. Suddenly the door cracked open only a few inches and Professor Kleitman peered out at me. Self-conscious and realizing I should have made an appointment, I blurted out, "Professor Kleitman, I would like to work in your lab."

Without missing a beat, he demanded, "Do you know anything about sleep?"

"Well—no."

"Read my book." And the door shut, not quite a slam.

Luckily for me, Kleitman was an excellent writer. His 429-page book, *Sleep and Wakefulness,* covered absolutely everything that was known about sleep up to 1939, its publication date. It is unfair from today's perspective to say that everything known about sleep back then was not very much. However, lacking the ability to perform all-night EEG monitoring, many of the things people had done were no more than questionnaires or brief samples of a single variable. But Kleitman's book was exhaustive and, as I said, very well written, making it much easier to read than most of my other medical books. The main point is that pure chance had delivered me from Walla Walla, Washington, to the doorstep of the only man in the world whose entire professional life was devoted to the study of sleep, and that having read his book, I may have known more about the field at that moment than anyone else but Kleitman himself.

The Dawn of Sleep Science
Sleep—and especially dreams—had played a central role in the culture of ancient peoples. Anthropologists speculate that dreams first

brought early humans the vision of the soul, an identity inside but separate from the body. Each night the body slept and the soul was revealed. Some believed that the soul left the body and went walking in the spirit world. Others believed that dreams provided sacred guidance for daily life, that the dreamer had to act out the dream the next day to remain safe and healthy.

Night itself was, and is, otherworldly, rubbing up against the unknown, close kin to death. An ancient concept with enduring influence was the idea that sleep is a short death, and death is a long sleep. In ancient Greece Hypnos, the god of sleep—from which we get the word "hypnotism"—and Thanatos, the god of death, were believed to be the twin offspring of the night. Sometimes small figurines depict them as young babies, each one suckling on a breast of Mother Night.

The theme that runs through most of history is the erroneous idea that sleep is not actively generated by the brain but is something imposed on the brain. The Greeks were the first known to attempt a scientific explanation of how and why we go to sleep. In the fifth century B.C. Alcmaeon proposed that sleep was caused by blood filling the brain vessels, and sleepers woke when the blood left their brain. Plato and Aristotle believed that vapors from food decomposing in the stomach rose to the brain to cause sleep. Aristotle's ideas about sleep held sway until the natural philosophers of the fifteenth and sixteenth centuries discovered them to be anatomically impossible. Strangely enough, new theories still concentrated on blood and "animal humors." According to the most popular theory of the eighteenth century, sleep occurred when blood flowing to the head put pressure on the brain—pretty close to what the Greeks had proposed more than 2,000 years before!

The nineteenth century brought new theories, but they were all based on the erroneous assumption that the brain shuts down during sleep. Natural philosophers believed that sleep occurred when there wasn't enough stimulation to keep the brain awake. The brain was like a machine whose handle needed to be cranked in order to operate. When the cranking stopped, the brain ground to a halt. In the 1830s one thoughtful observer summed up the idea with this statement: "Sleep is the intermediate state between wakefulness and death; wakefulness being regarded as the active state of all the animal and intellectual functions, and death as that of their total suspension."

Philosophers also tended to regard the act of falling asleep as a process imposed on a passive brain by the dark and quiet environment of nighttime. It wasn't until the middle of the twentieth century that sleep scientists found evidence that sleep is not something that just happens to us but that the brain puts itself to sleep. Until then the idea of passive brain seemed intuitively correct.

Research on sleep entered a new era in 1952, and in the intervening years we have learned more about sleep than in all prior history. What used to be rough speculation by natural philosophers now has become a solid science wherein we can record electrical brain waves and characterize them across the spectrum of consciousness and unconsciousness, from full alertness to drowsiness, through all the stages of sleep and dreaming.

What I regard as the watershed series of technological advances that were necessary for the dawn of sleep science were, first, the discovery of spontaneous electrical activity in the brains of animals by Richard Coton in 1875, and next the demonstration by German psychiatrist Hans Berger in the late 1920s and early 1930s that the brains of human beings also showed spontaneous electrical activity that could be recorded from the scalp. Given all the trials and tribulations I had in the early days with Kleitman trying to get decent brain wave recordings, I believe that Berger's demonstration with the primitive equipment available to him was nothing short of miraculous. He clearly identified the waking alpha rhythm and said that if a subject fell asleep, the rhythm disappeared and electrical activity was very low amplitude or sparse during sleep. I now believe that this was so in keeping with what Berger expected to see that he made very little effort to study sleep more thoroughly. The existence of spontaneous electrical activity in the human brain was confirmed by Lord Adrian in the 30s, and some of the wave forms that we know today were described. However, the technology continued to be too primitive and difficult to use. World War II interrupted things, but rapid improvement in technology was possible afterward because of wartime advances in electronics.

You might think that the mass of signals created by the billions of neurons in the human brain would create a chaotic, disorganized signal, like the frenzied din of a stock exchange. But brain signals are not like that. The nerves don't fire exactly in time with each other, but there is a definite pattern of nerve signaling, and the general swell and fade of nerve activity shows up on EEGs as the brain waves I mentioned earlier. Brain waves are not smooth when graphed on paper—there is still a lot of chaotic activity that makes the line look shaky—but the waves are unmistakably there.

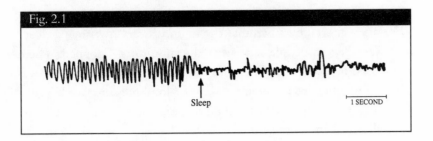

Fig. 2.1

Sleep

1 SECOND

Nathaniel Kleitman, the man who would later be my professor and mentor, was the first to devote the bulk of his entire professional life to the study of sleep. Kleitman was born in Russia but emigrated to Palestine before World War I to become a doctor. When war broke out, he was afraid the Turks controlling Palestine at the time would arrest him as a Russian agent, and he fled on the first ship available, which sailed to New York. Eventually he earned his doctoral degree in physiology and became a professor at the University of Chicago, where he set up a laboratory to study sleep in the early 1920s. Until then the study of sleep was a huge blind spot in the science of physiology; no one had made a career out of its study. Kleitman was the first in the world to set up a laboratory permanently devoted to the study of sleep. Next to his office in the physiology building was an old two-room chemistry lab with a door between the rooms. He set up a cot in one room where volunteers would sleep and left the other room for the observer. It was makeshift, but it worked well enough.

By the time I met Kleitman, he had lost any trace of a Russian accent, but in research he retained a certain Russian autocracy. He always dressed in black or charcoal suits, a no-nonsense scientist, guiding his laboratory with a firm hand and little small talk. He read every publication that mentioned sleep, an exhausting feat that most scientists didn't attempt. He also worked hard at research, laboring with thousands of others to build the house of science brick by brick, experiment by experiment, one observation after another. He got into sleep research by placing a few missing bricks in the edifice of physiology. Soon he was the expert—not just patching holes, but building a whole addition to the structure.

Everyone at the time, including Kleitman, erroneously believed that the brain needed a certain amount of external stimulation to maintain wakefulness. A number of experiments conducted in the 1930s were flawed by a bias that the brain was inactive during sleep. In general, when people fell asleep the monitoring stopped. There seemed no need to keep measuring the same thing. Much work was of the kind where someone interested in blood pressure would take a few samples during sleep and then assume these samples could be generalized to the entire night.

In Kleitman's Night Laboratory—the Discovery of Rapid Eye Movements

After I read his book and returned to his office, Kleitman accepted me. "Okay," he said, "you can help Gene Aserinsky, who is trying to record eye movements during sleep."

The previous spring Kleitman had given Eugene Aserinsky, a graduate student in physiology, the assignment of watching people's eye movements as they slept. Since Kleitman was meticulous about staying abreast of all developments in the sleep field and because he read fluently in six languages, he picked up on things that most others would surely have missed. He had read Italian reports that the onset of sleep in both infants and adults is accompanied by slow, rolling eye movements, which gradually disappear. Kleitman wondered if these eye movements might be an indicator of the depth of sleep, and might come and go as a function of a hypothetical 50- to 60-minute basic rest-activity cycle during sleep. Kleitman felt that such a basic cycle might ensure that infants would wake up to nurse when hungry enough.

Kleitman's first assignment for Gene Aserinsky was to observe body movement and eye motility in infants. I'm sure Kleitman expected that the result of this research would be a minor detail in the study of sleep. I think that Gene agreed with him, and was not wildly excited about just sitting and watching people sleep. For Gene, a physiology graduate student, sleep research was simply not on a par with the study of cell metabolism and other hot areas of those days. In addition, Aserinsky had a family to support and wanted to get his Ph.D. as quickly as possible and get a real job. As soon as he earned his degree, he left sleep research except for a few experiments over the years. Sadly, Gene was killed in 1998 when his car hit a tree.

Gene observed 14 infants in their cribs in their homes for several hours during the daytime. He solidly documented the existence of a regular cycle in body activity and eye motility with a period of 50 to 60 minutes. Amazingly, he did not detect an important fact: There were really two types of eye movements—slow and fast.

Because the rest/activity cycle was so clear in infants, Aserinsky and Kleitman decided that similar observations should be conducted in sleeping adults. However, there was a big difference between observing infants in the daytime and observing adults at night. Since the iris and pupil of the eye bulge out slightly, small eye movements can be detected even when the eyelids are closed by watching the bulge move. But sitting up through the entire night watching for movement under someone's closed eyelids is about as tedious a task as the human mind can conceive; especially when you are sleepy yourself. Fortunately, Kleitman and Aserinsky came up with an easier method of recording eye movements. When the eyeball moves it creates electrical signals, so if you put electrodes on the skin next to the eye you can record the signals on a polygraph, in the same way that you can record the signals from the brain.

To make the job easier and save paper, Aserinsky would turn the polygraph on for short periods and then turn it off for 10 or 15 minutes. If he saw an eye movement during the recording period, he made a note of it and turned the machine off. He was really getting some good data on slow eye movements, but something else began to catch his interest. Occasionally, when he monitored long enough, he would see the pens jerk rapidly back and forth. This wasn't the slower pen movements of the eye motion he was used to seeing, so he initially assumed it was just more of the electronic "noise" that the primitive vacuum tube amplifiers produced in discouragingly plentiful amounts. All the electronics used at the time were based on vacuum tubes, which could malfunction dramatically at the slightest touch. Even an insect wandering into the machinery could cause a problem; the first computer "bugs" were, in fact, real bugs that made their way into the racks of vacuum tubes in early computers.

So at first he wrote it off—he didn't think that the eyes could really be moving that rapidly. But when he saw this same pattern again on subsequent nights, he began to have doubts. Finally, when Aserinsky saw the rapid zigzag of the pens on the paper once again, he decided just to go and look at the subject and figure out what was causing the malfunction. He walked into the bedroom, shined his flashlight on the sleeper's face, looked at his eyelids, and saw that the eyes were in fact moving rapidly underneath. Meanwhile the rest of the body lay quite still, sound asleep. The machinery wasn't malfunctioning at all—the eyes were really moving. In the lab, Aserinsky and Kleitman started calling this "rapid eye movement" to differentiate it from the slow eye movements they had been studying.

I have often wondered what would have happened if rapid eye movements during sleep had not been discovered essentially by accident in Nathaniel Kleitman's lab in 1952. It seems possible, if not probable, that the concept of REM sleep and the discipline of sleep medicine would not exist today. Remarkably, REM sleep could have been discovered by anybody. As Al Rechtshaffen said, "If anyone had thought that sleep was important enough to stay up and study it, rapid eye movements could have been discovered at any time in all previous history." Rapid eye movements also can be seen easily in a sleeping baby or child, or even in a sleeping pet dog or a cat, if you know what you are looking for. I don't entirely agree with Al, however, because even when they are looking, people usually see only what they expect to find and they do not see what they assume for whatever reason could not exist.

When I joined Kleitman's lab that fall, Aserinsky didn't seem terribly excited by what he was documenting. He was not really sure that these eye movements were occurring every night, and Kleitman was skeptical about what they might mean. In addition, the nighttime observations were hard work, and I think they were putting some strain on Aserinsky's marriage, so he was glad to have a medical student who could take over most of the sleep recordings.

Meanwhile, I was unmarried, energetic, and incredibly excited that I was going to have the chance to be documenting something that had never been observed before. Aserinsky told me about what he had been seeing in the sleep lab and then threw in the kicker that really hooked me: "Dr. Kleitman and I think that these eye movements might be related to dreaming." For a student interested in psychiatry, this offhand comment was more stunning than if he had just offered me a winning lottery ticket. It was as if he had told me "We found this old map to something called the Fountain of Youth." In fact, he *had* shown me a kind of map, one that seemed to point the way along the "royal road" to the heart of Freudian psychology—and, I hoped, to the final answer to the "consciousness problem."

The Royal Road

In the early 1950s, Freudian psychology and its offshoots held a new intellectual monopoly on the study of the mind. Every other book or movie, it seemed, had some element of Freudian psychology or some character being psychoanalyzed. Cartoons and jokes featuring a goateed psychiatrist popped up in everything from *The New Yorker* to *Reader's Digest*. Freud's ideas promised the tools to create a better future, and psychoanalysts were a powerful force in the medical profession and popular culture. There was a belief that Freudian psychoanalysis could explain every aspect of our problems: fears, anxieties, mental illnesses, and perhaps even physical illness. Proponents were claiming that psychoanalytic techniques could cure all manner of psychological problems, neuroses, and even psychoses because the insight brought by analysis inevitably would lead to healing. It was even thought that we could apply psychoanalytic principles to whole cultures and societies, to cure the world of war, crime, ill will, and so on.

The problem with such grandiose aspirations was that psychoanalysis wasn't really a science. Psychoanalysts of the day were always talking about "the science of psychoanalysis," but there was little objective research basis for it. Psychoanalytic theory was largely metaphorical, more analogous to religious beliefs than a scientific discipline. Many papers in respected psychoanalytic journals would start out with something like "In 1917 Freud said . . ." as if they were quoting from holy scripture. Many of the scholars writing about Freud were prolific and imaginative about disseminating their ideas, but they did little actual research. Today this would never pass for hard science, but at the time it was extremely compelling.

In order to understand why dreams were so interesting to aspiring psychoanalysts of my day, it is important to understand a little about the man who changed the very way we thought about dreams and who so thoroughly dominated American psychiatry even long after his death. Sigmund Freud, a turn-of-the-century Viennese doctor, is often identified as the "discoverer" of the unconscious—the mass of the most primitive instinctual drives, impulses, desires, and feelings that are not illuminated by the spotlight of conscious thought. Freud postulated that during most of our waking moments we deal with these "unthinkable" desires and impulses by repressing them. Ultimately these thoughts must come out, said Freud, which they did through dreams. In his 1905 book *The Interpretation of Dreams,* Freud proposed that dreams disguise forbidden thoughts or desires by cloaking them in other forms. The fantastical quality of dreams also works to protect sleep, since dreaming the forbidden in a straightforward way might shock us awake. Dreams therefore represent "the royal road to a knowledge of the part the unconscious plays in mental life," wrote Freud. To discover what these repressed thoughts or feelings represent, a psychoanalyst must decipher the dream symbols and events.

So you can see why, when Gene Aserinsky told me, the aspiring psychoanalyst, "We think these rapid eye movements might be related to dreaming," I was doubly blessed. Not only would I get the chance to look into the nature of consciousness, I would be studying the very root of unconscious motivation in dreams. The study of dreams was far from the world of "real" physiological research for Aserinsky, who was perfectly content to allow someone else to continue down this particular road.

One of my first assignments was to awaken people during the night and ask them if they remembered dreaming. We didn't have the money to pay volunteers, so they were almost always other medical students whom I recruited through word of mouth or through my classes. I would arrange to meet them at the entrance to Abbot Hall at about 9:00 or 10:00 P.M., and we would walk up to Kleitman's lab. There were two rooms that had once been chemistry laboratories, and the lab benches and desks were still there. The cot where people slept was underneath a fume hood, where the previous residents had vented the noxious chemicals they worked with. Of course, the rooms were cleared of any chemicals, but it still wasn't the cheeriest place to sleep. Sleep-deprived students, however, usually had little problem falling asleep here.

The other room housed the EEG machine and was where volunteers would be prepared for the night's recording. I used a special glue to fix electrodes to their scalp and forehead, then placed a cap on them to hold it all in place. I made sure to explain to subjects that currents could not pass back down the wires and give them a shock—this was a common, unspoken fear, and I didn't want it to interfere with their sleep. After they went into the bedroom and lay down in a bed under the fume hood, I turned off the lights (save a single dim one) and slipped away to the adjoining control room. There I kept the EEG machine on long enough to watch them going to sleep, then I turned it off and waited. It was alternately boring and eerie sitting in a deserted building at night, with only a prostrate body in the next room for company. Every once in a while the old creaky elevator would arrive on our floor and no one would get off, which really spooked me.

Since we had not yet realized that rapid eye movements occurred at regular, predictable intervals, I would just turn the machine on at random, never leaving it on for too long so that we wouldn't waste paper. If I got a hit—jiggling pens on the paper—I would cross into the next room, gently shake the subject's shoulder, softly call out his name in the nearly dark room and say, "Were you dreaming just now?" I tried to say it with a little urgency so that the significance of the question would get through the subject's sleep-addled brain. Then the answers would come pouring out: long descriptions of dreams that we captured on our old reel-to-reel tape recorder, to be transcribed later. Even short dreams could have very long explanations—think how much longer it can take to describe a movie sequence than to watch it—so at the end of the night we usually had the basis for 20 to 30, occasionally 50 or more, pages of dream descriptions.

I believe that the study of sleep became a true scientific field in 1953, when I finally was able to make all-night, continuous recordings of brain and eye activity during sleep. The most profound point to make is that for the first time, it was possible to carry out continuous observations of sleep without disturbing the sleeper. In addition, science is largely quantification, and this work was the beginning of studying sleep as a whole for its own sake and of describing and quantifying its overall patterns through the night. Others had noticed that there were changes in sleep patterns, but all-night recordings showed me how long each type of sleep tended to be and the shift from one type to another. After carrying out all-night recordings in a large number of individuals, I began to become convinced that periods of rapid eye movement were part of a 90-minute basic sleep cycle. Everybody, without exception, had the same pattern of sleep. This was a major discovery. In some cases, the eight-hour pattern from one night's recording could be superimposed almost perfectly on the pattern of another night.

Two other amazing observations awaited me in these all-night recordings: There were distinct stages of sleep during the night, which I called stage 1, stage 2, stage 3, and stage 4 sleep. Furthermore, I observed that rapid eye movements did not take place during any of these stages, but constituted a fifth distinct stage, which I called REM sleep. At the time, I made up these names casually, having no idea that the same names would still be used almost 50 years later. Simply making up the names for sleep stages is something I would never have the audacity to do now. Scientific progress is much more formalized today, and I probably would have to hold some kind of consensus conference on nomenclature first.

It is hard to convey how exciting it was to be doing this work. Here I was, a mere medical student, holed up in a nearly deserted building, making one surprising discovery after another. And knowing that I was the only one in the whole world who was looking at this aspect of human existence only added to the thrill of discovery. I imagine that this must have been how the first man to discover gold in California must have felt in 1848, when he looked at the mill race at Sutter's mill and saw it littered with gold nuggets—at that moment, he was the only one in the world who knew that a fortune was his for the picking. For me, I was gathering a scientific bonanza, and the rewards were intellectual rather than monetary, but the excitement was just as great.

As I began my own research into brain activity in people during

REM period, it quickly became clear that these recurring periods of sleep itself changed over the course of the night, with subjects having more frequent and longer periods of rapid eye movements toward the end of the night. Over the next few years I looked for rapid eye movements during sleep in all sorts of people to see if they were something that absolutely everyone experienced. I looked at schizophrenic patients, children, people of different races. Everywhere I looked, I found this intriguing sleep state. Even people who are blind from birth experience REM sleep, though the content of their dreams does not contain visual images.

One of the first groups I checked for rapid eye movements were infants, which Gene Aserinsky had observed and found only what we now know are slow eye movements. Kleitman and I had engaged in several discussions about at what age dreaming might begin and rapid eye movement might begin to occur. I had recorded a five-year-old child and had seen rapid eye movements. Gene had recorded in his 10-year-old son. So I thought it might be a good idea to go back to the crib. After about five minutes of watching a four-month-old baby, there were the rapid eye movements as plain as could be. I then got permission to hang around the newborn nursery in the Chicago Lying-In Hospital. Within a very short period of time, it was very obvious that rapid eye movements occurred during sleep of newborn infants. I think it says something about how strongly preconceived ideas can affect perceptions. By my calculations, Gene spent about 1,000 hours observing infants and never perceived a rapid eye movement. I might have fallen prey to the same blindness, but once the scales of dogma had dropped from my eyes the rapid eye movements were completely obvious.

At first we were not allowed to record the sleep of a representative of the largest group in the world—women. It seemed the whole idea of studying someone in bed got people's imaginations running. In the 1950s studies of sleep were always conducted on male volunteers for fear of shocking those ignorant of just how unsexy it was to do sleep research. I proposed testing a woman for REM sleep, but Kleitman was absolutely opposed. He feared scandal for either the laboratory or my career. Finally, after much negotiation, he allowed me to test my girlfriend, as long as Gene was there as "chaperon." As soon as the recording began, Aserinsky fell asleep on a couch.

Shortly thereafter I observed that at least one woman also had rapid eye movements during sleep.

I obtained my M.D. in 1955, and while all my classmates went on to their internships I stayed behind to begin a $3,000-a-year research fellowship. Shortly thereafter I met Pat Weber, the woman who would later become my wife. She volunteered to be recorded on 20 consecutive nights to see if sleep patterns were the same every night in a single individual. It isn't true, however, that I married her to get a cooperative subject.

As I continued to include an occasional woman in my sleep studies, there were always people who thought something untoward was going on. After I had earned my Ph.D. degree in 1957, I moved to New York City and I began work at Mount Sinai Hospital. By 1959 we were parents and I wanted to spend more time with my family, but doing research nearly every night and sleeping during the day did not allow us much time together. We were lucky to find a large apartment; I was able to set up half as a laboratory and the other half was our home. (I was actually able to get a grant from the National Institutes of Health to pay for half the apartment.) This worked out nicely, but the eyebrows started rising after a Barnard student responded to my classified advertisement for study volunteers. This woman, who happened to be a member of the Rockefeller Center's dance troupe, the Rockettes, was so delighted to be paid for sleeping that she told several other Rockettes, who also became research subjects. Thus, the following became a common scene: In the evening a lovely woman, still in theatrical makeup, would come to my apartment building and ask the doorman for my room. The next morning she would reappear in the same clothes, sometimes accompanied by an exhausted and unshaven Howie Roffwarg—a psychiatric resident at Columbia Presbyterian Medical Center—who had spent the night monitoring the machines. I was impressed that the doormen who saw this scene day after day managed to contain their curiosity. For a long time they managed to stay stony-faced, like the guards at Buckingham Palace. But then one day the doorman could stand it no longer and asked me, "Dr. Dement, what goes on in your apartment?" I suppose I could have satisfied his curiosity—but I couldn't resist the impulse just to smile broadly and say nothing.

While still in Chicago I found that during REM the brain acts as if it were awake, even though the rest of the body lies still. While the eyes dart back and forth, EEGs show that the neurons in the brain are amazingly active, as if the brain were living the dream while encased in its motionless body. In people the similarity between the brain in REM sleep and the brain awake is striking.

At the same time, I also was studying REM sleep in cats, and I found that the dreaming feline brain is so active that there is no discernible difference between sleeping and waking activity. The first time I recorded this phenomenon, I could hardly believe it. In fact, no one else could either. I wrote a paper on REM sleep in cats and had it rejected five times before it was finally accepted for publication. Everyone said, "This can't be the recording of a cat asleep—it is obviously awake." Even though I assured the journal editors that the cat was absolutely asleep, they concluded that, being a mere medical student, I must have made some dumb rookie error, like mixing up my recordings. Ultimately the paper was published, and in fact that first article later became one of the most cited scientific papers in biomedical research.

The journal editors' mistake is really not so surprising, in light of the history of sleep research. The idea that the brain is active during sleep, not turned off, flew in the face of thousands of years of prejudice. People reacted as if I were claiming that we don't need air to breathe.

Gradually, experiments convinced me that everyone experiences the regularly occurring periods of rapid eye movements and more active brain-wave patterns, and that these periods are an entirely different state of existence. Prior to this we regarded the rapid-eye-movement periods as a recurrent lightening of sleep, or possibly part of a vestige of the rest/activity cycle documented in infants. We even called the stage 1 brain-wave patterns "emergent stage 1" as opposed to "descending stage 1" at the onset of sleep. What really made the difference were observations that muscle tension tended to disappear entirely during REM periods in humans and cats. The work of Michel Jouvet in Lyons, France, showed that muscle activity was actually inhibited. We tested this out using electrically induced reflexes in humans, and I think I can safely say that by 1960 the tiny band of scientists worldwide who were studying sleep agreed that there are two fundamentally different kinds of sleep: REM sleep and non-REM sleep. Even though everyone thinks of sleep as one thing, REM and non-REM are as different from one another as both are from wakefulness.

A Need for Dreams

Of the three of us in the Kleitman lab—Kleitman, Aserinsky, and myself—I was the only one who took Freud's writings about dreaming seriously. I had read and reread *The Interpretation of Dreams,* and I was overcome with excitement that REM sleep might hold the key to understanding dreaming and perhaps mental illness. Once I had answered all doubts and concerns about the universality of REM sleep, I began studies in "dream deprivation." It was actually REM deprivation, but I called it dream deprivation because I believed at the time that dreaming was always associated with and only with REM sleep.

The big question in my mind then became "Do we need REM sleep, and what does it accomplish?" Freud believed that if taboo impulses and desires are not expressed or released through dreams, the psychic pressure will build up, leading to neurosis and to psychotic episodes in which the patient's view of reality is extremely distorted. In other words, dreaming is the safety valve of the mind. I hoped to prove Freud right about the connection between dreams and mental illness; I ended up contributing to the evidence against Freud's theory that began to pile up in the 1960s.

I participated in one of the first scientifically observed studies of very prolonged, total sleep deprivation, an experiment that seemed to support Freud's ideas. In January 1959 a New York disk jockey named Peter Tripp decided to raise money for the March of Dimes by staying awake for 200 hours, which is eight days and eight hours. He made daily broadcasts from a glass booth in Times Square, where people gathered to watch. He managed to stay lively and entertaining at least during his broadcasts, but toward the end of the marathon he began to suffer from paranoid delusions and had some auditory and visual hallucinations.

As I said earlier, the dogma of the time was that sleep may have different stages, but sleep is a single, unitary state, varying only in depth indicated by the changing brain-wave stages. My job was to record brain waves and eye movements when Peter Tripp ended his marathon and went to bed. At the time I was sort of dancing around the notion that sleep consisted of two entirely different states but wasn't quite ready to embrace the idea fully.

One of the reasons I wanted to participate in recording Peter Tripp's recovery sleep, although the event was basically a publicity stunt, was that it could provide a large and unambiguous sample of very deep sleep. If REM periods were merely a periodic lightening of sleep with no particular uniqueness, they should disappear altogether for at least the first few hours when sleep would be extremely deep. If, on the other hand, REM periods were qualitatively different from the remainder of sleep, if they had a different function, they should not disappear and perhaps they even would increase. About 30 minutes after I started recording, Tripp had one of the longest REM periods I had ever recorded, and over the course of the 10 hours I was able to keep everything operating in the hotel environment he had substantially more REM sleep than normal. It was as if the loss of REM sleep during the marathon had led to a REM sleep pressure that was spilling over into wakefulness as the psychotic symptomatology. This led me to formulate of the hypothesis that if people were not allowed to have REM sleep, they would start becoming mentally unstable. These ideas were right in line with Freud's theories, and were accepted excitedly by the psychiatric community of the time.

I immediately set out to deprive people of REM sleep in the lab to see what would happen. I started these experiments with Charles Fisher, a Mount Sinai psychiatrist and Freudian psychoanalyst who was studying dream recall during the day. We called the procedure "dream deprivation," and this is how it worked: For five consecutive nights I would continuously monitor volunteers' sleep, watching for the first signs of REM sleep. At that point I would shake them by the shoulder and say their name. As soon as they were definitely awake, I let them go back to sleep. Usually it took a substantial amount of time, 30 minutes or so, for someone to go from falling asleep to their next REM period, so they were able to get some non-REM sleep before the next interruption.

I saw immediately that the brain values REM sleep on its own. When the brain is deprived of REM periods, it tries to compensate by having longer REM periods and having them sooner. We called this REM pressure, and it was right in line with what we had seen in Tripp's recovery sleep. The problem for me was that by the third or fourth night, REM pressure would increase to the point where the REM periods would start right after the subject fell asleep. I kept having to wake people almost right after they fell asleep. After a whole night of interrupted sleep, the subjects were not too happy to have me waking them every five minutes. The volunteers, usually graduate students or unemployed actors, would start to get really angry and tell me they were getting sick of this. I often pleaded with them to stick with it, trying to play on their natural competitiveness and toughness—as well as their altruism by emphasizing their contribution to science. Mostly I succeeded, but sometimes I just had to give up and let them drift off to dreamland, consoling myself with getting a record of their recovery sleep.

These studies seemed to confirm Freud's ideas that dreams are vitally important. If they were not, why would the brain try so hard to compensate when deprived of them? In the next few years our REM-deprivation findings made me a celebrity in psychiatric circles. I began to talk about dreaming as a kind of nighttime psychosis, saying at one point "Dreaming permits each of us to become quietly and safely insane every night of our lives," which was really an elaboration of Freud's ideas about dreaming as a safety valve. From our early experiments with dream deprivation, it seemed a short step to showing that if we stopped dreaming long enough, the dream pressure would erupt as psychosis in waking life.

After I moved to Stanford University in 1962, I continued studies of REM deprivation in both humans and cats. I observed humans who voluntarily stayed up for days on end; they often became confused, bad tempered, and tremendously sleepy, but never clearly psychotic. Depriving cats of REM sleep was also arduous, but we found ways to do it that were gentle and effective at the same time. We carried out the procedure in successive durations up to 70 consecutive days. At this point, the size of the REM sleep makeup leveled off. The cats actually became more active, and their basic drives (food, sex, etc.) were enhanced. But these cats showed no sign of a deterioration in other behavior that could be interpreted as a true mental or physical impairment.

We have never found conclusive evidence that depriving people of dreams causes mental illness. Although dreams may play some part in keeping our mental equilibrium, and sleep itself indisputably does so, we realized we would have to look elsewhere for the source of the kind of mental illness that Freud studied. Regarding Peter Tripp's experience, we now know it is significant he was being given large doses of Ritalin, an amphetaminelike drug, to help him stay awake. At the time, amphetamine-induced psychoses were not well known, so no one suspected that the drugs might be the real cause of his paranoia and hallucinations.

By the mid-1960s sleep scientists were turning away from this part of dream research and taking much more interest in the mechanisms of sleep itself. Although in most ways the effort to back up Freud's theories with scientific data did not bear fruit, the flurry of interest in dreaming, REM sleep, and REM deprivation and their psychoanalytic implications were sufficient to inspire several scores of psychologists and psychiatrists to get involved in sleep research. I am absolutely convinced that had this excitement not occurred, the discovery of REM sleep and its relation to dreams might have been largely ignored and the impetus for further sleep research might have died on the vine.

The Birth of Sleep Medicine

Although REM sleep and its exploration were fascinating and important, in some ways it was a decade-long delay in addressing something more important: the integration of sleep research into the practice of medicine. As late as 1970, the practice of medicine ended when the patient fell asleep. Medicine occupied itself wholly with diseases and disorders that could be seen and diagnosed in waking patients. If physicians thought about sleep at all, their thoughts tended to reflect a prejudice that sleep was always good, always healing. There was a general attitude that sleep was a boundary that doctors should not cross, that nothing bad could happen when the patient was soundly asleep.

On the other hand, because my intense interest in sleep was becoming known beyond my own laboratory, I occasionally would be sent someone with a sleep problem. My interest was always captured even though I never knew exactly what to do. A few years before I left New York for Stanford, Charles Fisher sent me a patient whose diagnosis was narcolepsy, a sleep disorder characterized by extreme daytime sleepiness and sudden, brief attacks of muscle weakness. I did a sleep test on him, and the results were sufficiently interesting to make me want to do more studies. When I arrived in Stanford in January 1963, I searched high and low for another narcoleptic patient, querying all my medical center colleagues. Finally, in desperation, I put a tiny want ad in the *San Francisco Chronicle* describing the symptoms of narcolepsy, though not naming the illness. I was absolutely astounded to get about 100 letters in response to my ad—more than half of which were absolutely valid. We continued the research we had begun in New York and began to identify more and more individuals with the illness.

This episode really opened my eyes about medicine's blindness to sleep disorders: None of the victims had ever been diagnosed. On average, the narcoleptics had been living for 15 years with severely debilitating symptoms and had sought help from an average of five different physicians. None of the doctors realized these patients had narcolepsy. Until they were diagnosed, many of these narcoleptics thought they were crazy or lazy. They were incredibly relieved to find out what their problem was and start treatment.

What further opened my eyes to the lack of sleep awareness in medicine is what happened when I referred a few patients back to their local physicians, and their doctors simply ignored the problem, didn't know what to do, or didn't believe our recommendations.

By 1964, we were providing ongoing care for well over 100 narcolepsy patients in our geographic region and thought it would be nice to get paid for it, so we opened a narcolepsy clinic. We hoped to generate a revenue stream independent of grants from the National Institutes of Health, and, to be honest, after years of research I had developed a longing to take care of patients as a real doctor at least part of the time. In a sense, this was the first sleep disorders clinical service, but it lost so much money by the end of the first year I had to close it.

In 1970 a new and dangerous sleep disorder reared its head. Awareness of narcolepsy had grown, and patients were being referred who were described as narcoleptic but who had none of the typical symptoms. Their sole daytime symptom was incredible sleepiness and "sleep attacks." We discovered that most of these patients had another sleep disorder, called "apnea," in which their breathing was disrupted severely at night, depriving them of most of their night-time sleep. Once again the medical community had been blind to the problem, and in this case even actively resisted recognizing it.

Also in 1970, I decided to formally reopen our narcolepsy clinic as a general sleep disorders clinic. In addition to attempting to manage narcolepsy patients, optimize their treatment, and provide a diagnostic test, we offered our services to any and all patients with insomnia. At the time, we did several things: crucial all-night sleep recordings looking for a sleep-onset REM period at the beginning of nighttime sleep; a single nap recording in the daytime looking for a sleep-onset REM period; and occasionally 24-hour recordings, although these were generally under a research protocol.

Dr. Christian Guilleminault had spent six months at the Stanford Sleep Center sort of by happenstance in 1970. In 1971 Dr. Vincent Zarcone and I decided that we needed a neurologist to be involved in our sleep disorders program and we both thought of Christian, who had returned to France. At the First International Congress of Sleep Research, which met that summer in Brugge, Belgium, Vince and I persuaded Christian to return to Stanford. There is no question that this determined the future role of Stanford University in sleep disorders medicine. As every sleep specialist knows, Christian Guilleminault has been a giant in every aspect of the field and was crucial in the early development of a sleep apnea clinical practice, surmounting all sorts of obstacles and conducting his clinical research and care of patients with boundless energy.

One of the results of all our efforts in sleep medicine was that our little group at Stanford was accused of "ruining" sleep, of taking it away from people, because we dared to point out that sleep was not always healthy, not always good for you. It could be pathological and even life threatening. And again I, along with my Stanford sleep colleagues found ourselves virtually alone in the world in applying what we had learned about sleep to clinical practice.

The year of 1975 was pivotal. The Second International Congress of Sleep Research took place in Edinburgh on the centennial of the discovery of brain waves. At this international meeting, a few individuals who were interested in our sleep disorders clinical practice had a luncheon meeting to discuss some of the issues, particularly how to standardize the evaluation of patients. Many of us, including some of the world's outstanding narcoleptologists, assembled later in the summer to thoroughly review the state of narcolepsy research and to study pathophysiology and treatment possibilities at the First International Symposium on Narcolepsy convened by Pierre Passouant, Christian Guilleminault, and myself at La Grande Motte, France. At this event, the first consensus definition of a sleep disorder was approved unanimously. The American Narcolepsy Association, a patient volunteer organization, also was formed in 1975.

I have some photographs from La Grande Motte that frequently remind me of not just the meeting, but an evening at the casino. It had been announced that there would be a special entertainment. As we were all seated at tables, more or less facing a small stage, a very handsome young couple in Shakespearean garb presented themselves. "Ahh, how wonderful," I thought, "Shakespeare in French." Then the couple proceeded to take off all their clothes and carry out a ballet which seemed to portray symbolically a gymnast's approach to making love. I will never forget Madame Passouant turning to my wife afterward, and asking, "And did you enjoy the entertainment?" "I'm really not used to this sort of entertainment," my wife replied. "Oh, thank heavens," said Mme. Passouant, "Neither am I."

Twenty years later, one of the French participants in the international meeting visited Stanford. Though he was working in an entirely different area, I reminded him that we had previously met at La Grande Motte. He gave me a very blank stare. "The narcolepsy symposium," I added. The stare grew blanker. "It was the meeting with the very special entertainment. Surely you remember the very, very special entertainment," I persisted. Recall! His eyes lit up, "Oh yes," he smiled, "Oh sure." I eschew stereotypes, but with the French, its not easy.

In the fall of 1975, an even dozen clinical sleep researchers interested in the diagnosis and treatment of sleep disorders met at Chicago's O'Hare Airport. Several of these researchers had been at the informal meeting in Edinburgh that summer. The group agreed that clinical sleep disorders had advanced to the point where a more formal approach was desirable. The Association of Sleep Disorders Centers (ASDC) came into being over the next year. I was elected the first president and for the next twelve years I worked very hard to foster the development of this new clinical discipline and its professional organization. The goals of the organization were the enhancement of patient care, introduction of standards and standardization in clinical practice, and formulation and development of a standard diagnostic classification system.

Certification standards and guidelines for sleep disorders centers were developed, and the first examination of candidates to qualify for certification as "sleep specialists" was held in December 1977, in Cincinnati. In the autumn of 1978, the first edition of the scientific journal *Sleep* was published. This effort was arranged entirely by Christian Guilleminault and me, and I had to come up with a payment of $25,000, quite a large sum in 1978 dollars.

The ASDC *Diagnostic Classification of Sleep and Arousal Disorders* was published in the fall of 1979 after three years of extraordinary effort by the small group of dedicated individuals who comprised the "nosology" committee. On December 17 the Surgeon General of the United States, my friend Dr. Julius Richmond, announced the inauguration of "Project Sleep: The National Program on Insomnia and Sleep Disorders" at a small press conference in Washington, D.C. To quote the surgeon general, this project was to be "a major educational and research effort aimed at increasing the level of knowledge of physicians, their patients, and the public about the nature of insomnia and sleep disorders and their treatment. I was appointed chairman of Project Sleep, and had very high hopes for what might be accomplished.

In spite of what many people believe, a lot can be changed by an election. The administration that was elected in 1980 promptly eliminated Project Sleep even though it was making good progress. As we approach the millennium, the only folks in the entire world who understand the vast landscape of sleep disorders and the incredible things it contains are a few thousand sleep specialists. Today, if someone asks me what I do and I answer, "I take care of people with sleep disorders," they invariably reply, "What's that?" or "You mean people who can't sleep?"

Even though the benefits of sleep medicine are only minimally available to the public, I feel that founding sleep medicine has been my proudest accomplishment, the one that I most want to be remembered by. As I have pointed out, the struggle to bring what we know about sleep to the public and get the medical community to be knowledgeable about sleep continues to be an obsession for me. Again, for a long time I found myself alone in this mission.

Ultimately, however, I may be recognized more for the research that began in the mid-1970s and continues even now. This work was the next great phase of sleep research: understanding what drives the great daily cycle of sleep and wakefulness. What determines when we feel awake, alive, alert, and when we feel drowsy, listless, or sleepy? The answers affect how we act, feel, and think every day of our lives. That is what I want to tell you about in the next two chapters.

Chapter 3

Sleep Debt and the Mortgaged Mind

THE NIGHT of March 24, 1989, was cold and calm, the air crystalline, as the giant *Exxon Valdez* oil tanker pulled out of Valdez, Alaska, into the tranquil waters of Prince William Sound. In these clearest of possible conditions, the ship made a planned turn out of the shipping channel and didn't turn back in time. The huge tanker ran aground, spilling millions of gallons of crude oil into the sound. The cost of the cleanup effort was over $2 billion. The ultimate cost of continuing environmental damage is incalculable. Furthermore, when the civil trial was finally over in the summer of 1995, the Exxon Corporation was assessed an additional $5 billion in punitive damages. Everyone I query in my travels vividly recalls the accident, and most have the impression that it had something to do with the master's alcohol consumption. No one is aware of the true cause of the tragedy. In its final report, the National Transportation Safety Board (NTSB) found that sleep deprivation and sleep debt were direct causes of the accident. This stunning result got a brief mention in the back pages of the newspapers.

Out of the vast ocean of knowledge about sleep, there are a few facts that are so important that I will try to burn them into your brain forever. None is more important than the topic of sleep debt. If we can learn to understand sleep indebtedness and manage it, we can improve everyday life as well as avoid many injuries, horribly diminished lives, and premature deaths.

The *Exxon Valdez* disaster offers a good example of how sleep debt can create a tragedy and how the true villain—sleep indebtedness—remains concealed. I am sure that I was just as shocked as anyone when I learned about America's worst oil spill. The TV coverage of the dead birds and seals filled me with outrage over the environmental devastation. One of my friends went to Alaska and participated in the cleanup. He brought back photos and a big jar of crude oil. If you haven't been exposed to crude oil, keep away from it. It isn't the purified stuff that goes into your car. It's awful. It stinks to high heaven. You want to vomit.

When I watched the public debate what to do about the spill, I had no idea that it would have a special meaning for me a year later. The National Commission on Sleep Disorders Research finally mandated by the Congress was convened for the first time in March 1990, and 20 commissioners were assembled in Washington, D.C. After the first meeting I decided to visit a friend, Dr. John Lauber, who had been confirmed by the Senate as one of five members of the National Transportation Safety Board. He told me that the board would very likely identify sleep deprivation as the "direct cause" of the grounding of the *Exxon Valdez*.

I had worked with John a few years earlier on a study of the layover sleep of pilots on intercontinental airlines. He was head of human factors research at NASA-Ames and at the beginning of the layover study knew little about "sleep debt." At the end of the study, he was one of the few real experts in the world. Two months after the visit with John, he sent me the NTSB's final report.

The report noted that on the March night when the *Exxon Valdez* steamed out of Valdez, there were ice floes across part of the shipping lane, forcing the ship to turn to avoid them. The captain determined that his maneuver could be done safely if the ship was steered back to the main channel when it was abeam of a well-known landmark, Busby Island. With this plan established, he turned over command to the third mate and left the bridge. Although news reports linked much of what happened next to the captain's alcohol consumption, the captain was off the bridge well before the accident. The direct cause of America's worst oil spill was the behavior of the third mate, who had slept only 6 hours in the previous 48 and was severely sleep deprived.

As the *Exxon Valdez* passed Busby Island, the third mate ordered the helm to starboard, but he didn't notice that the autopilot was still on and the ship did not turn. Instead it plowed farther out of the channel. Twice lookouts warned the third mate about the position of lights marking the reef, but he didn't change or check his previous orders. His brain was not interpreting the danger in what they said. Finally he noticed that he was far outside the channel, turned off the autopilot, and tried hard to get the great ship pointed back to safety—too late.

For several years I would ask every audience that I addressed if there was anyone in the audience who had not heard the words *"Exxon Valdez."* A hand was never raised. Then I would say, "Who knows what caused the grounding?" Many hands would be raised, and the answer would always be "alcohol." Thus I could never exploit the potential impact of this catastrophe in getting knowledge about sleep into the mainstream, because of the media emphasis on the captain's drinking. When the report finally came out, there was no real interest. Even at the trial, in the summer of 1995, the true cause of the accident received little attention. What everyone ought to be talking about is how to deal with sleep deprivation and how to avoid it in the transportation industry and throughout all components of society, saying over and over again "Look what it caused." But instead, the poor captain has been hounded for nearly a decade.

An even more dramatic tragedy was the explosion of the space shuttle *Challenger*. After a year-long investigation, the Rogers Commission declared that in the absence of adequate data on O-ring function at low temperatures the decision to launch the rocket was an error. Those of us who saw this catastrophic event on television over and over and over know the ghastly consequences of that error. But not well known at all is the fact that the Human Factors Subcommittee attributed the error to the severe sleep deprivation of the NASA managers. This conclusion was only included in the committee's final report, which only noted that top managers in such situations are generally the ones who sacrifice the most sleep.

Was this the most costly case of sleepiness in history? The parents of any teenager who has died while asleep at the wheel might not agree. Even the most careful drivers are at risk, because we simply do not tell people—not even young people in the driver-training courses required in many states—how to recognize signs of dangerous sleepiness.

Of course, even children are at risk. For example in the past several years I have received many reports of school bus accidents where the driver fell asleep. Unfortunately, it may take another *Exxon Valdez* or Three Mile Island before the sleep community can mobilize public opinion to do something about this issue. Thus, I find myself in the bizarre circumstance of simultaneously fearing and at the same time hoping for another highly visible disaster.

Just last year I stepped up to the plate to fulfill this responsibility to my Stanford students. Drowsiness, that feeling when the eyelids are trying to close and we cannot seem to keep them open, is the last step before we fall asleep, not the first. If at this moment we let sleep come, it will arrive instantly. When driving a car, or in any hazardous situation, the first wave of drowsiness should be a dramatic warning. Get out of harm's way instantly! My message to the students is "Drowsiness is red alert!" I delivered and explained this message over and over in my 1997 undergraduate course "Sleep and Dreams," and the students got it. I am confident few will ever drive drowsy.

Everyone can recall a jolt of heart-stopping panic in the face of peril—when we realize a cab seems about to jump the curb we're standing on, or when we lose track of a child in a crowd. The response is instantaneous. We act. We should have a similar response the instant we feel drowsy at the wheel.

Ignorance About Sleepiness

Although I consider the pervasive lack of awareness about sleep deprivation a national emergency, it is difficult to indict any single culprit for this reprehensible neglect. Even though being sleepy obviously leads directly to sleep, and even though how tired you feel is an awfully good indication of how poorly you slept the night before, daytime sleepiness was not studied directly until fairly recently. It just didn't seem to be a part of the process of sleep itself.

For my part, I didn't seriously address the topic of sleepiness for many years, partly because I had been consumed by a decades-long fascination with REM sleep, but mainly because there was no way to measure it. Thus, the stunningly predictable connection between the lack of sleep and the desire for it—a connection that must have been obvious since the dawn of history—went without any serious scientific consideration until well into the 1970s.

True, there had been many studies of sleep deprivation over the years. Concern over the "confessions" by American prisoners about using germ warfare during the Korean War caused a surge of interest in the subject, because it was rumored that sleep deprivation was the method used to extort the confessions. However, for all intents and purposes, those studying sleep deprivation were looking in the wrong place, trying to measure changes in performance on various kinds of tests and looking for signs of mental breakdown, such as hallucinations, delusions or outright psychotic behavior. I myself had carried out literally years of work on sleep deprivation emphasizing the selective deprivation of REM sleep with similar outcome expectations. However, when we were trying to develop a better treatment for narcolepsy, we needed to measure subtle changes in the overall level of daytime sleepiness, and we were very frustrated because we had no tool to do this.

As you will see, we did find a tool, and learned of the enormous prevalence of daytime sleepiness in the average person. Since our level of daytime alertness is probably the number-one determinant of how we will function mentally—learning, school performance, everything—I wondered what psychologists might have to say about the sleepiness/alertness dimension. To my everlasting amazement, I couldn't find a single reference to sleepiness in the indexes of the 10 leading textbooks of introductory psychology, or in any other psychology text. The word "sleepiness" was even absent from 1963's second edition of my mentor's monumental tome, *Sleep and Wakefulness,* which was then in the library of every one of the small band of sleep researchers.

Academia's—and, for a time, my own—gigantic blind spot for sleepiness as a major determinant of waking function became baffling to me. I now think the continuum of sleepiness and alertness as the stage upon which all human behavior is acted out. Since we now can claim with confidence that where we are on this stage, from the high peak of optimal alertness to the deep trough of extreme drowsiness, is the single most important determinant of how well we perform, the total absence of this subject from psychology textbooks or any other educational materials is incomprehensible. Although the scientific knowledge has been available for more than two decades, students are still not acquiring crucial knowledge about sleepiness, sleep debt, and sleep deprivation in any of our educational institutions.

I really can't blame anyone for the long delay in measuring sleepiness because it is such a difficult quality to pin down and dissect. The instinct of a good scientist is to quantify, and how tired a subject feels used to be considered nearly impossible to measure. If you and your spouse are both up in the middle of the night with a sick baby, for instance, how can you decide which of you is really more tired and ought to get first claim on sleep? Can you accurately quantify your sleepiness?

In the early days of sleep research, rather than talk about sleepiness or alertness itself, researchers measured the ability of sleep deprived people to perform a task, such as stacking blocks in the right order or solving word puzzles. They called this measure "performance failure" or "fatigue." The problem with this approach is that a person faced with a task can temporarily shake off fatigue. We all do this. Every morning, no matter how exhausted, we rouse ourselves out of bed and start the coffee machine. Or late at night, when we'd much rather be asleep, we can force ourselves to concentrate on homework or paying bills. So sleep-deprived test subjects presented with a task changed the conditions of the test by arousing themselves and masking the severity of their sleepiness, the very thing that researchers were trying to measure.

The feeling of being tired and needing sleep is a basic drive of nature, like hunger. If you don't eat enough, you are driven to eat. If you go long enough without food, you can think of nothing else. Once you get food, you eat until you feel full and then you stop. Thus, the subjective responses of hunger and satiation ensure that you fulfill your overall daily requirement for calories. In essentially the same way, your sleep drive keeps an exact tally of accumulated waking hours. Like bricks in a backpack, accumulated sleep drive is a burden that weighs down on you. Every hour that you are awake adds another brick to the backpack: The brain's sleep load increases until you go to sleep, when the load starts to lighten.

In a very real sense all wakefulness is sleep deprivation. As soon as you wake up, the meter starts ticking, calculating how many hours of sleep you will need to pay off that night. Or, to continue the load metaphor, it tallies how many bricks you will have to shed to get back to zero. Generally, people need to sleep one hour for every two hours awake, which means that most need around eight hours of sleep a night. Of course, some people need more and some need less, and a few people seem to need a great deal more or less. From the work we have done, we must conclude that each person has his or her own specific daily sleep requirement. The brain tries to hit this mark, and the farther you are from getting the number of hours of sleep you need, the harder your brain tries to force you to get that sleep.

How Tired Are You? The Multiple Sleep Latency Test

In 1970, in the same month that I opened the Stanford University Sleep Disorders Clinic, my wife and I began a year as resident fellows in one of Stanford's all-freshman dormitories. As part of the residential education effort, I devised a number of projects for small groups of my freshmen students, one of which was called the 90-minute day. The purpose of the study was to test the vital need for REM sleep. One of my fellow sleep researchers had previously published a study, never confirmed, that awakening people at the onset of REM periods and substituting 20 minutes of mild exercise for REM sleep seemed to replace the need for the REM period. In our 90-minute day protocol, we would let the subject sleep for 30 minutes—that is, keep them in bed for 30 minutes—and then keep them out of bed for 60 minutes. Throughout the 24-hour day, this would allow the opportunity to get a full eight hours (16 times 30 minutes) of sleep. But since the first period of REM sleep does not occur until about 60 minutes of non-REM sleep have elapsed, we felt that if REM sleep was not vitally necessary, it would never appear. There were about five students in the group and one was designated as the subject who had to go to bed every 90 minutes around the clock for five consecutive days during spring break. The other five students monitored the sleep periods and wake periods in shifts during that time.

We were somewhat surprised when we found that REM sleep filled several of the 30-minute "nights" the subject was in bed. The only time I had ever seen sleep-onset REM periods in normal sleep—periods of REM sleep occurring immediately after sleep starts—was in newborn babies. I actually had the experiment repeated with five additional subjects in our university sleep laboratory and we obtained the same result. This was exciting evidence in support of the vital necessity of REM sleep, but I didn't see a more important possibility for another five years.

By 1975 Christian Guilleminault and I were pretty sure that excessive daytime sleepiness was the most important symptom in sleep disorders medicine. We had written several original papers on disorders of excessive sleepiness and we were getting desperate for a precise objective measure. It turned up where we weren't even looking. Because of my interest in narcolepsy, I persuaded the formidable Mary Carskadon to repeat the 90-minute-day protocol.

Mary was someone I had known for a long time because she was one of my wife's cousins. Mary was a social worker in Washington, D.C., and when I heard she was looking for another job, I immediately offered her a position in our new clinic. At first she did mostly clerical work—scheduling patients and so on—but soon she was taking data that others had gathered, pulling them together, and analysing them and publishing in scientific journals, and eventually entered the Stanford Ph.D. program in neuroscience. Now she is a professor at Brown University.

After repeating the 90-minute-day experiment, Mary and I were sitting at a table looking at a plot of results from one volunteer and suddenly we saw it! A lightbulb turned on simultaneously in both our brains. The amount of time it took the subject to fall asleep during the successive 30-minute periods in bed fluctuated exactly in rhythm with the subject's own feelings of sleepiness. The objective measure of daytime sleepiness that had never before existed was staring us in the face—sleep latency, or the length of time it takes to fall asleep. This may not seem like an earthshaking epiphany, but conceiving and developing an objective measure of sleepiness was perhaps one of the most important advances in sleep science.

Mary and I dubbed the new test the Multiple Sleep Latency Test, or MSLT. We arbitrarily decided to measure the speed of falling asleep every two hours during the daytime and, to minimize the possible horrendous boredom of lying in bed awake for long periods, we decided that the maximum duration of a single test would be limited to 20 minutes. We had the subjects go to the bathroom, then put them to bed in a quiet dark room and told them to close their eyes, relax, and try to sleep. We removed every source of arousal we could think of so that the strength of the underlying tendency to fall asleep would be clearly revealed. Further, we terminated the test and woke the subject immediately after he or she fell asleep, so the subject didn't get any sleep during the test (which could change their level of sleepiness on subsequent tests). We scored the test by noting the number of minutes it took the subject to get to sleep, from 0 to 20. If the person did not fall asleep in 20 minutes, we ended the test and gave him or her a score of 20, which denoted maximum alertness at that time of the day. Individual sleep latency measurements were taken at 10, 12, 2, 4, and 6 o'clock.

Once we had the MSLT test, we investigated the effect of missing two nights' sleep on daytime alertness. Our volunteers' MSLT scores fell close to zero after the first night—meaning that they fell asleep in less than a minute—and stayed at the same level during repeated tests for the entire 48 hours. With another group of volunteers we decided to vary the amounts of sleep over the course of one night. Some subjects slept 10 hours, some 2 hours, and others slept various amounts in between. This allowed a few volunteers to get as much sleep as they normally needed, others obviously far less. When we tallied the individual sleep latency scores from the next day's five tests, we found a direct linear relationship between the average amount of sleep lost and the average change in MSLT scores. In other words, the less sleep subjects got, the more rapidly they fell asleep—in direct proportion to the amount of sleep lost. We realized with great excitement that we could accurately measure a person's sleep load in a way that we never could with performance tests.

After we gathered more data we decided that a score of 0 to 5 signified an extreme sleep tendency. People's own internal arousal processes, or some external demand (such as playing sports or driving a car) can make people feel pretty good and not sleepy at all. But this temporary arousal is a dangerous state, because sleep can overtake the brain the moment the arousal ceases or the person relaxes. When this happens in someone with narcolepsy, we call it a "sleep attack," although the term can just as well fit anyone who is suddenly overtaken by a large sleep debt. We often refer informally to the range of scores from 0 to 5 minutes as the "twilight zone," because in this range, physical and mental reactions often are very impaired. A score of 5 to 10 minutes is borderline, while a score of 10 to 15 indicates a manageable sleep load. A score of 15 to 20 represents excellent alertness.

Sleep Debt: Nature's Loan Shark

Once we made the breakthrough advance that gave us a precise and reliable objective measure of our tendency to fall asleep, the MSLT, Mary and I were poised to make another major discovery: The brain keeps an exact accounting of how much sleep it is owed. In our first study, we restricted the sleep of ten volunteers to exactly 5 hours each night for seven nights and observed that the tendency to fall asleep increased progressively each successive day. For the first time in the history of sleep research, we discovered that the effect of each successive night of partial sleep loss carried over, and the effect appeared to accumulate in a precisely additive fashion. In other words, the strength of the tendency to fall asleep was progressively greater during each successive day with exactly the same amount of sleep each night. For some time Mary and I referred to this as an increased sleep tendency, and it was clear that the increase did not dissipate without additional rest. How people recover from various levels of sleep deprivation after getting sleep has not been well studied. However, current evidence suggests that the accumulated lost sleep must be paid back at some time, perhaps even hour for hour.

We use the term "sleep debt" because accumulated lost sleep is like a monetary debt: It must be paid back. Regardless of how rapidly it can be paid back, the important thing is that the size of the sleep debt and its dangerous effects are definitely directly related to the amount of lost sleep. My guess is that after a period of substantial sleep loss, we can pay back a little and feel a lot better, although the remaining sleep debt is still large. The danger of an unintended sleep episode is still there. Until proven otherwise, it is reasonable and certainly safer to assume that accumulated lost sleep must be paid back hour for hour. Therefore, if you miss 3 hours one night, you must sleep 11 hours the next night (3 plus your normal 8) in order to feel alert throughout the day.

Your sleep debt may have accumulated in small increments over many days. For example, during a five-day work week where you needed 8 hours each night and instead got 6, you would build up a sleep debt of 10 hours (5 times 2). From this perspective, sleeping in until noon on Saturday is not enough to pay back the 10 lost hours plus your nightly requirement of 8; you would have to sleep until about 5:00 P.M. to balance the sleep ledger. Of course, most people won't sleep that long, and in fact it is difficult to do because of the alerting process of the biological clock, which I will talk about more in the next chapter. More likely, you will sleep in an extra hour or two and get up feeling better. But the debt is still there, demanding to be paid. Later that day you'll start feeling the effects of the sleep debt again. And if you borrow more sleep time over subsequent nights, you won't just stay sleepy, you'll get even sleepier. As your debt grows, your energy, mood, and cognition will be undermined.

There is another important way that sleep deprivation can occur and sleep debt can accumulate. As you will learn later, several sleep disorders are characterized by very severe and impairing daytime sleepiness. In such patients we typically see hundreds of brief interruptions of sleep in a single night. In spite of this, careful tabulation of the intervening short periods of sleep can add up to what ought to be a satisfactory amount of total sleep.

Several groups of sleep researchers have carried out studies on normal volunteers which have clarified this situation. In these studies, subjects were awakened every minute or so throughout entire nights, and the next day's alertness was evaluated using the MSLT. The nocturnal awakenings were brief, 5 to 10 seconds, and subjects usually returned to sleep immediately. Although there were usually several hundred interruptions, the cumulative total sleep can add up to normal amounts. Nevertheless, daytime sleepiness is markedly increased, as if there had been no sleep at all, or very little.

Interrupting sleep every minute or so all night long is a heroic experimental manipulation. I am happy to report that the results of these particular experiments have been very consistent. Accordingly, we may conclude that the restorative value of sleep is severely curtailed if sleep periods are not allowed to continue for at least several minutes. If 10 to 15 minutes of sleep are allowed to occur before an interruption, this effect is greatly lessened. These studies have led to the concept that there are minimal units of restorative sleep. In other words, it is as if the bank that keeps track of sleep debt doesn't accept small deposits.

In one of our first studies we evaluated the clinical usefulness of the MSLT by comparing narcoleptics and normal sleepers. The results were fabulous. The MSLT sharply distinguished patients and normals. However, the MSLT scores of a few normal volunteers were in the pathologically sleepy range (1 to 5 minutes). This latter group tended to be college students. For a while we thought that these younger "normals" were in the early stages of the narcoleptic sleep disorder, not yet manifesting the other symptoms. But it was hard to imagine why Stanford University would attract so many budding narcoleptics. We tested a few more students, allowing a baseline normal amount of sleep (8 hours a day) and carefully measuring their sleep tendency day to day with the MSLT. Nearly all of the students appeared to be pathologically sleepy! I should not have been so surprised, because I have been watching students fall asleep in class ever since I was a college student myself.

The obvious explanation finally occurred to Mary and me: The students needed more sleep. To prove this we did studies where we extended their nightly hours in bed to 10, and over several days, the MSLT score steadily improved. Now that we know about sleep debt, we can only imagine how many thousands of observations on human behavior have been made over the decades on chronically sleep-deprived subjects whom researchers thought were "normal." Since people are so severely affected by a large sleep debt, its presence can potentially alter the results of almost all research measures, from I.Q. tests to observations of drug side effects. The baseline studies of all human research, regardless of their nature, now must include measures of daytime sleep tendency, so that the variable degree of chronic sleep loss does not contaminate every study.

Despite the fact that "sleep debt" has entered common parlance (some researchers also call it "sleep load" or "sleep tendency"), many people don't fully understand the concept. Again and again I hear people complain that they sleep a full night, even an extra hour or so, and still feel just as sleepy or even sleepier than before. "Well," they think, "I must be sleepy because I am sleeping too much." The fact is that you don't work off a large sleep debt, which is what most of us have, by getting one good night's sleep.

In 1985 I testified before the Congress on the dangers of sleepiness. The problem with testifying before congressional committees is that members of the Congress have a mind-numbing number of issues before them every day and, if they attend at all, run in and out of committee hearings, read over other material, or whisper with pages and aides. I had noticed that a really effective witness would do something dramatic to get committee members' attention. So when I came before the committee I stood up and stated, "Gentlemen, our national sleep debt is a greater threat to our country than the national monetary debt." I was pleased to see that several of the previously distracted committee members sat up and began to take notice. Then I explained how widespread sleep debt is and why it is a vital public health issue. Today I have the dubious satisfaction of being vindicated. Our government has been able to balance the national budget, but our national sleep debt is bigger and more dangerous than ever.

People also sometimes ask me if the exact accounting could mean that they are still carrying around sleep debt from all those all-nighters years earlier in college. We don't know what happens to sleep debt in the long term. You may have paid off those sleep-deprived periods when you got sick shortly afterward and slept 18 hours at a stretch. Or the brain may lose track of sleep debt accumulated months or years earlier.

Although it is clear that some occupations appear to be associated with daily sleep loss over very long periods of time, we can never be sure that there are not occasional nights with extra sleep, or unintended naps. Prolonged partial sleep loss is most likely in some seasonal occupations, harvest for example, where work goes on seven days a week and during all daylight hours. But we don't know for sure what happens. We know that most people completely collapse after three or four days of total sleep loss, which would add 24 to 32 hours of sleep debt to whatever they already had. Some people say they have been in jobs or situations where they never got enough sleep, and surely their sleep debt would have been in the hundreds of hours. Why didn't they collapse?

When I was in high school, I would get up between 2:00 A.M. and 3:00 A.M. (for a couple of months in the spring) to go out in the field and cut asparagus, seven mornings a week. Being a teenager, I didn't habitually go to bed at 6:00 P.M. to get enough sleep. Even if I lost only 2 hours a night, that would be at least 100 hours of debt over the several months. I remember falling asleep in class, only to face a very angry teacher, and falling asleep on the couch at home many times. So I may have paid back some of the debt in short catnaps, but I still would have had so much sleep debt that I don't know how I kept going.

A final answer to this issue can't be obtained until precise studies over long periods of time are carried out. Right now we know only that the brain keeps an accurate count of sleep debt for up to two weeks, because that's the longest controlled laboratory experiments have lasted. The next question is usually "Why don't you do experiments to find out?" I can't think of any research that is more important or more needed by our society. It is just a question of funding.

Getting funding for sleep research is often difficult. In the first place, the vast majority of people are still unaware of the research on chronic sleep loss and of the concept of sleep debt. These include people who award grants. It is very difficult to obtain grant funds from people who don't know about or don't understand the implications of your research. In the second place, these studies are much more expensive than purchasing a few chemicals and a few test tubes. To do a proper long-term sleep study, you must recruit volunteers who are willing to live in a laboratory environment, however comfortable, for months at a time; you must feed and house them and pay for three shifts of technicians to monitor them and record exactly how many hours of sleep they get. This represents millions of dollars of grant money that researchers are not likely to get from the government or drug companies, because sleep debt is not directly associated with any disease. The irony, though, is that in the end, the number of people killed or maimed in accidents caused by sleep deprivation may exceed the number killed by far better-funded diseases. There are likely many other negative consequences of sleep deprivation—sleep debt is known to lower productivity and increase a tendency to be angry or violent.

Arousal: The Mask of Sleep Debt

Because the alertness-sleepiness continuum is a complex function of sleep debt, biological alerting, and environmental stimulation, we are generally very bad judges of our sleep tendency. How likely we are to fall asleep is the combination of two opposing forces: our sleep load minus our level of alerting. We may be so excited or stressed by external stimulation that we don't perceive a huge sleep debt. Recall that we even can feel pretty good when our MSLT score is well into the twilight zone.

In 1988 my good friend and colleague Tom Roth and his team at the Henry Ford Hospital's Sleep Disorders Center and research lab in Detroit studied a large group of people who specifically claimed that they were never sleepy in the daytime. They first put each of them to bed for eight hours—a good night's sleep, most people would agree. And the people in the group thought so too—they said they felt great. Yet when their daytime alertness was tested the next day, more than 80 percent actually were not optimally alert, as shown by low MSLT scores. Of those, about one quarter tested as pathologically sleepy, falling asleep in five minutes or less every time they were given the chance. Somehow, 1 out of 5 people who said they felt fine were actually so in need of sleep that they posed a great danger to themselves or others. Out of all those who said that daytime sleepiness wasn't a problem, only about 1 in 10 were actually at peak alertness. And the situation may be much worse with regard to people who say they do feel sleepy. In population surveys carried out by the National Sleep Foundation, 75 percent of adults said they experience daytime sleepiness and 34 percent said sleepiness interfered with their daytime activities.

Perhaps the sleep-deprived people who say sleepiness isn't a problem actually feel sleepy, but don't think it's a big deal. Certainly many people think it's "normal" to feel sleepy during the day. Our automatic reaction to sleepiness is to fight it by seeking out stimulation—driving to the store, working harder, or taking a stretch. Many of us habitually make ourselves do something more active when we start to feel sleepy, which masks our underlying sleep debt. This stimulation can take us from moment to moment through the day because we live in perpetual motion, moving from one task to the next, pushing ourselves to accomplish what we must. Only when we can't find something stimulating are we forced to confront our hidden sleep tendency. At these times the sleep debt that has been kept at bay comes flooding back through the body and mind.

Driving Under the Influence of Sleep Debt

People *must* learn to pay attention to their own sleep debt and how it is affecting them. Not doing so, and misunderstanding the rules of sleep debt and arousal, can be extremely dangerous. A friend of mine, also a Stanford professor, once participated in a bicycle race around Lake Tahoe. He got very little sleep during the race, but then he slept about nine hours a night for the two nights he stayed at the lake after the race. He woke up on Sunday morning feeling rested, ready to pack up and drive home. But as he was coming down the winding mountain road he began to yawn and his eyelids felt heavy. He told me that he was a little surprised because he thought he had gotten plenty of sleep. If someone had been with him, he probably would have traded places, but it did not occur to him to pull over and take a nap. As he drove on, it became harder and harder to keep his eyes open, and he began to be concerned. At that moment he saw a sign for a restaurant only several miles farther down the road. "Good," he thought, "I'll be able to get some coffee." Right after that he fell asleep, just for a moment, and awoke with a terrible start to find that he had drifted into the oncoming lane. He jerked the wheel to the right, but the road curved to the left, and the car went over a 30-foot ledge. The next thing he knew he was upside down, suspended by his seat belt, the car impaled on a jagged rock that had sliced through the roof and into the empty passenger seat next to him. He sustained serious cuts and bruises, and his right arm was completely paralyzed, but miraculously he was alive.

When he told me the story later, he still didn't understand how he could have been so sleepy. "But Bill, I got two full nights of sleep before I left Tahoe." Not knowing about sleep debt, he could not know that a few hours of extra sleep does not alleviate the sleep debt accumulated over the preceding nights or weeks. He was driving alone without the stimulation of conversation, along a route he knew fairly well. In short, there was little to act as a dike against the sea of sleep debt that he had built up. Ironically, his awareness of how terribly drowsy he was feeling may have forestalled sleep in the minutes before the crash. When he saw the sign for the restaurant up ahead and knew that he would soon get coffee, he relaxed and let that worry go. A few moments later he was hurtling off the mountain road. If the idea that drowsiness is supremely dangerous had been burned into his brain, he would have stopped driving no matter how difficult or inconvenient.

Fatal Fatigue: Alcohol and Sleep Debt

As I will emphasize in Chapter 5, older children never feel sleepy during the day. They were the only group we studied in sleep camp who never fell asleep in the twenty minutes allotted for the individual sleep latency tests. And of course, children are usually not sleep deprived. Putting all our results together, we can state with confidence that if you feel sleepy or drowsy in the daytime, then you must have a sizable sleep debt. Sleep debt is the physical side of the coin, and the feelings of sleepiness or drowsiness are the psychological side. As an analogy, dehydration is the physical side of the coin and the feeling of being thirsty is the psychological side. To carry the analogy a little further, if we have thoroughly quenched our thirst, we cannot immediately feel thirsty. But if we are becoming dehydrated, the desire to drink may be diminished if we are involved in something very interesting or demanding. At some point, of course, thirst becomes overwhelming. Likewise, we cannot feel sleepy in the daytime if we do not have a sleep debt, but we may not feel sleepy if we are doing something that excites us. If we have a very strong tendency to fall asleep and we reduce the stimuli that are keeping us awake, we will very soon begin to feel sleepy and will inevitably fall asleep, intentionally or otherwise.

But all those interested in traffic safety and all those who wish to have a long life as well must take note. When a crash is attributed to alcohol, the real culprit, or at least a coconspirator, is often sleep deprivation. In studies that are second to none in importance, the powerful interaction between sleep and alcohol was revealed by the outstanding sleep research team at Henry Ford Hospital Sleep Disorders Center. A group of volunteers slept 10 hours a night for one week, 8 hours a night during a separate week, and on a third schedule simulated a social weekend by getting 5 hours of sleep for 2 nights. In the morning after completing each schedule, all of the volunteers were given either a low dose of alcohol or a placebo. Then their degree of impaired alertness was evaluated utilizing the

MSLT and performance tests. When the subjects were given the low dose of alcohol after the 8-hour schedule, they became slightly more sleepy than when given placebo. After the schedule of 2 nights with little sleep, the exact same dose of alcohol the next morning made them severely sleepy, barely able to stay awake. However, the exact same dose of alcohol after 10 hours of sleep every night for a week had no discernible effect. In other words, alcohol may not be a potent sedative by itself, but it becomes very sedating when paired with sleep debt. It is tempting to speculate that all sedatives, particularly sleeping pills, interact with sleep debt. This area deserves much more research. I will, however, describe some very spectacular findings related to this issue in the next chapter.

The implications of this are far-reaching. People are well aware of the dangers of drinking and driving, but they don't know that a large sleep debt and even a small amount of alcohol can create a "fatal fatigue." People can be just fine driving after a single drink one day (when they have little sleep debt), and be a hazard to themselves and others if they have that same drink on a day in which they have a large sleep debt. A fact little known by the public at large is that in nearly every accident linked to alcohol consumption, sleep debt almost certainly plays a major role.

In one state traffic agency, researchers are trying very hard to understand traffic accidents designated as alcohol-related even though the alcohol in the tissue is far below any level thought to be impairing.

Uncovering Sleep Debt

We can get an idea of how much sleep debt the average person carries around from reviewing two landmark experiments that were conducted 20 years apart. The first of these experiments was carried out almost four decades ago by investigators at the United States Naval Hospital in Bethesda, Maryland. At the time, there was no idea whatsoever about sleep debt, but there was a great deal of interest in the possibility that sensory deprivation might cause disorientation, hallucinations, and psychosis. To test this hypothesis, the naval hospital investigators required subjects to stay alone inside silent, dark cubicles 24 hours a day for one entire week. The cubicles were insulated against sound and maintained at a constant temperature and humidity. The subjects wore thick gloves to minimize their sense of touch, and they took liquid nutrients through a straw. They were not able to move about; they could only lie awake or fall asleep.

Volunteers must be incredibly motivated to participate in this sort of experiment. The reader may wonder why anyone would submit to such an ordeal. The subjects were navy personnel and were rewarded with leave for participating. Even so, many people wouldn't be psychologically capable of handling the boredom and isolation. The naval volunteers were screened to ensure that they were not the type to fall apart easily; their rigorous navy training involving months at sea was no doubt a factor in their ability to endure.

Over the seven days and nights, the subjects' brain waves were monitored constantly. With absolutely nothing to do, the group slept a lot the first day—averaging more than 16 hours of sleep time out of 24. A few slept 20 hours. Thereafter, on each successive day their average amount of sleep decreased, which I interpret as a consequence of working off sleep debt. By the final day, in spite of the complete absence of environmental stimulation, the subjects were able to sleep only an average of about 8 hours. But prior to this, they obtained a total of about 25 hours of extra sleep (and by extra sleep I mean the hours of sleep more than 8 hours per day). This 25 hours would be about the amount of sleep debt they had when they entered the study.

More recently psychiatrist Thomas Wehr and his colleagues at the National Institutes of Health in Bethesda, Maryland, embarked on an equally ambitious experiment. They decided to put a group of volunteers on a sleeping schedule that would simulate life in the winter before electricity or gas lamps, when folks pretty much went to sleep after the sun set and rose when the sun came up. Wehr put the volunteers on a regimen of 14 consecutive hours of bedtime per day for weeks on end and monitored how their mood and feelings changed over that time. Two volunteers stayed on this schedule for 14 weeks.

As in the navy study, the experiment at the NIH involved a lot of effort and expense for the scientists, and a good measure of devotion and hardiness on the part of the volunteers. The 16 volunteers had received a complete psychological evaluation designed to exclude anyone prone to depression or other mental disorders.

The volunteers first spent 8 hours in bed per night for one week, a common amount in our modern era and typical of summer sleep in centuries past. Then they began spending 14 hours in the dark, in bed. They were allowed to have a normal day outside the National Institutes of Health (but no naps!) and were required to arrive at the NIH every day at 4:00 P.M. They were then given a short test of their mood and wired with temperature and sleep probes. At 5:00 P.M. they went to their separate bedrooms—windowless chambers without lights. They could not read, listen to music, or do any other activity that might keep them awake artificially. Like the navy subjects, they could only lie in bed in the dark. At 7:00 A.M., 14 hours later, they rose and were brought out of their rooms, unwired, given another psychological test, and at about 8:00 A.M. allowed back out into the wide world. But for only eight hours.

You might think that this sort of existence would drive people crazy, but in fact the volunteers were happy with the routine. Like those in the navy experiment, they slept a lot at first, an average of more than 12 hours per day. But by the fourth week they had settled down to a steady-state average of 8 hours and 15 minutes of sleep. Some people slept a little more, some a little less. The longest sleeper regularly got about 9 hours of sleep, and the shortest sleeper got about 7.5 hours of sleep.

As in the navy study, my interpretation of the results is that the subjects were carrying sizable sleep debts when the baseline week began, and they may have accumulated a little more sleep debt during the baseline week. When given extra hours of darkness and deprived of stimulation that normally would override sleep debt, they had nothing to do but pay off that debt. Slowly, as the sleep debt was worked off, they slept less and less, even though they had the opportunity to keep sleeping long hours. Eventually subjects in both experiments adopted a steady state of close to 8 hours' sleep per day, which probably represents their actual daily sleep requirement. In other words, when they had no carryover sleep debt, the time spent awake during one day added up to a debt that required 8 hours of sleep to pay back. In Wehr's experiment volunteers who seemed perfectly normal when they entered the test worked off an average of about 30 hours of sleep debt—the equivalent of 2 lost hours a day for two weeks!

The subjects' mood and level of energy also improved tremendously over the course of the NIH study. The crucial variable for mood was not the amount of light but the size of each person's sleep debt.

The neat thing about Wehr's experiment was that it was really not a sleep experiment. Tom Wehr has done quite a lot of good research on seasonal changes in psychological function—changes brought on by changes in temperature and day length. People with seasonal affective disorder, for instance, get depressed during the winter. So if there were any preconceptions about what the experiment would show, they would have been all in the opposite direction of the actual results. In other words, although mood was expected to deteriorate with the very sizable reduction in light exposure, a very significant improvement occurred. The fact that any experimental bias was completely negated in this way makes this result very strong.

Finally, this remarkable study illustrates the principle that a small amount of sleep debt is good, indeed is necessary, for sleeping efficiently. As subjects' sleep debt was paid back, it took them longer and longer to fall asleep. Furthermore, as their sleep debt became very low, the subjects tended to wake up in the middle of the experiment and lie awake for 4 hours until they accumulated sufficient debt to fall asleep again. Most likely we need the sleep debt accumulated during our waking 16 hours, plus a little extra, in order to fall asleep in 5 or 10 minutes and sleep through the night. The idea that a little sleep debt is good is a revolutionary concept. But we are not saying that if a little is good, a lot is great.

We may assume that Wehr's subjects had no sleep debt at all when they left the laboratory in the morning during the final weeks of the study. When they went to bed at night, they had only the sleep debt of 10 hours being awake. This very small sleep debt was associated with light, fragmented, and very inefficient sleep. Indeed, recall that they were awake in bed an average of 5 hours and 45 minutes a night. The latter weeks of the Wehr study represent a situation in which carryover sleep debt is zero. Clearly, we must go to bed with the debt from 16 hours of wakefulness plus some amount of carryover sleep debt in order to fall asleep quickly and to enjoy deep continuous efficient sleep. The challenge then becomes to find a perfect balance in which we get the daily amount of sleep we need but have a large enough carryover sleep debt to achieve it in the most efficient manner. Remember that all wakefulness is sleep deprivation. Another important principle is that we cannot sleep if we have no sleep debt whatsoever. When the Wehr subjects woke up in the morning spontaneously, if they were then asked to go back to sleep, it is almost certain that this would have been completely impossible.

Potentially one of the most important consequences of excessive sleep debt is highlighted by additional research carried out by Tom Roth and his colleagues. In the experiment mentioned earlier, Roth and crew tested the mental performance of some of his subjects who had scored near zero on the MSLT. Then they required the subjects to spend 10 hours in bed for seven consecutive nights in order to pay off their debts. Afterward the subjects were retested. Lo and behold, their mental performance improved. The results showed a direct correlation between the quality of mental performance and the level of sleep debt. What this means to me is that millions of us are living a less than optimal life and performing at a less than optimal level, impaired by an amount of sleep debt that we're not even aware we carry. The implications for productivity and performance in every area of life and every component of society are staggering.

It's hard to communicate how rare experiments like Wehr's are in sleep research. In fact, they are essentially nonexistent because neither the navy study nor Tom Wehr's study were designed specifically to understand some aspect of sleep. Even though the volunteers were out of the lab during the day, just getting the space to house them during the night is very costly. Empty lab space is always rare in research institutions, and especially rare for sleep research. Getting the use of 16 rooms for more than a month takes a fair amount of clout. And for studying sleep, the rooms cannot be just any rooms— they have to be outfitted with monitoring equipment, and still be comfortable and technicians have to be paid to monitor the volunteers every night. It would be extraordinarily difficult to get a grant to do such an experiment. Both the navy experiment and Wehr's NIH experiment were possible because the researchers involved were staff scientists of national research institutions. We would all like to see more of these experiments conducted, but I fear that will happen only when sleep research is a much higher national priority.

These experiments demonstrate that individuals thought to be completely normal can be carrying a sizable sleep debt, which impairs their mood, energy, and performance. If you haven't already done so, I think it's worthwhile to ask yourself how your sleep debt is affecting you. How often do you think about taking a quick snooze? How often do you rub your eyes and yawn during the day? How often do you feel like you really need some coffee? Each of these is a warning of a sleep debt that you ignore at your peril. I can't overemphasize the dangers of unintended sleep episodes or severe drowsiness. I hope this information can save your life.

I know that people often are driven to stay up late and get up early, that the demands of modern life push us to stay up past our biological bedtime. But I also know it's not too onerous to avoid accumulating sleep debt. The Wehr studies suggest the likelihood that people can avoid dangerously high sleep debt by adding a relatively small amount of sleep to their normal sleep schedule. People who have lowered their sleep debt usually report that they gain a new sense of well-being. That may just mean not watching the news at night, or putting off some other nonessential pleasure, like the bedtime crossword puzzle. I bet most people would give up many late-night diversions if they could feel truly awake throughout the day—fresh and full of hope, senses wide open, the mind receptive to people and ideas.

Chapter 4

The Human Animal
and the Biological Clock

MANY READERS HAVE heard of the "biological clock" and "circadian rhythms," and even more have heard about jet lag. Very few, however, know how these processes really work. Many of the puzzling symptoms of jet lag, for instance, are explainable only when you understand the true workings of the biological clock.

Let's imagine you are taking a trip from San Francisco to Paris 9 time zones to the East. First you lose a great deal of sleep getting ready for the trip. Then you don't sleep well on the plane, and when you arrive in Paris, you tramp around the Louvre all day long. Obviously, you have accumulated a huge sleep debt. It's so bad you have trouble staying alert through your first dinner in a very famous three-star restaurant. You are so tired, you skip all your evening plans, turn off the lights, and collapse into bed at 10:00 P.M. without even taking your clothes off.

But then the impossible happens. You closed your eyes and slept for a time, but they pop open at 3:00 A.M. and you feel wide awake. There is no question that you are tired, but no matter how hard you try to relax and think peaceful thoughts, sleep does not return. At 4:00 A.M. you take off your clothes and in desperation soak in a hot tub in search of that delicious drowsy feeling. It doesn't come. Where did the huge sleep debt go? With only five hours of sleep, you should be even more sleep deprived. Maybe there really is no such thing as sleep debt.

At 7:00 A.M. you quit trying. Petit déjeuner (breakfast) is available. You get up, dress, and begin your day. Sure enough, at about 11:00 A.M. the effect of not sleeping hits you like a ton of falling luggage. You fall asleep in the taxi on your way to lunch, and when you arrive at the restaurant it feels like the middle of the night. All you want to do is sleep. After lunch you go back to your hotel. Into bed for a nice long nap. When you open your eyes it is 10:00 P.M. You completely slept through your dinner engagement. Oh, well, back to sleep. And sure enough, your eyes pop open, you are wide awake, and the clock says 3:00 A.M.

I took a trip years ago with my family that was much like this. We had the same awful problems, but after several weeks we adjusted to the European clock. My most vivid memory, however, is from the day we got home. I was out in the park with my young children. At just about 1:00 P.M. (10:00 P.M. according to her body time), my 15-month-old daughter, Elizabeth, standing up close to and facing a large tree, actually put her forehead against it and fell asleep. To this day, it is hard to believe that she didn't fall down.

Being so tired and sleeping through dinner in Paris proves that sleep debt does exist—but a second, powerful unseen mechanism is also at work.

Over millions of years, our bodies have developed a remarkably precise biological clock that ticks like a metronome to regulate sleeping and waking. The clock is an internal chronometer that marks time by basic molecular mechanisms that scientists now are beginning to unravel. Since before the birth of our species, the daily rising and setting of the sun and the seasonal flux of light's transit into darkness have shaped this molecular timepiece, until the clock itself has become a tiny mirror of the celestial clock. The rotation of our planet as it spins its way around the sun is represented in miniature within our cells. And each day the sun tweaks its earthly ambassador into alignment.

From my personal perspective, by far the most important function of this biological clock is that it is a major determinant of our daily cycle of sleep and wakefulness. It also synchronizes a vast array of biochemical events in our bodies. It is the maestro conducting the complex symphony of chemical, hormonal, and nerve cell activities that promote our daily fluctuation in feelings and actions. Even the mind's ebb and flow of consciousness as we pass from night to day and back is a product of the march and retreat of biochemical events under the command of this master timekeeper. We eat, think, exercise, wake up, and sleep best when we heed the rhythm of our internal clock. Individuals who are out of synchrony with their clocks, such as shift workers who never fully adjust to nighttime work and daytime sleep, underperform both physically and mentally, as study after study has confirmed.

Ours is a timepiece of such remarkable precision that people often wake up a few minutes before their alarm clocks go off. Rats with no clue to external time climb into their exercise wheel and start running at the exact same minute every day. People who have struggled with drowsiness most of the day will often start to feel more alert at the same time every evening, despite the large additional accumulation of sleep debt over the course of the day. This precise time mechanism plays a fundamental role in the wide variations of sleepiness and alertness that we experience throughout every day, keeping us alert during the daytime and allowing us to sleep during the night—as nature intended.

For the jet traveler, the alarm just went off at the wrong time. But unlike your average alarm clock, our traveler could not turn it off and go back to sleep.

What is not so easily explained is the apparent absence of any impact of the traveler's huge sleep debt. Where was it at 3 A.M. in Paris? Did it, as so many people seem to think, dissipate like smoke? Absolutely not! It is still there and getting larger. Even though it is the middle of the night in Paris, where a large sleep debt is pressing our traveler down, it is stay-awake time in San Francisco; consequently, his biological clock will initiate a period of "clock-dependent alerting." Our understanding of both clock-dependent alerting and sleep debt has provided the pillars for a very simple and elegant model of what governs why we are awake during the day and asleep at night; in fact, it can further account for periods of alertness or drowsiness whenever they occur. For my grandparents, who farmed the land at the turn of the century, this elegant cycle probably played itself out over and over every day of their lives. In today's incomparably more chaotic society, this model can also be greatly extended to account for periods of inexplicable drowsiness and inappropriate wakefulness whenever they occur.

The Biological Clock and the Opponent-Process Model

In 1985 we at the Stanford Sleep Center were very fortunate to persuade Dr. Dale Edgar to join us as a postdoctoral fellow. Although he is now a faculty member, at the time Dale had just received his Ph.D. from the University of California at Davis, where he had carried out a very important series of observations on the sleep and wakefulness in squirrel monkeys before and after eliminating their biological clocks. In order to minimize the effect of environmental stimulation, Dale studied his monkeys while they were maintained in constant dim light, sound insulation, constant temperature and ad-lib food and water. In an absolutely unchanging environment, the normal monkeys behaved as if there were a sunset and sunrise or some sort of daylight schedule. They would wake up and stay awake for 15 to 16 hours, and then go to sleep for 8 to 9. The complete absence of all the effects of the earth's rotation did not appear to make any difference except that the robust cycle of sleep and wakefulness was a little longer than 24 hours. The inescapable conclusion is that an internal pacemaker or biological clock controls this profound daily oscillation. This continuing cycle manifested in constant conditions is therefore called freerunning and it belongs to a class of rhythms or cycles that have a period approximating 24 hours. Such cycles are called circadian rhythms. This term was introduced by University of Minnesota biological rhythm pioneer researcher Franz Halberg and is a combination of the Latin terms for "around," "near," or "close to" (circa) and "day" (dias). We now know that circadian rhythms can be seen in almost every function in the body, from basic cell processes to activities of the whole body.

Most of circadian rhythm research in mammals is done in rodents, but one of the problems with rodents and other small mammals is that they are what is called polycylic—they wake up and go to sleep many times during the day. Not only does this tend to obscure the difference between total sleep time during the day and total sleep time during the night, but it also seems to support people's assumption that the biological clock is active both in putting us to sleep and waking us up. This is obviously very different from how we primates sleep. Species that tend to be more awake during the night are called nocturnal, and those that tend to be more awake during the day are called diurnal. Primates are diurnal and also have the capacity to remain continuously awake for an entire daytime period and sleep the entire night.

As Dale found, squirrel monkeys, like humans, remain awake for about 15 to 16 hours, with perhaps a brief nap or two during this period. Then they tend to sleep almost continuously for 8 or 9 hours. After uninterruptedly recording brain waves and other variables for about a week, Dale put the monkeys' biological clocks out of action. When he repeated the same continuous recordings, he saw a profound change. Instead of remaining awake for hours and then sleeping for hours, the monkeys were continually falling asleep. Their periods of wakefulness become very short and evenly distributed throughout the entire observation period. Over a number of days of continuous brain wave recording, it was absolutely clear that the dramatic circadian rhythm of sustained sleep and wakefulness had completely disappeared. The remarkable increase in total daily sleep time experienced by the squirrel monkeys in the absence of their biological clocks requires explanation. Since there was no clock-dependent alerting to keep the monkeys awake, they fell asleep very frequently and their sleep was equally distributed around the clock in smaller, lighter fragments that totaled 12 to 13 hours per day. Thus, in the absence of the 15 to 16 hours of wakefulness, the sustained eight- to nine-hour period of consolidated sleep was also lost. This suggests to me that primates, including man, are able to compress their daily need to sleep into eight hours because they sleep more deeply and much more continuously than if there was no daily period of sustained wakefulness.

I was very interested in Dale's work and was eager to study his Ph.D. thesis. It was, however, more than 400 pages long, and I had enough time only to flip through it and study the most interesting charts. Fortunately, one result almost jumped off the page. My years as a sleep doctor had prepared me to recognize its overriding importance instantaneously. In addition to the loss of circadian rhythms of sleep-wake, body temperature, and drinking, the total sleep time of the clockless animals had *increased* 4 to 6 hours per day, without exception. There was no ambiguity. This was a stunning result, because it meant not only that the biological clock is not necessary for sleep but that it normally promotes wakefulness and actively opposes sleep. In fact, we could conclude that the only role played by the biological clock in our daily cycle is to promote and maintain alert wakefulness. Furthermore, this role is expressed only at certain times. The Stanford group has designated this profound function as clock-dependent alerting. At certain times each day, our brains are powerfully stimulated by our biological clocks. At the other times, the stimulation subsides or is turned off.

It would be difficult for me to describe fully the excitement that these results engendered at Stanford. A number of things that were previously not so clear became crystal clear, such as why a traveler would become wide awake in the middle of the night even though he has a huge sleep debt that should keep him asleep for several days. Our discoveries have resulted in the creation of what I regard as a most useful, and, if I may say, most beautiful model to understand how we human beings have the capacity to get the sleep we need and function at an optimal or near-optimal level throughout our waking, daytime hours. It also explains how we can be flexible, losing a little sleep and making it up without serious daytime impairment, and maintaining an optimal synchrony of our sleep-wake cycle to the environmental cycle.

Dale and I have named this the opponent-process model. It is similar to an earlier model proposed by the Swiss sleep researcher Alex Borbely but has important differences. The opponent-process model allows us to understand clearly why people tend to fall asleep or stay awake at any particular time of the day or night. It will explain why people usually can stay awake or fall asleep when they want to and why sometimes this is impossible. Finally, it provides the basis for the personal insights that have enabled some of us to include sleep in the effective management of our individual lives and schedules.

As we have learned already, the brain in every human being possesses a process that is active 24 hours a day. Its sole function is to induce and maintain sleep. It does this by regulating sleep homeostatically: When an individual obtains less sleep than the needed amount, the homeostatic process increases the tendency to fall asleep; conversely, when extra sleep is obtained, the homeostatic process decreases the tendency to fall asleep. This ensures that an individual has the same amount of sleep each day on the average. In its own way, this process appears to have a precision similar to the biological clock in terms of keeping a precise record of the accumulated sleep debt. Theoretically, since all wakefulness is sleep deprivation, sleep debt can be zero for only a brief time. As soon as sleep debt is zero, the sleeper awakens and starts accumulating sleep debt again. In general, homeostasis means maintaining a constant internal environment. Body temperature, caloric intake, and sleep are all regulated homeostatically. After Dale's work we also knew that the brain of every human being possesses an entirely separate process, clock-dependent alerting, whose function is to induce and maintain alert wakefulness.

The biological sleep drive that causes us to fall asleep and to remain asleep through the night is continuously active, even when we are awake. In fact, when we are awake, the homeostatic sleep drive is steadily increasing. Opposing this sleep tendency is the alerting action of the biological clock. In contrast to sleep homeostasis, the process in our brain that fosters wakefulness and sustained alertness is not active continuously. For humans and other diurnal animals, the clock-dependent alerting process is active in the daytime and inactive at night, with lowered activity in the early afternoon. The push and pull of these opposing processes allows us to stay up all day and sleep all night. In summary, the main reason we do not fall asleep as soon as we have been awake for a few hours is that the homeostatic sleep drive is strongly held at bay by the independent internal stimulation of the biological clock. The main reason that we can sleep through the night is that we have accumulated sufficient sleep debt during the day so that the unopposed homeostatic sleep process is free to operate all night long.

It can be said that the biological clock is the primary regulator of the daily cycle of sleep and wakefulness. Its active alerting function maintains wakefulness all day long and it permits sleep by turning off and allowing the sleep process to operate unopposed throughout the night.

Dale and I and other members of the Stanford group postulate that the daytime clock-dependent alerting occurs in two waves, one in the morning (starting when you wake up) and the other late in the day (starting typically in the late afternoon, around 4:00 or 5:00 P.M.). We further postulate that clock-dependent alerting is substantially stronger during the evening period than in the morning period. This is a beautiful mechanism, because as sleep debt accumulates while we are awake during the day, a stronger stimulation is required to keep us awake and alert into the evening. If preteen children (who have optimal alertness all day long because they always get the sleep they need each night) are partially sleep deprived, their morning alertness will become impaired fairly quickly, but the evening alertness is strong enough to persist.

On the other hand, after we have slept through the night, our sleep debt is at its lowest ebb and the stimulation needed to waken us doesn't need to be as strong. Furthermore, the weaker clock-dependent alerting allows extra sleep to be obtained more easily. In other words, when we still have a large carryover sleep debt at the time we usually get up, we can sleep till noon. In the case of the San Francisco traveller waking up too early in Paris, we can safely assume that 3:00 A.M. (or 6:00 P.M. in California) was about the time that the strong clock-dependent alerting was well under way.

In the early afternoon, between the two peaks of heightened clock-dependent alerting, the clock slacks off in its efforts to keep us awake. The result is post-prandial drowsiness, which most people wrongly attribute to the aftereffects of eating lunch. In reality, people are only feeling their accumulated sleep debt, unopposed by clock-dependent alerting. Some of us completely "bottom out" during this time. In many cultures, people cope with this early-afternoon dip by retiring immediately after lunch for an afternoon nap.

To better understand the interaction of the biological clock and sleep debt, imagine again the family you met in Chapter 1, this time on the night before the mother's annual report is due. The report is nowhere near the shape she would like it to be, so she decides to pull an all-nighter. As the night drags on, she finds herself feeling worse and worse—not just a little sleepy, but drugged by drowsiness and really awful physically. She feels stiff and hollow, her stomach is upset, and she has more and more trouble concentrating. But something unexpected occurs as the hour nears 6:00 A.M. She has been awake continuously for 24 hours and is despairing of ever finishing the report, but she starts to feel a little better. Her concentration begins to improve, her typing gets a little faster, and she feels a bit more optimistic. Even parts of the report that seemed substandard just a few hours before starts to look pretty good. As light enters the window she is actually fairly cheerful, and she finishes formatting and printing a little ahead of time. Her fatigue is lifting, her spirits rising with the sun—all because of the action of her biological clock.

Once the afternoon dip in alertness hits, however, she will feel terrible again, barely able to drag herself through the rest of the day. Then, in the early evening, despite the huge amount of sleep debt that she has accumulated over 36 hours of wakefulness, she will start feeling better again. She may not feel totally alert, but the alerting action of her biological clock will diminish the impact of her heightened sleep drive. When the clock's alerting action naturally falls off in late evening, the full load of sleep debt will hit her hard and she will fall asleep quickly. During the night she will pay back the sleep debt she had accumulated during the last 24 hours, but do little to diminish the carryover sleep debt she has from previous days.

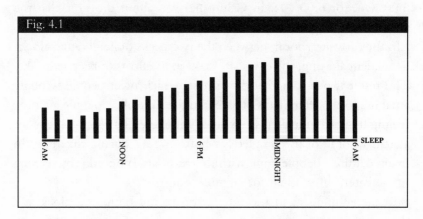

Fig. 4.1

We can graphically represent the sleep debt accumulated by one man during the course of the day. (See Figure 4.1.) We will assume that he has slept a full night and has zero sleep debt when he gets up at 8:00 A.M., although this is not the norm. The graph shows his sleep debt rising steadily throughout the day. When he goes to bed at 12:00 A.M., his sleep debt falls again (at twice the rate he accumulated it) until he is back to zero at 8:00 A.M. after eight hours of sleep.

Now let's look at how he is affected by his biological clock. (See

Figure 4.2.) His clock has two waves per day, with peaks at about 9:00 A.M. and 9:00 P.M. That is to say, at 9 in the morning and 9 at night, his inner clock has revved up his body's alertness, with the greatest maximum in the evening. At 3:00 A.M. and 3:00 P.M., by contrast, there is a lot less internal alerting going on.

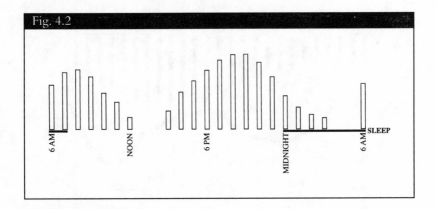

Now we put these two effects together: the alerting effect of his biological clock (upward arrows) and the sleep inducing effect of sleep load (downward arrows). (See Figure 4.3.) Throughout the morning the alerting is greater than the day's sleep load, and he feels awake and alert. Then the biological clock begins to dip down. By midafternoon his accumulating sleep load is greater than his alertness, and for a while he feels sleepy.

Although the clock-dependent alerting has dropped—as it does for many people—at 3:00 P.M., the day is only half over. Not enough sleep load has accumulated to make him overwhelmingly sleepy. He can make it through. After 3:00 P.M. the biological clock's alerting mechanism becomes active again, and just after 6:00 P.M. it is catching up with the ever-rising level of sleep load. For a time the man begins to perk up. By 9:00 P.M. the clock's alerting function is again at its peak. But now, unlike during the previous alertness peak at 9:00 A.M., he has a heavy load of sleep load opposing his clock's waking effect. The result is that, in spite of heavy sleep debt, he feels just about as alert at 9 P.M. as he did at 9 A.M. After 9:00 P.M. clock-dependent alerting begins its downswing, even as sleep load keeps rising. The result is a sharp drop in alertness and a rapid onset of intense sleepiness and waves of drowsiness. Keep in mind that the figures represent a simplified version of one individual. Your experience may be quite different.

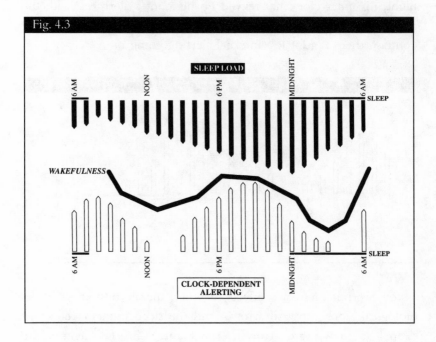

Dale Edgar recently seized the opportunity for a different set of obeservations which have provided, in my opinion, a beautiful confirmation of the wakefulness maintaining role of the biological clock. He was able to participate in a study of the Alaskan black bear in its natural habitat before, during, and after hibernation. In contrast to true hibernators whose body temperature drops almost to freezing, the body temperature of bears drops only slightly and their winter "vacation" closely resembles normal sleep.

According to Dale, the preliminary results show that before hibernation, bear sleep and wake periods are highly consolidated. During hibernation, this consolidated circadian organization of sleep disappears and the total sleep time increases by 4 to 5 hours. Dale told me he thinks clock-dependent alerting might be temporarily suspended while bears are in their caves. This is because, he says, they sleep all around the clock in shorter bouts in a manner that closely resembles the squirrel monkeys without biological clocks mentioned earlier.

In my opinion, the strongest experimental evidence for the existence of clock-dependent alerting in humans comes from a variant of the Multiple Sleep Latency Test (the standard MSLT described in some detail in Chapter 3). However, at the time we collected the data, we didn't fully understand their significance. The vast majority of studies in our laboratory utilized five sleep latency measures in one day because requiring the subjects to interrupt whatever they are doing every two hours and go to bed can be somewhat tedious and many people must go home at the end of the afternoon. But in the Stanford Summer Sleep Camp, Mary and her crew pushed the envelope and added two additional tests at 8:00 P.M. and 10:00 P.M. We called this approach the "extended MSLT." Invariably, the sleep latency was longer than previously (alertness improved over previous tests that day) in the 8:00 P.M. test and even longer (alertness most improved) in the 10:00 P.M. test. Occasionally subjects were completely unable to fall asleep during the last test.

After centuries of assuming the longer we are awake, the sleepier we will become and the more we will tend to fall asleep, we were confronted with the surprising result that after 12 hours of being awake, the subjects were *less* sleepy than they had been earlier in the same day, and at the 10 o'clock test, after more than 14 hours of wakefulness had elapsed (they generally got up at 7:30 in the morning), they were even less sleepy. That wasn't the way it was supposed to work—or so we thought twenty years ago. Mary and I cautiously attributed these results to some sort of circadian rhythm effect but we really didn't understand them. To be perfectly honest, I simply ignored a finding that contradicted my strong belief that our feeling of sleepiness and our tendency to fall asleep ought to increase the longer we are awake. Nonetheless, I was uncomfortable, and every once in a while I would say to myself, "This has got to be explained." Now we know that there is a strong evening period of clock-dependent alerting. The extended MSLT results are not only perfectly understandable, but they provide strong confirmation of the role of the biological clock in the opponent process model. Think about it. The higher MSLT scores at the very end of the day show that the biological clock can dramatically reverse a whole day's worth of accumulated sleep debt.

Because the effects of the clock-dependent alerting are so important, I want to remind you of the basic principles we know: the process of clock-dependent alerting is entirely independent from the process underlying the homeostatic sleep drive. It is an independent timed process arising from the biological clock, which opposes our tendency to fall asleep. When the biological clock is eliminated, the homeostatic process continues to operate in a normal fashion. Animals without a clock can be awakened, stimulation will keep them awake, though for much shorter periods of time than normal animals, and their sleep tendency to fall asleep increases in direct proportion to the time they have been awake. Thus, by keeping us awake all day, the biological clock ensures that we will be able to sleep through the night.

I recently discovered a dramatic example of reversing sleepiness in my own office. A young man who graduated from Stanford last year is now my number one assistant. Our desks are at opposite ends of a large room. During the afternoon, he often looks very tired. He used to maintain a conventional schedule, arriving at 8:00 A.M. and leaving around 5:00 P.M. each day. One day not too long ago, it was around 4 or 4:30 P.M., and I was very irritated by the disorganization and clutter in the office. I was pushing my young assistant hard to go through piles and get things filed out of sight, when it became clear that I was pushing too hard. He looked so tired that I said, "Never mind," and returned to my desk.

About thirty minutes later, he was suddenly standing over me, demanding to know where to file three or four documents. "We've got to get these things done," he muttered, and he was moving around the office with an alacrity he had not shown before. His eyes were bright, he was talking faster and more precisely than usual, and of course it dawned on me. "Do you realize what has happened?!" I roared. "Your clock-dependent alerting has finally kicked in." He hadn't taken a cold shower, he had had no coffee, he hadn't taken amphetamines. Responding to an unseen force, he became more wide awake and alert than I had ever seen him. Ordinarily, I suppose this took place while he was driving home, and probably has prevented an accident many times. Those of us who hire students do not realize our loss. Just as their brains are starting to work at peak alertness, they leave.

I wonder how many of my fellow professors have any clue that this is happening. Since the revelation, my assistant has been spending a lot more time in the office after 5:00 P.M. We arranged a schedule in which he comes to work at 9:00 A.M., thus catching up on his sleep in the morning, and I have him do personal errands and things requiring very little energy and intelligence in the late morning and after lunch. Then as my day is winding up, his late afternoon enthusiasm motivates me to work another hour and accomplish quite a few additional tasks. This situation has proved to be an exceptional one for us, but I am left with a feeling of how the conventional schedules, sleep debt, and clock-dependent alerting deprive other employers or cheat them from getting their money's worth.

It is very rare to encounter a college student who is tired and wants to go to bed at 8:00 P.M., and conversely, is bursting with energy at 8:00 A.M. However, they do exist. The sleep and biological-rhythms community calls them "larks," and differentiates between "owls" and "larks." Owls, of course, experience peak alertness in the evening. We now use these terms somewhat carelessly, a morning person being a lark, and a night person being an owl. When the tendencies are a little more extreme, there are some formal criteria for these terms.

Keep in mind that the graphs presented in this chapter that show sleep debt and clock-dependent alerting represent an idealized version of a typical pattern. As you begin to pay attention to your own feelings, you may find your pattern is quite different. As I have indicated, peak clock-dependent alerting can occur in the morning as well as in the evening. Since I am immersed in an environment of students, however, my experience with larks (except for myself) is much smaller. Interestingly, I do not recall a single MSLT test out of hundreds where a clear peak of alertness (long individual sleep latencies) occurred in the middle of the day. It probably happens but is rare. When an adequately large database of MSLTs has finally been accumulated, I am sure we will see some interesting individual patterns.

In Search of the Biological Clock
The notion of an internal biological clock has historically provoked both curiosity and disbelief. For ages, it was commonly accepted that people fell asleep as night came on, because of decreasing stimulation. Around the turn of the century, Russian scientist Ivan Pavlov

had shown in his well-known experiments that when dogs were repeatedly fed dinner right after a bell rang, they eventually salivated thereafter whenever they heard the bell—regardless of the presence of food. This was called a "conditioned reflex." By the early twentieth century nearly all scientists had a vague idea that humans—like Pavlov's dogs—fall asleep because they are conditioned by the setting sun, the evening meal, the quiet of the night, or other cues. This conditioned reflex theory of sleep, combined with the reduction of stimulation, was favored by Kleitman in the 1930s. Although some sleep researchers today still believe conditioning may help open the door to sleep, they do not see it as the major influence.

The first clear demonstration of the existence of an internally determined daily oscillation in activity was offered by Jean Jacques d'Ortous de Mairan in 1729. He studied a plant called a heliotrope, which opens its petals in the daytime and closes them at night. When de Mairan put the plant in darkness for 24 hours, he noticed that the plant still opened and closed its petals on the same schedule. He suggested that the plant was following an internal clock, rather than just the outside light. Unfortunately little attention was paid to his discovery for more than two centuries.

Nathaniel Kleitman himself was aware that the daily sleep/wake rhythm was not entirely dependent on an increase or decrease in external stimulation. In 1939 he noted that passengers sailing to Europe from the United States tended to sleep a little later each day and often missed breakfast. On the return trip to the United States, passengers woke up a little earlier each day, sometimes having skipped dinner the night before, but never missing breakfast. This "boat lag" occurred on the eastward trip to Europe as the ship set its clocks forward and again on the trip home when it set the clocks back. The passengers' internal clocks, on the other hand, lagged behind the time set by the rising and setting sun. Kleitman attributed the passengers' persistence in staying with their previous schedule to conditioning.

When I entered medical school in the early 1950s, it was clear that the human body makes an effort to maintain a regular rhythm of sleep and wakefulness on its own. By this time, some posited an internal clock governing the ebb and flow of sleep. Others, like Kleitman, held to the conditioned response theories that the hour at which we wake or sleep is dictated by innumerable combinations of such factors as social interactions, noise, electromagnetic fields, and meals.

Oddly enough, in the early days the small and scattered group of scientists who were interested in biological and circadian rhythms generally were not concerned with sleep itself. And the tiny group of sleep researchers were certainly not concerned with circadian rhythms. Both groups of researchers acted as if they lived in different countries; only with the development of sleep medicine did the two communities really come together to understand how the biological clock orchestrates the daily cycle of sleep and wakefulness and how it is involved in causing sleep disorders.

The Max Planck Cave and the 25-Hour Day

After more than a decade of describing 24-hour cycles in sleep and wakefulness, as well as a host of other bodily activities, Kleitman addressed the question of whether these cycles could be modified. In his initial attempts, he chose to study a period of 21 hours and a period of 28 hours. This was simply because eight 21-hour days and six 28-hour days conveniently and precisely occupied one week (168 hours). He soon realized that the ordinary laboratory environment was not satisfactory and made arrangements to spend one month living in the Mammoth Cave, Kentucky. When Kleitman and a colleague descended into the huge cave, their story attracted enormous attention from major news media. It was the first time that human sleep patterns were studied in complete isolation from environmental influences.

The two scientists spent a month far underground, sleeping on bunk beds and passing the time by analyzing their body temperature and motility data. When they emerged from the cave at the end of the month, the bearded and bedraggled duo were greeted by a horde of reporters and newsreel cameras. The experience was a media blockbuster (the wonderful Movietone newsreel can still be seen on videotape), but the scientific results were inconclusive. The two sleep researchers spent one whole month living on a 28-hour day. The temperature and body motility cycle of one appeared to adjust, and after one week he slept quite well, during the regular nine hours in bed. The other researcher (Kleitman) could not adjust and his temperature rhythm appeared stuck at a 24-hour periodicity. He slept poorly. Had both individuals demonstrated an apparent fixity of the 24-hour rhythm, Kleitman might have been turned in the direction of postulating an internal clock. However, the ease with which his colleague adapted to the 28-hour schedule led Kleitman to conclude that "there is no foundation for assuming that some cosmic forces determine the normal 24-hour rhythm, aside from rest, movement, food intake, and sleep."

It wasn't until the late 1960s that scientists at the Max Planck Institute in Germany succeeded in developing an artificial living space in which they could isolate subjects from all possible environmental cues about the time of day. In order to shield against light and noise, they built a room underground, wrapped the whole structure in copper wire to insulate it from changing electromagnetic fields, and took other extraordinary precautions. They even required male research assistants to shave at odd hours so that the sight of a man with a five-o'clock shadow wouldn't influence the subjects' biological rhythms.

Once the subjects were completely isolated from every possible clue about what time it was, they were allowed to keep their own schedules. They could turn the lights off and go to bed whenever they wanted and back on after they had slept. The German scientists observed that, yes, subjects still kept a regular cycle of sleeping and waking. At last they were able to demonstrate that the rhythms of sleeping and awakening are set by an internal pacemaker.

The Max Planck researchers made another crucial observation in their human volunteers. Our biological day didn't seem to be exactly 24 hours long. Subjects who were isolated from the external world and allowed to sleep whenever they chose eventually settled into a daily cycle close to 25 hours long. Subjects inside the isolation facility therefore went to sleep and woke up a little later each day. Their "days" and "nights" drifted out of sync with the real day and night of the outside world. After a month or so, the subjects came out of isolation feeling a little bit like Rip Van Winkle; more time had passed in the outside world than they had experienced in their sheltered world. At last scientists were able to see the timing of the internal human clock, free of environmental influences.

The slightly longer biological day is often blamed for what has been variously called Sunday night insomnia or Monday morning blues. On the weekends, many of us go to bed late and let ourselves sleep in on Saturday and Sunday morning. The idea is that the biological clock tends to push in this direction as well, since its natural period is slightly longer than 24 hours. On Monday morning, we are exhausted, struggling against the urgings of our biological clock to sleep a couple more hours.

There is a tendency for the biological clocks to gradually drift back and run later. People who have trouble getting to sleep at night and getting up in the morning, for instance, may have a clock shift: The biological clock has come to act as if midnight were actually 9:00 P.M. and 6:00 A.M. were 3:00 A.M.

This tendency is very common in young people, and in my opinion is almost always present in college students. In the early days of the Stanford Sleep Disorders Clinic, we began to see such people, typically high school–age children brought to the clinic by their parents because they had insomnia. We quickly realized that although they had trouble falling asleep at their scheduled bedtimes, the problem of staying asleep was completely absent when the alarm went off in the morning and they had to be dragged from their beds. An extreme case of clock shifting came to our attention in 1975, when we were approached by a Stanford graduate student who was frustrated because he would lie awake all night and then finally fall asleep as others were beginning their day. Most physicians at the time would treat people like him as if they had a psychological problem, such as anxiety disorder, fear of the dark, or a resistance toward a parentally imposed bedtime. I was convinced, however, that we were seeing a *biological* problem—a biological clock out of sync with nature. I talked to our circadian rhythm expert, Chuck Czeisler, who had come to the laboratory as a medical student in 1974. To get the graduate student back on track we designed a system that took advantage of the longer natural biological day. Instead of trying to wake him an hour earlier each day, we requested that he stay up a few hours later each day. The first day he went to sleep at 9:00 A.M. instead of 6:00 and slept for a solid eight hours until he awoke at 5:00 P.M. The next day he went to sleep at 12 noon and woke at 8:00 P.M.

After seven days we had him going to bed at 10:00 P.M. and sleeping until 6:00 A.M., and we decided to stop the therapy right there. He was able to stick to this schedule with no problems.

Here is an old riddle: Which tells better time, a broken clock or one that is slow two minutes per day? Answer: The broken clock, because twice a day it tells the correct time. Our biological clocks are slow—each cycle is slightly longer than the time it takes Earth to spin once on its axis—and slow clocks aren't much use. It is Earth itself that must act as a metronome, a timekeeper setting the tempo of our days. The bright light of morning and its dimming at dusk must synchronize our clocks each day, calling us awake and lulling us to sleep.

The Role of Light

Although many laboratory animals were known to be exquisitely sensitive to light, for a long time biological rhythm researchers believed that light had no effect on humans' biological clocks. This was a result of the experiments carried out at the Max Planck Institute that led researchers there to conclude that social interactions were the most important controlling *Zeitgeber,* or time cue. Throughout the 1970s and 1980s, however, Chuck Czeisler at Stanford and Al Lewy at the Oregon Health Sciences University began accumulating evidence that bright light, like sunlight, can reset the circadian cycle. In fact, we now know that light is the most powerful time cue our bodies have.

Because dim light (such as electric room lights) has a much more subtle effect on the biological clock than bright light has, its ability to influence the clock wasn't revealed until the early 1990s, nearly 20 years after Dr. Czeisler first tried to prove it. In 1976, Chuck went on a tour of the isolation chamber at the Max Planck Institute. As he and a guide were walking through the rooms where the famous clock experiments were done, Chuck asked, "What's it like when it's dark in here?"

The German scientist who was his guide said: "It *is* dark in here."

Seeing how light it was in the room and thinking he was misunderstood, Chuck repeated the question a little louder, "What's it like when it's dark in here?"

The guide repeated, also a little louder and little irritated: "It is dark in here."

It turned out that during the "dark" periods, the Germans shut off the overhead lights but left on the desk lights and floor lights. These provided enough light to make it unnecessary to turn on the overhead lights during the tour. Excited by the implications of this revelation, Chuck rushed back to his laboratory to find out how people were affected when they were exposed to absolute light-and-dark cycles, just like the ones used in the animal experiments.

These experiments showed that human circadian cycles could be affected by dim light such as the desk and floor lamps left on during the earlier experiments. The subjects experienced cycles of dim-light periods and absolute darkness and it was found that their clocks could be reset by using the dim lights as cues. Even though the experiments followed the same protocol as the previous animal experiments, other biological rhythm researchers were not convinced. They believed that the action of turning off the lights was in fact a social interaction between the subjects and the scientists, even though a machine was responsible for switching the lights on and off. The German investigators argued that, unlike the animals used in previous studies, the human subjects could reason that the lights were switched off at night and turned on in the morning, thereby nullifying Czeisler's hypothesis that the light had any biological effect.

Somewhat disgruntled but still very determined to prove he was right, Chuck decided to finish medical school and develop a new protocol for his experiment that would prove light had a biological effect on the circadian clock. This took about 10 years, and in 1986 or 1987 he proved beyond any doubt that bright light had a tremendous resetting effect. In light of this newfound data (no pun intended), the researchers who had earlier argued against Chuck did a complete 180 degree turn and claimed they had always believed that bright light would have such an effect since we are, after all, animals ourselves.

Once the idea that bright light had a biological resetting effect, Chuck went on to prove, finally, that dim light also had an effect. He used the same protocol as he did in the bright light experiment, but he decreased the intensity of the light slightly. He repeated this over and over, each time decreasing the intensity of the light, and after nearly 20 years, since he first tried to show that dim light could reset the human circadian clock, he was successful. The sleep and biological-rhythm community was surprised by his results, especially by how little light was actually necessary to significantly effect the clock. In the shade of a tree during the noonday sun, we experience way over 10,000 lux of light (one lux is the light of one candle). A 100-watt bulb, held 10 feet away, bathes us in about 190 lux of light. In his experiments, Chuck and his colleagues showed that as little as 180 lux could reset the clock. The effect was weaker than that of bright light, which is why it wasn't spotted earlier. But for those of us who are exposed to room light much more than bright light (those working in offices during the winter, for instance), our cumulative dose of dimmer room lights probably has more effect on us than our exposure to bright lights.

The implications of this finding are far reaching. First of all, we now know that all the use of electric lights in the evening, which we previously thought had no effect, can have a profound effect in lengthening our biological day and shifting our clocks. Simple activities like checking our e-mail or reading at night have the potential to fool our bodies into delaying our biological onset of sleepiness. As Chuck likes to say, "It's almost as if we have flown westward for three time zones every evening."

The second major conclusion is that most of the experiments completely isolating people from natural light had to be redone. Nearly all of them had been set up so that people were ostensibly free of any outside effects on their biological clock. But now Chuck knew that the light in the room did affect the subjects' rhythms. He and his colleagues undertook the admirable and difficult task of carrying out the cave experiments while controlling for light exposure. What they found was that the room lights in previous experiments had been making people stay up longer. In Chuck's subjects, the natural period of the biological clock averaged 24 hours and 10 minutes, rather than the nearly 25 hours that had been documented before. Other experiments by Chuck have now confirmed this result.

Of course, this doesn't change some of the implications of previous experiments. The period of the biological clock is still longer than 24 hours, and even if our internal circadian day is substantially closer to 24 hours than 25, we operate under conditions that are much more like the original experiments than the revised ones. In other words, being surrounded by electric lights in the evening pushes our biological clocks around, so that in everyday life our light-bathed bodies try to live a 25-hour day. Once we use electric lights, our clocks start lagging about an hour every day.

Early in 1998 I read about an intriguing study published in a medical journal and subsequently reported in *The New York Times*. My reaction to reading the article was a mixture of incredulity and amazement at the complexity of our biological clocks—and the continuing ability of sleep research to overturn our presumptions. Instead of exposing their subjects' eyes to light, sleep researchers at the Cornell Circadian Rhythm and Sleep Laboratory delivered the light to the skin on the back of the knees. Incredibly, they measured significant changes in the subjects' circadian rhythms as a result of this seemingly innocuous light exposure. If other investigators confirm this result, it suggests to me that some of the skin on our body is sensitive to the alerting action of light. It would be amazing if this one spot on the back of the knees represents a unique light-sensitive patch of skin. I believe that the skin does not represent a separate or autonomous biological clock but rather acts on the brain's biological clock via signals carried in the blood or nerves. In any case, this finding represents a completely unexpected development in sleep and biological rhythm science.

There is an enormous amount of research in hamsters, guinea pigs, and other rodents which describes in detail the mechanisms of resetting the biological clock. Though there is far less research on clock resetting in humans, in my opinion it is just as convincing. The biological clock can be reset by exposure to light, the presence of melatonin in the blood, and vigorous, repetitive physical activity. While the role of activity is clear and powerful in rodents, its role is less clear in humans.

A very important aspect of resetting the biological clock is that the clock can only be reset at certain times. These times are specific portions of the circadian rhythm. Depending upon the time (referred to as the phase of the rhythm) the resetting stimulus is delivered, the clock will be reset to an earlier time or a later time, and the change will be either larger or smaller. Obviously, clock resetting cannot be done carelessly. It is sufficiently complex that specific individual instructions should be followed. It is important to note that the clock responds to light exposure at night and not in the middle of the day.

In general, light exposure in the evening and into the first part of the nocturnal hours will have an increasing potency in delaying the clock. For example, typically the first wake-up signal would occur and hour or so later than normal. At approximately the middle of the night, there is a sudden shift in the direction of the resetting response such that now light exposure in the latter hours of the night and early morning will advance the clock, so that the wake-up signal it emits will occur earlier than normal.

The clock resetting effect of melatonin is essentially the opposite of light. If melatonin is ingested in the morning, it should delay the biological clock, and if ingested after the evening, it should advance the biological clock. When the resetting sensitivity of the biological clock is systematically tested at a number of different points around the circadian cycle, the result is called a phase response curve. This curve will show how much of a response to expect depending on the nature of the stimulus, when it is delivered, and in which species.

With just the right laboratory conditions, Chuck Czeisler has shown that over a three-day period, the biological clock can be reset to any time desired. Though it is another story, Chuck has been very involved in resetting the biological clocks of astronauts so that they are optimally alert when they need to perform at their absolute peak.

Clockworks

In 1972, two separate laboratory teams headed by Robert Moore and David Zucker identified the locus of the biological clock deep in the brain in two pinhead-size clusters of nerve cells called the suprachiasmatic nuclei, or SCN. There are about 10,000 nerve cells in these tiny clusters, which is a very small fraction of the human brain's trillion neurons. These few cells strongly influence about 10 million other brain cells, which in turn have jurisdiction over the cycles of trillions of cells throughout the body. The two SCN sit in the midline of the brain, directly above the optic nerves, which are two great neural cables carrying electrochemical signals from the eyes to the visual portions of the brain. The SCN uses this position to monitor levels of light entering the eyes and to adjust the rhythmic fluctuations of body temperature, hormone release, and metabolic rate.

The discovery of the SCN enabled scientists to prove on a cellular level that, even though light has a resetting effect on the biological clock, that clock can function independently of any light alerting. At the Mitsubishi Institute in Tokyo, Shin Ichi Inoue and Charles Kawamura isolated tissue from the suprachiasmatic nuclei in animals, maintained it in culture, and recorded its electrical activity. They found that the electrical activity of the isolated tissue displays the same circadian cycle as shown in the isolated intact organism.

It may seem a wonder that something nonmechanical can measure time so accurately, down to a few minutes over the course of 24 hours. Although we are most familiar with mechanical timepieces, a clock can be anything that measures how things change at a steady rate, such as the flow of water in a water clock or the passage of sand through an hourglass. Both the water clock and the hourglass are accurate, nonmechanical timekeepers. The most efficient clocks, though, are based on oscillation—such as the swinging of a pendulum, the vibrations of the crystal in a quartz watch, or the deterioration of atoms in an atomic clock. These oscillations can go on for a very long time without running down. But the biological clock is no pushover in comparison. Mice and rats that have been maintained in constant conditions for their entire life span demonstrate robust circadian oscillations until senility sets in.

The timekeeping mechanisms of the biological clock seems to be based on the movement and chemical interactions of molecules in the SCN. In this case the oscillation is the slow ebb and flow of the molecules as they move in and out of the nuclei of SCN cells. Scientists now have identified genes that appear to be the main components of the biological clock in fruit flies. The genes create proteins that regulate the very genes that make them. The clock proteins build up inside the cell until they reach a critical mass. Once enough clock protein builds up in the cell, it travels to the cell nucleus and turns off its own production. As the existing proteins disintegrate naturally, their ability to suppress their own production fails, and their production begins again. This sets up a natural oscillation of protein production and disintegration.

We don't know whether the biological clock works exactly the same way in mammals, but it is probably based on the same principle. In May 1997 Joseph Takahashi and other scientists at Northwestern University reported finding in mice a gene similar to the one in fruit flies. They named the gene CLOCK because it produces a protein crucial to the regulation of circadian rhythms. Takahashi's studies indicate that the body's internal timing system determines much more than simply the biochemistry of our sleep-wake cycle. It is a master clock that regulates a great many body systems and cycles, such as the fertility cycle, across months and seasons. The Northwestern University scientists found the CLOCK protein not only in the SCN but also in the cells of the testes, ovaries, kidneys, and most other body organs. Perhaps we are on the way to a detailed understanding of the breadth of the biological clock's influence on our behavior.

The Electric Cave of Modern Life

The more we learn about the science of sleep, the more apparent it becomes how radically the course of modern life has diverted us from our bodies' natural rhythms. In virtually every aspect of contemporary living—from electric lights to all-night television to split shifts at work—we are literally punching the clock that maintains the synchronicity of our mind and body. In just a few decades of technological innovation we have managed totally to overthrow our magnificently evolved biological clocks and the complex biorhythms they regulate.

Before the invention of electric lights, our internal clocks kept us irrevocably tied to the rhythms of nature. As diurnal (rather than nocturnal) animals, humans are not adapted to surviving in the dark, so finding a safe place to ensconce ourselves through the hours of darkness was a good formula for survival. The control of fire was a critical development in human evolution. Fire offered an aura of illumination, a small island of relative safety in a sea of darkness. It was the first step that humans took in exempting themselves from the natural order. Night could be staved off. A small bit of the day's light could be borrowed to hold back the darkness.

Much later, the use of oil lamps afforded an even more controlled use of light indoors. People could stay up late and read or do other work. "Burning the midnight oil" became an expression for hard work well into the night. But fire is not daylight. Wood fires and oil lamps are fairly dim and cast a reddish-orange light that is bright enough to see by, but not bright enough really to wake someone up and reset the biological clock. Further, burning oil far into the night was expensive and thus rare, with most tasks wisely left for the next day. When darkness fell, work ceased. The introduction of gas lamps in the mid-nineteenth century did not appreciably change the situation, for they too relied on naked flame that spread a dim, candlelike pool of light around a room. If you visit one of the historical "gas lamp districts" in some cities, you can still get a feeling for the relative paltriness of light produced by gas.

Our loss of sleep time and natural sleep rhythms is the tragic legacy of a single and profound technological advance—the light bulb. When Thomas Edison invented the incandescent bulb in 1879, he became a modern Prometheus, taking fire from the gods and giving it to humans. Yet Edison accomplished something Prometheus could not imagine, because he separated the light from the fire and offered it for our infinitely more convenient and flexible use. Never before had people seen light that did not come from some sort of fire. Soon after the invention of the light bulb, a parade in New York featured dozens of men proudly wearing large, single light bulbs on their heads. The image seems comical to us now, but at the time it was astounding to see people wearing fire on their heads. Stunts such as the parade of lights were used to demonstrate the safety of this new light source and to allay our innate fear of fire. After Edison, light without fire was easily available with the flick of a switch.

Although the first incandescent lights were fairly dim (and grew dimmer as the carbonized filament deposited soot on the inside of the bulb), they led to brighter and brighter bulbs, such as the tungsten bulbs introduced in the 1910s. Now people could work late or read for pleasure into the wee hours. Bright electric lights not only let people stay up longer, but they also were bright enough to mimic the daylight and significantly shift people's internal biological clocks. When bedtime shifted to 10:00 or 11:00 P.M. instead of 8:00 or 9:00 P.M., midnight was no longer the middle of the night. The natural order was upset. No longer would people sleep nine hours and slowly wake at dawn. Late hours and alarm clocks made the twilight slumber of slow awakening practically extinct.

The incandescent bulb marked the beginning of the modern era of sleeplessness, and Edison was by no means ignorant of the implications of his breakthrough. A restless genius and experimenter, Edison believed that too much sleep was bad for you. "The person who sleeps eight or ten hours a night," he declared, "is never fully asleep and never fully awake—he has only different degrees of doze through the 24 hours." Edison thought that people got twice as much sleep as they needed and that the extra sleep made them "unhealthy and inefficient." Edison was quite proud of working until dawn on many a night, a practice he started in one of his first jobs as a railroad telegrapher on the night shift. When he was well into his 70s, he boasted that he slept only four hours a night; however, there is strong anecdotal evidence that Edison was a prodigious daytime napper, whose total sleep approached the normal eight hours.

In his emphasis on productivity and efficiency, and his equation of sleep with the sin of sloth, Edison embodied the energetic and boisterous spirit of the late-nineteenth-century Industrial Revolution. However, his invention of bright electric lights threw a dangerous wrench into the human clockworks. Over millions of years our bodies and minds had evolved to use sunlight as a Universal Standard Time, as the infallible index against which we reset our internal clock. Our daily activity and even our seasonal need to breed or put on weight for cold weather are driven by the hours of darkness and light. Our whole pattern of existence is based on a genetic code formed by the cumulative experience of millions of human ancestors who knew only the light of the sun and whatever dim illumination could be rendered from burning fat. Edison's bright electric lights gave us supernaturally long days, as if we are always living in summertime Alaska.

To some extent, we all have set up house in an electric cave, each of us master of his own schedule. None of us is bound tightly to the rising and setting of the sun. We have grown so accustomed to living year round in an artificial summer of light, with long days and short nights, that it is hard to imagine life before electric lights and modern work schedules. But our bodies haven't forgotten. They are the product of millions of years of genetic adaptation. Can we really believe that in 100 years our bodies can so easily change needs buried deep within the workings of each cell? What are we leaving behind when we create our own sunlight and determine the beginning or end of our day with the flick of a switch?

I think it's telling that so many of us find the modern habit of hiking into the wilderness and camping out under the stars so deeply satisfying. We leave behind the bright lights of civilization and allow ourselves to revert to a more primitive pattern of sleep. Night falls and we start feeling sleepy. Far from the sea of illumination that surrounds every city, most campers soon douse the lantern. With the stars as our only night-light, we are rocked in the welcoming arms of Mother Nature back to the dreamy sleep of the ancients. It's little wonder we wake the next morning feeling so refreshed and alive.

Chapter 5

The Circadian Rhythm of Life:
Growth and Aging

ON THE ROAD to Athens, a Greek myth tells us, the Sphinx asked travelers this riddle: What walks on four legs in the morning, two legs at midday, and three legs in the evening? The correct answer, given by Oedipus, was Man—early in life he crawls on all fours, in childhood and adulthood he walks on two legs, and in old age he uses a cane. Sleep poses a similar puzzle, because like the strange creature in the Sphinx's riddle, sleep patterns are very different at the beginning, the middle, and the end of life. How much we sleep, when we sleep, and the proportion of REM to non-REM sleep, all evolve and change as we move through our lives.

Perhaps more important, our attitudes about sleep and our habits of sleep also change. The misconceptions and bad sleep habits we acquire early in life can cause health problems at any age. For instance, misunderstanding about the sleep needs of teenagers is having a severe effect on the education of our nation's youth. Teens have their own biological rhythm, and forcing them to adapt to an adult timetable is counterproductive, causing problems both in learning and behavior. And too many adults behave like overgrown children when it comes to regulating their own sleep habits, even when their chronic daytime fatigue tells them that something's wrong. The consequences of these behaviors range from increased traffic fatalities to decreased productivity and job satisfaction.

Consider how our changing view of sleep through life parallels how we deal with another strong biological drive: hunger. When we are infants we eat whenever we want to, and our parents make sure we get the nutrition we need to keep growing. When we are young children we often want to have candy and other treats, but good parents keep us in line most of the time and enforce good eating habits. A few incidents of unrestrained candy bingeing puts a dent in the idea that candy is always a great thing to have. When we get to be teenagers, though, it seems childish to be told what to eat all the time. Mothers keep reminding us to eat healthily, but being a member of the unofficial Teenage Liberation Front means eating junk food whenever we want. Most parents frown on this but realize that their kids eventually need to make their own eating decisions. By the time adulthood hits, most of us have acquired a lot of bad eating habits. Pressured by school and work and running our own lives, we grab snacks when we can and don't worry much about eating from each of the basic food groups.

At least we are taught the facts of healthy nutrition in school, and we know what is good for us, even if we don't always put it to practice. But as a nation of sleep illiterates, few of us even grasp the importance of healthy, age-appropriate sleep. So when we get insomnia or when we fall asleep at the wheel, we can't figure out why it's happening, or we come up with the wrong explanations for these events. Sleep education is light-years from achieving parity with teaching about nutrition or physical fitness. Sleep becomes the stepchild of our lives, pushed aside by social and work demands. The only time most of us catch up on sleep is when our bodies break down and force us to rest.

Appreciating our personal sleep need and circadian rhythm is a two-step process. First, we have to remain attentive to our body's unique circadian patterns and know how they tend to change over the lifespan. Second, we have to respect those rhythms and adapt our lives to them. As with any force of nature—the tides, the seasons, or the process of aging—we defy our circadian rhythms and sleep indebtedness at our own peril. When we harmonize our lifestyle with our body's master clock, we maximize the quality of our life—physically, mentally, and emotionally.

The Earliest Sleep

Sleep begins well before we are born. It is hard to say exactly when we begin to oscillate between the worlds of sleep and wakefulness, but certainly this oscillation is present in all premature babies. Like sleep at every developmental stage after birth, sleep in the womb has its own unique characteristics. We can tell from looking at premature infants, and by studying the motions of babies in the womb, that once a pregnancy is well along, the fetus spends most of its time asleep—about 16 to 20 hours per day. Interestingly, the fetus is more active while asleep than we are, which explains why pregnant women can feel kicking at almost any hour.

After we discovered the connection between REM sleep and dreaming back in Chicago in the mid-1950s, we began to ask "At what age does dreaming begin?" Nathaniel Kleitman thought that REM activity and dreaming would develop along with consciousness, so that as children grow older and became self-aware, they would begin to have more and more REM sleep and dreams. In other words, REM sleep should be absent in neonatal life.

In the summer of 1955, my wife-to-be had some friends with new babies. One baby was about two months old, and the other was about three months. I asked if I could watch the babies sleep, and when I did so I recognized the presence of rapid eye movements almost instantly. At that point I decided not to fool around and obtained permission to spend time simply watching infants' eyes in the neonatal nursery at the Chicago Women's Lying-In Hospital. Here I had about 50 subjects who were just as likely to be sleeping during the day as during the night. What astonished me was that every single infant showed copious rapid eye movements, and in about an hour our entire perspective on the development of rapid eye movements and dreaming was drastically altered. For anyone who thinks it is amazing that neither parents nor pediatricians nor nurses nor anyone else ever observed these movements, I would like to remind them that REMs were uncovered by a machine, *not* by a human observer. Humans often do not see what they are not looking for, and because no one felt anything important was going on during sleep, they weren't looking.

Since newborns infant can't talk, we can't really confirm that they dream—but very young children can and do talk about their dreams. I remember this in my own daughter, when she was less than two years old. Talking is unusual during REM sleep, so I was surprised one morning when I walked into the room where she was sleeping to hear her say "Pick me, pick me." I looked at her eyes and saw some typical rapid movements. I immediately woke her and she said, "Oh, Daddy, I was a flower."

Such experiences make me absolutely certain that dreaming begins long before a child has the ability to talk about it, or even to know the difference between dream and reality. Dreaming is a form of awareness, an ability to put together sensory information and thoughts in a way that mimics what happens when we are awake. As soon as babies are able to make sense of the world on a primitive level, the same sensibility ought to be associated with REM brain activity and what might qualify as dreaming. Whenever it is suggested that newborns might dream, the response is almost always "What in the world would they dream about?" My only answer is that there is a growing body of evidence that the fetus in the womb responds to stimuli and can be conditioned. Thus, some very primitive experience may be repeated or rehearsed in fetal REM sleep.

In Chicago I had observed rapid eye movements during sleep in infants, but I hadn't yet done brain wave recordings on infants. In fact, only two kids in the whole world had been recorded all night: Gene Aserinsky's 10-year-old son, and a little girl, age 5, who lived across the hall from me when I was at the University of Chicago. I persuaded the girl's mother to allow an all-night recording, but it took several visits to the laboratory to convince the girl. I told her that it would be fun to sleep in this place, and reassured her that her mother would stay with her all night. Even then she was anxious. I taped the reference electrodes to her earlobes with ordinary adhesive tape. A little glitch occurred in the morning when she would not let me take the electrode tape off her earlobes because pulling on the little hairs hurt. She would not even allow her mother to pull the tape off. I finally cut the wires and left the electrodes on. "There," I said, "Now you have very special earrings." She beamed and went home happy.

Dr. Howard Roffwarg holds a special place in my heart as my first real sleep research colleague. He spent many nights with me in my apartment/laboratory on Riverside Drive, and we hit it off as collaborators and became close friends. Howie became passionately committed to sleep research almost as quickly as I had. Howie was really the first person I worked with on a continuing basis who shared the excitement of the new findings in sleep research.

One of the things that really excited us was the question of what was really going on during babies' sleep. We persuaded several couples within our circle of friends to allow us to attach electrodes to their babies and to record their sleep for a few hours. As I recall, the babies were close to three months of age. We were very impressed with the ease of distinguishing the differences between REM and non-REM sleep. We also were impressed with the large amount of REM sleep, although our small sample would not allow a firm conclusion. I was delighted with the beauty and clarity of babies' sleep spindles.

At that point it became clear that we needed a much more precise quantification and description. In 1960 mothers and infants stayed longer in the hospital than today, which was a plus. Persuading mothers to allow "experimentation" on their new babies was something else altogether. Many mothers refused, but the procedure itself was of course harmless and our enthusiasm convinced a sufficient number. So, for the first time, neonatal sleep was studied systematically. We were surprised to find how much REM sleep infants have. Typical newborns spend about eight hours in REM sleep—about 50 percent of their daily sleep. More recent studies suggest that near-term fetuses actually spend about 60 to 80 percent of their sleep time in REM sleep. Most adults, on the other hand, spend about 25 percent, or about two hours a night, in REM sleep. This percentage actually drops over the course of our lives, so that by old age we enjoy relatively little REM sleep—only 15 to 20 percent of the time asleep.

Circadian sleep cycles also begin before birth by passing across the placenta. Even though the fetus isn't exposed to light from outside the womb and can't tell when it is night or day, the mother is communicating this information to her baby. Steven Reppert and his group at Harvard University have found that these signals from the mother actually will stimulate the fetus to mirror its mother's circadian cycles. Most of this group's work is done on mice and rats, which mirror their mothers' circadian patterns pretty closely. They have found that the mothers' fluctuating melatonin levels signal the biological clock in the fetal brain, preparing the babies for the rhythms of life outside the womb. Although we don't do the same experiments on pregnant women, scientists have found that other primate mothers also set their offsprings' circadian clocks while they are still in the womb.

We now know the fetus signals the mother when its body is mature and ready to be born and actually starts the labor process. But the mother has some say in the process. All mammals tend to give birth during the time they normally would be asleep, possibly to make sure the birth happens "at home," and therefore safe from predators. The mother's circadian rhythm seems to act as a gatekeeper, inhibiting birth during the day and promoting it at night. This is why women often go through "false labor" the night or two before actual labor begins: The mother's circadian rhythm is opening the gate to a nighttime delivery, even before the baby's biochemical push to be born is strong enough.

In 1957, while I was an intern on my obstetrical service tour of duty, it was very obvious that babies were born much more frequently at one time of day than another. Things would always be very quiet in the afternoon and early evening. Perhaps only a few, or even none, of the delivery rooms would be occupied, and I would begin to hope I would be able to get some sleep. It never happened. As each evening wore on, more and more women in labor showed up, and by the middle of the night, we were always frantically busy. Only later did I learn that nighttime birth was a fundamental part of the circadian modulation of our lives.

Sleeping Like a Baby

Immediately after birth there are only two sleep stages, REM and non-REM sleep. REM sleep is sometimes called active sleep in babies, because the muscular paralysis that always accompanies such sleep is not fully developed. Non-REM sleep, on the other hand, is often called quiet sleep, because the baby is, well, sleeping like a baby: perfectly still, quiet, and limp. Although this quiet sleep clearly is neither wakefulness nor REM sleep, it is initially void of the specific kinds of electrical signals that help us differentiate stages 2 through 4, which begin to appear soon after birth.

Normal infants' sleep is one of the few areas in which there is now a great deal of data on sleep states and stages. This is because since the early 1970s, the National Institutes of Health has supported sleep studies on normal infants as part of its mission to find the cause or causes of sudden infant death syndrome (SIDS). The several laboratories funded for infant sleep research have found that at birth, infants usually sleep 16 to 18 hours per day, distributed evenly over six to seven brief sleep periods. The cycle of each usually includes both REM and non-REM sleep. This is possible in part because the sleep cycle is shorter—infants can pass directly from wakefulness to REM sleep. Infants also alternate between REM and non-REM sleep every 60 minutes or so, instead of the 90 minutes that adults take to cycle from REM sleep, through the other sleep stages, and back to REM sleep.

A regular, set pattern of sleeping and waking in newborns is typically absent or very weak. Dazed parents groggily note this night after night, when the baby wakes time after time for feeding or comforting. For a while parents have to adapt their own sleep cycle to the baby's irregular sleep, taking catnaps and rising out of deep sleep to attend to the little one's needs. Parents who know something about sleep get a new appreciation for the importance of the circadian clock and the power of sleep debt.

Many parents think their infant's sleep is totally random. But a closer look reveals that there is usually a pattern to newborns' sleep. Nathaniel Kleitman was one of the first to observe this back in the 1930's. Kleitman asked parents to keep careful track of when their babies were awake and when they were asleep. They tracked newborns' activity over 50 weeks and recorded the data for each day in a single line.

The solid line represents times when the baby seemed to be asleep, and breaks in the line are times when the baby was awake. A dot represents a feeding. When each line—each day's record—is stacked with all the others, it looks like Figure 5.1.

Fig. 5.1

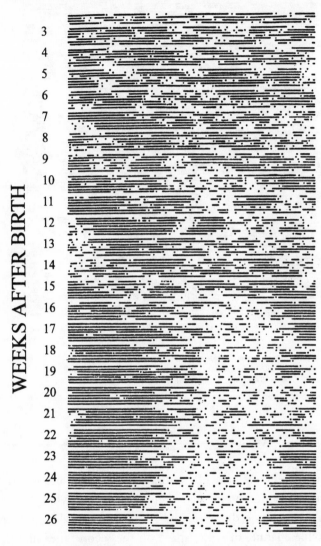

WEEKS AFTER BIRTH

3
4
5
6
7
8
9
10
11
12
13
14
15
16
17
18
19
20
21
22
23
24
25
26

24 02 04 06 08 10 12 14 16 18 20 22 24

MIDNIGHT   NOON   MIDNIGHT

Fig. 13. Consolidation of sleep-wakefulness rhythm in an infant: black lines indicate sleep, dots indicate feeding, and white patches indicate wakefulness. From the jacket of N. Kleitman's *Sleep and Wakefulness*, 2d ed. (Chicago: University of Chicago Press, 1963).

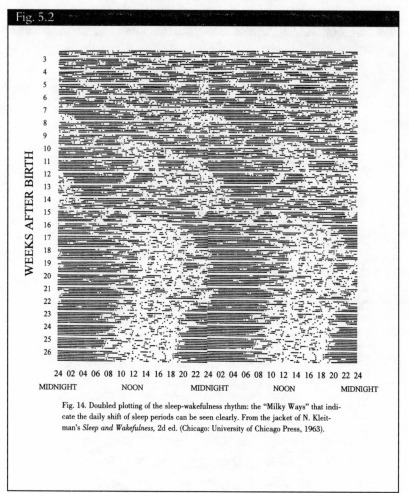

Fig. 5.2

WEEKS AFTER BIRTH

24 02 04 06 08 10 12 14 16 18 20 22 24 02 04 06 08 10 12 14 16 18 20 22 24
MIDNIGHT   NOON   MIDNIGHT   NOON   MIDNIGHT

Fig. 14. Doubled plotting of the sleep-wakefulness rhythm: the "Milky Ways" that indicate the daily shift of sleep periods can be seen clearly. From the jacket of N. Kleitman's *Sleep and Wakefulness,* 2d ed. (Chicago: University of Chicago Press, 1963).

The number of weeks since the infant's birth is indicated by the numbers at left. Since white space represents times when the baby was awake, we can see that after the seventeenth week, the baby is leaving a wide channel of white space on the record, meaning she is awake mostly from about 10:00 A.M. until 8:00 P.M. In the middle of this channel are some short black lines, indicating naps. The fact that the white channel is roughly vertical shows that the baby is waking and going to sleep about the same time each day. When the graph is duplicated and placed one next to the other, it is a little easier to see the "channels" of wakefulness. (see figure 5.2).

Notice that before the seventeenth week there is no such vertical channel of white in the sleepy black background, but there are rough, slanted channels. These angle downward, from left to right across the page. If you look carefully, you can see that they are even present (barely) in the first weeks after birth.

The fact that the channels are slanted left to right in the early weeks means that the infant's most wakeful time is about 10 minutes later each day, about an hour later each week. This pattern is very much like what we see in experiments in which people are isolated from external time cues. As the weeks go by, the white channels get wider as the baby starts sleeping longer and being awake longer. This is caused by the consolidation of sleep periods. Then, around the fortieth week, something else really striking occurs. The slanting white channel on the chart goes vertical—at last the baby has started waking and going to sleep at about the same time each day.

Sleep-starved parents rejoice when the baby first sleeps through the night, which they consider five or so hours of sleep without an awakening. When parents have been getting up every hour or two for weeks on end, five hours seems like a long slumber. (In my own case, our first child, Cathy, was what was then called a "colicky baby." I was extremely envious of those fortunate parents whose babies slept through the night fairly soon.)

No scientific experiments have been done on how best to train an infant to sleep, but I can make a few conjectures. I doubt that a regular pattern of sleeping and being awake can ever be imposed on infants immediately after birth or that anyone should even try. Their biological clocks seem to need to mature more before they can keep track of the time of day. But the same kinds of cues that work for us should work on infants' clocks as they are maturing. Light in their rooms during the morning and dim light in the evening, as well as a feeding and activity schedule that is as regular as possible, should help put the biological clock in tune with the 24-hour day once it has matured enough to kick in.

Sleep in Children

By the end of the first year, the overall number of sleeping and waking hours has changed relatively little. The infant still sleeps 14 to 15 hours a day. Except for one to two daytime naps, the sleep periods have shifted to the night and the waking periods to the day. By about 18 months of age, most toddlers are taking only one nap.

By the end of the second year, children sleep about 50 percent of the time. Somewhere between 2 and 5 years of age, the other nap fades away. Children slowly sleep less and less until their daily sleep measures about 10 hours, which holds steady until they reach puberty. Remember that this 10 hours is the amount of actual sleep they get, not just the hours they spend in bed. Many children go to bed and spend time playing, reading, or goofing off before they actually get to sleep, and after they wake up in the morning.

Scientific curiosity led me to study the sleep of infants, but our work with older children and adolescents was the beneficial product of the always burdensome and often more desperate part of science. Most people think that scientists carry on their research by focusing on the next important problem in their field and then simply begin attacking it. So, the awful truth is that many of us spend huge amounts of our time applying for grants—the lifeblood of research—in effect "selling" our research to review committees before we start any work at all. This process is structured to be as fair as possible, but it is inevitably influenced by fashionable research topics and essentially political directives about getting money to certain geographic areas or certain types of colleges or researchers. Many private foundations only fund research that has to do with one special area, such as diabetes, so someone studying basic cell metabolism might have to "spin" the grant proposal, emphasizing the importance of cell metabolism to diabetes research. Researchers who need grants try to read the prevailing signs, then cast their nets upon the waters and hope that they can catch a grant that will sustain what they consider their most promising work. When the nets come up empty, there is a crisis.

That is what happened to me in 1975, when my major source of funding, a large multiyear program grant from the National Institutes of Health, was not renewed. I had been led to believe it would be—the Stanford Sleep Center was in its glory years of sleep research, having just made major discoveries in sleep disorders and basic sleep research. If a large grant is not going to be renewed, an investigator usually is given an indication long before so that contingency plans can be made, but I got the news only one month before our money ran out. I was stunned, and deeply pained that I had to lay off all but a few of my 20 employees. I thought my sleep research career might well be over. Finding another source of funding soon enough seemed impossible. Demoralized, I began a permanent shut down of my whole program. I was saved by a grant from the Spencer Foundation. The only major restriction on the money was that the research had to be on children. This turned out to be a true blessing in disguise. It led directly to a very interesting and valuable research program on sleep in children and adolescents, but I must admit that before the crisis I had no plans whatsoever to study children.

The Spencer grant resulted in the creation of the Stanford Summer Sleep Camp, which I mentioned in Chapter 3. Mary Carskadon and I set up the camp to do a multiyear study of what sleep is like in preteens and how it changes through adolescence. Although some kids dropped out and others were added, basically the same group came back summer after summer during 10 years of study. We started with 10-, 11-, and 12-year-olds and finished the study with 18-, 19-, and 20-year-olds. Mary ran the sleep camp very effectively. You can imagine the difficulty of gathering good scientific data while keeping 40 to 50 adolescents in line during a summer camp away from their parents. She was good at it and continued to investigate adolescent sleep when she took a position at Brown University.

One of the major findings in the first summer of the camp in 1976 was that preteens tend to be very well rested. When we gave the MSLT test, we would put kids to bed in their darkened bedrooms during the daytime, ask them to try to go to sleep, and clock the time it took them to succeed. As I remember, all of the kids were off the scale, never able to go to sleep in the 20 minutes we allotted for each of a single days five tests. During the rest of the day they were like puppies, bursting with energy; at night they slept about 10 hours. With regard to sleep and wakefulness, this is truly life's pinnacle of perfection. Think about it—completely wide awake and bursting with energy all day long, and then deeply, soundly, and continuously asleep for the entire night. Of course, the home environment and the parents must encourage adequate sleep at night and be sure the necessary time in bed is scheduled. In most families this is easy because prepubertal adolescents are generally much more interested in daytime activities than late night. They get up with a song on their lips, eager to play games, get to school, eat breakfast—the list is endless.

As a sleep researcher I thought I would inevitably encounter nearly every problem related to sleep and sleepiness, but my work had inadvertently kept me from seeing one that nearly every parent knows all too well. Because I went into the sleep lab almost every evening, and because wives did most of the child rearing in the 1950s and 1960s, I usually wasn't around to put my kids to bed and didn't see their bedtime behavior. When I spent a lot of time with my grandchildren, I finally was able to witness what I had only read about: Children really can get cranky and irrational, act out, and, paradoxically, become more active and energetic when they are sleepy. While many kids are very good about going to bed, others will get "wild," causing trouble, being rambunctious, and resisting going to sleep. They insist they aren't sleepy even though it is obvious they are. (I find that kids will say they are tired only to avoid doing something, which I call sudden fatigue syndrome.) They finally crash and fall asleep so soundly that it is extremely difficult to wake them. Since the sleep camp started I have taken a much more active interest in understanding childhood and adolescent sleep patterns and problems.

For preschoolers, the effects of delaying bedtime by even half an hour can be subtle and pernicious. Ever more cases of attention deficit/hyperactivity disorder (ADHD) are being diagnosed in elementary schools and junior high school, and I think there is a good possibility that some of these kids are really just sleepy. Their reaction is to resist the sleepiness and become more active, but at the same time they become less attentive, less focused, and generally more troublesome. This pattern begins to fade in older children as they learn to recognize their sleepy feelings on a much more rational level and accept the need for sleep. But the desire for joy and excitement never really leaves us completely. Even most adults love to feel excited, love to feel "up" and energetic. The resulting desire to stay up past our biological bedtime is a subtle but important part of our sleep behavior most of our lives, and it needs to be considered carefully when evaluating our sleep needs.

The Physical Side of Puberty

When puberty strikes, the hormones rage, the heart beats faster, and parents' blood pressure rises. "It was like some alien moved into our house," one of my younger colleagues said of his son's entrance into puberty. "It seemed that one day our wonderful boy was replaced by this resentful, surly urchin."

In a way, teens are different people. Under the influence of a rush of hormones, the brain is being remade. Some nerve networks grow and become dominant, others shrink and atrophy. Over the course of puberty, the cerebral cortex undergoes a last great bloom of neural rewiring. Nerve connections keep changing throughout adulthood, of course, but the scale of the change during puberty is unmatched again until very old age, when neurodegeneration starts undoing the brain organization that has been built up over a lifetime. Teenagers actually begin to see the world differently—the same old symbols and objects begin to have entirely new meanings. One of the most obvious changes is the way that heterosexual boys and girls look at the opposite sex. My grandson, who is now ten years old, doesn't want to have anything to do with girls. I look at him and think, "Oh boy, is he in store for a big change." In a few years he will feel completely different about girls—not because he is taught to, but because his testes will have started pumping out testosterone, and the hypothalamus and the sexually dimorphic nucleus in his brain will be calling the shots.

These hormonal developments are integrally tied to changes in teenagers' sleep, where one of the first signs of puberty is found. The onset of puberty is heralded by a rise in the amount of growth hormone that is secreted into the bloodstream at night. Teenagers have long been warned that smoking and other bad habits can stunt their growth, but they are not taught that sleeping less can too.

Some sex hormones also have a close relationship with the sleep cycle during puberty. These hormones—testosterone, follicle-stimu-lating hormone (FSH), and leuteinizing hormone (LH)—are re-leased in small amounts during childhood, but the release does not take place at any particular time of the day. During puberty, how-ever, all three hormones are produced in much larger amounts, and all three are released mostly during sleep in both girls and boys.

Melatonin is the hormone that seems to communicate the pulse of the biological clock to every cell in the body, and is a crucial factor in the body's maturation: A decrease in melatonin levels signal the body to begin puberty. If peak levels of melatonin stay high, puberty will not begin. The danger is that kids, imitating their parents by taking melatonin for sleep, may inadvertently delay their sexual development by taking melatonin as a sleeping pill. Indeed, my colleague Dale Edgar has heard an anecdotal report of a girl who took melatonin regularly and didn't hit puberty until she was 15, a few years later than normal. This particular girl may not have reached puberty until this late anyway, but the story is troubling. Obviously, melatonin usage needs more research, but even more immediately important is a publicity campaign to alert parents to this potential danger.

The Teen Sleep Crunch

Like many new college freshmen, Aarthi Belani is a Stanford student who is happy to be able to select class times that will allow her to get enough sleep. This is a wonderful contrast to most of her high school years. Like many across the country, Aarthi's high school in Edina, Minnesota, started at 7:20 A.M. After staying up and studying until one or two in the morning, she would set her alarm for 6:30 A.M.— the last possible minute that she could get out of bed, rush to get ready, and still make it to school on time. Some of her classmates got up as early as 5:00 A.M. "It was terrible," she says now. "My first-period class was chemistry, and literally three fourths of the class fell asleep at some time during the period." Needless to say, little learning occurred in class. Neither teachers nor students were happy with this state of affairs.

But unlike most other American high school students, Belani and her classmates in Edina got a break when the school heeded a University of Minnesota study on school start times. The study, chaired by psychologist Kyla Wahlstrom, pulled together scientific information on teenagers' sleep needs and patterns and then applied these findings to high school students. Wahlstrom showed that sleep loss affects how students learn. Lack of sleep increases the chance that students will have automobile accidents, that they will use drugs, that they will be violent or aggressive, or that they will develop chronic sleep disorders. Just as important, Wahlstrom publicized something that was originally discovered by Mary Carskadon and me back at the Stanford Summer Sleep Camp: Adolescents are even more impaired by sleep loss than are the rest of us.

We found this as the kids in our multiyear study moved into adolescence. Before the study, everyone thought that teens would need less sleep than younger children. In fact, as they hit 13, 14, and 15, these kids were still sleeping the same number of hours as when they were younger. In addition, their scores on the MSLT showed them to be very sleepy. We were astounded to find not only that their sleep time was not changing, but also that even this amount of sleep seemed insufficient. At first, Mary and I thought this showed that teenagers need about an additional hour or hour and a half of sleep per night. This was before we fully understood the subject of sleep debt, and we hadn't realized how much sleep debt nearly every teenager is carrying around all the time. Our teen subjects probably came into our study with a large sleep debt, so that even full nights of sleep would not make up for the sleep their bodies were owed. Our current position is that teens need at least as much sleep as children do. Even with full nights of sleep, they will feel sleepy during the day if they are carrying a large sleep debt. I would like to see more research done to clarify this point, although it would probably take another multiyear study to pin down the truth.

What we had guessed, and what Mary's work at Brown proved, is that there is a change in the biological clock during the teen years. Adolescents tend to be classic night owls, staying up late and sleeping in late. This pattern is caused by a biologically driven shift in the circadian cycle that gives teens a troublesome kick in alertness at about the time the folks around them (younger and older) are getting sleepy and going to bed. Most teenagers will not start feeling sleepy for an hour or more after adults do.

Aarthi Belani reports that she always started perking up in the early evening. "Between 7:00 P.M. and midnight I felt wide awake, and I couldn't really go to sleep if I wanted to. My best studying was between 11:00 P.M. and 1:00 A.M." She would sleep late on weekends to try to make up for her shortened sleep, but of course this would only reinforce the shift in her circadian rhythm, making it harder to get to sleep at a reasonable time on Sunday night and harder to get up and feel awake and aware on Monday morning.

Meanwhile, though adolescents' biological sleep need not decreasing, their social limitations on sleep are changing. An essential part of getting older is becoming more independent, more able to make more decisions for oneself. Teens generally are allowed more leeway than younger children to stay up later and decide on their own sleep time. Staying up late becomes a coming-of-age emblem, a sign that the teen is more responsible and more of an adult. In one survey of American high school students, only five percent said that their parents set a bedtime for them.

There are a couple of problems with all of this. One is that few parents know their own sleep needs, much less know that their teens need just as much sleep as, or more than their preadolescent brothers and sisters. The other problem is that teens are given more permission to determine their own bedtimes just as their clocks are pushing them to stay up later. They feel great in the evening, so why sleep? But society still determines that they get up early, so the result is that they get much less sleep than they should.

The best recent statistics reveal that 53 percent of people ages 18 to 29 say they suffer from daytime sleepiness; the incidence decreases to 33 percent in adults over 30. The indications are serious. Seventy-two percent of people 18 to 24 report that they have driven while drowsy during the past year, which explains why more young people die in accidents caused by fatigue than caused by alcohol.

The Minnesota project was able to establish that biological and social changes of adolescence make early morning a bad time for learning. While most school districts in Minnesota could not delay the start of school for a variety of reasons, Edina did change, and so far the results have been dramatic. When the school start time was changed from 7:20 to 8:30 A.M., district officials reported that students were far more awake and engaged in class, and the number of behavioral problems went down.

"The difference was like night and day," Belani now says of her senior year, when school start times were changed. "In my first-period course no one was sleeping, and everyone felt more alive and able to absorb the lessons." Now that she is at Stanford, Aarthi is trying to get more sleep. But a freshman dormitory is an exciting place (especially if it houses Chelsea Clinton and her Secret Service detail, as Belani's does). The noise, the bull sessions, and the music all make it difficult for her to get to sleep before midnight. Her solution is to schedule her classes no earlier than 9:00 A.M., and on two days of the week her earliest class is at 11:00 A.M.

Back in Edina, Minnesota the only people who have problems with the new schedule have been students with after-school jobs or athletes. But nearly everyone has adjusted. And most important, they have done better in school. Student scores on standardized tests were measurably higher for the eleventh and twelfth graders after a year under the new schedule.

Sleep in Adulthood and Middle Age

We tend to think of aging as something that happens to us after, say, 50 years of life. Gerontologists and athletes know better. Both are careful observers of how the body changes as the years go by, and both know that aging starts very, very early. Some measures of physical performance start to decline in the early 20s. Athletes know that they have a very short career at the highest levels of competition. If they manage to keep playing into their mid- to late 30s, they count themselves extremely lucky. If they do keep playing, they usually have to take extra care not to injure themselves and to treat all injuries more carefully. In fact, once the bloom of adolescence is over, we get only a short period in our late teens and early 20s to enjoy the fruits of adulthood in all its ripeness before our bodies start the slow process of falling apart. The muscles lose strength and mass. We begin to gain fat. Our skin begins to lose resiliency and firmness. Researchers have found that fertility can start declining measurably in many women during their early 30s. Bones start to lose mass. We get injured more easily and take longer to recover. Nature is telling us that, as far as she is concerned, we've had our day in the sun, our chance to snag a mate, and she won't waste much effort on us anymore as we drift toward middle age.

Sleep also changes as we age. As adolescence ends, the amount of sleep we get declines slightly and continues to decline slowly into old age. I used to say that it was our ability to sleep—not our need for it—that declines as we get older. Recently I have revised my stand, concluding from the latest data that the amount of sleep we need actually does decrease somewhat as we get older. This data came partly from recent research on middle age.

It will surprise no one that the definition of middle age often depends on the age of the beholder. I once asked the students in my class to raise their hands if they thought that people 50 years old and over were middle aged. Every one of about 500 hands went into the air. Well, what about 40? I could see no difference in the sea of hands that were raised. I gulped. Well, how about 30? Clearly more than half the hands went up. Twenty-five? At last a clear drop: About 10 percent of the hands stayed up.

My own definition of middle age is the age at which individuals are so busy with earning money, building a family, and trying to succeed in whatever they are doing, that they cannot be induced to spend time in a sleep lab. For this reason, data on what constitutes normal sleep and daytime alertness in middle age have been until recently essentially nonexistent. For a number of years, Drs. Dan Kripke and Sonia Ancoli-Israel and their colleagues have been carrying out important population studies in the San Diego, California, area. They recently reported their findings on a large sample of middle-aged adults, who spent an average of five consecutive nights in the sleep lab, with instructions to make no changes in their sleep routine or any other aspect of their daily existence. The results were somewhat surprising to me. The average amount of sleep for ages 40 to 65 was about 7 hours per night, which is a fair amount less than older teens and those in their 20s.

Is this the amount that those in middle age really need, or are they shorting themselves on sleep during the experiment? The final arbiter of this question would be a test of daytime alertness over a long period, but this is an extremely expensive (although straightforward) approach if you want to examine large numbers of individuals. Nonetheless I believe that Kripke and Ancoli-Israel's tests of normal, daily sleep are likely to be pretty close to the individuals' true daily need. They support the idea that sleep need is already declining slightly in middle age. But we really don't know yet. Middle age still presents one of the biggest gaps in our knowledge of sleep over the lifespan, one that I think it is very important to fill. Those in middle age probably need this information more than any other age group, because their lives are so incredibly busy—which is, ironically, the same reason it is so hard to gather the data.

Even though adulthood slowly brings relatively small reductions in normal sleep need, young adulthood and middle age are the times when the greatest number of sleep problems occur. Many of them are caused by lifestyle factors. In young adulthood we have to make a difficult switch from a night-owl student schedule to one more suited to the working world. Keeping our old schedule on weekends for parties and nights out only makes this transition more difficult. Parents taking care of infants have their sleep schedule thrown into disarray again and again. Long hours or shift work on the job also throws a wrench into the gears of the circadian clock. A recent survey showed that over 80 percent of Americans believe you cannot both be a success at work and get enough sleep. The shifting sleep schedules and stresses of adult life can be a major contributor to bouts of insomnia.

On a physical level, the typical middle-age weight increase can contribute to a narrowing of the throat and obstructed breathing during sleep. Menopause brings hot flashes, increased nighttime urination, and hormonal volatility, all of which interfere with healthy sleep. Men's changing hormonal profile in midlife, sometimes called male menopause, also can take its toll.

Recognizing the impact of stress, aging, and other life changes on our circadian rhythms is the critical first step in addressing sleep problems. The important second step is taking sleep disorders seriously enough to change our lives—and, when necessary, seeking medical attention.

Sleep in the "Golden Years"

In 1979 Mary Carskadon and I expanded the Stanford Sleep Camp to include a group of elderly people. The sleep-camp environment allowed us to extend sleep studies in "normal" older people to include daytime sleep tendency as we had in children and adolescents. Our findings in over forty carefully screened, healthy men and women ranging from 65 to 88 was somewhat surprising. Over 40 percent of these normal elderly sleepers had some form of sleep apnea, and a majority of the group suffered from extraordinarily frequent "microarousals"—unremembered very brief awakenings lasting only three seconds or less, but recurring between 200 and 1,000 times per night. Because the arousals were so short, their total nightly sleep time was only somewhat reduced. However, the MSLT testing showed a clear relationship between the frequency of brief arousals and the daytime sleep tendency. Even so, very few of the MSLT scores were in the "twilight zone," mean score less than 5. As described in chapter 3, interrupting sleep this often in young adults had a much stronger effect on daytime sleep tendency. These results from the Stanford Summer Sleep Camp are part of the growing but still sparse scientific evidence that sleep need does decrease with age.

Other lab studies also have found that the release rate of growth hormone after the night's first period of stage 4 sleep grows smaller and smaller as the years go on—as does the amount of stage 3 and 4 sleep. Without further need to make us taller, growth hormone mostly takes on the important work of repairing and renewing cells and tissues. But we've seen that many people in their 60s and beyond have very little stage 4 sleep left at all, and comparatively little growth hormone is being released at night.

The circadian pattern of sleep also continues to change as we get older. In adolescence the sleep phase tends to shift so that we are more owllike, but as we get older we become more larklike, falling asleep earlier and getting up earlier. Chuck Czeisler at Harvard University found that older people wake earlier because their circadian dip isn't as deep as that of younger sleepers'. Normally our bodies have such a tremendous sleep load from being awake all day that it is easy to overcome circadian alerting, remaining asleep beyond 4:00 A.M. or 5:00 A.M., when circadian alerting hits its lowest point and starts to rise. One result of this change is that people get less sleep time after age 65 than they did before. As with middle-aged sleepers, new data on elderly sleepers seem to indicate that they need an hour or two less sleep per night than those in their younger years. For a long time we said that elderly people need just as much sleep as younger adults. This was partly because we were trying to get out the word that a lot of seniors' sleep problems may be due to actual sleep disorders like restless legs syndrome and apnea, and that these problems shouldn't be attributed to normal aging. As I mentioned before, although the dangers of unrecognized sleep disorders in the elderly are as real as ever, elderly people do seem to need a little less sleep.

We've also looked at how aging affects sleep in animals. One very interesting result, discovered by Dale Edgar, is that the sleep drive decreases noticeably in animals as they age, suggesting that the human sleep drive may also weaken as we get older. This may be one reason that older people are more easily awakened—because sleep debt works less hard to keep them asleep. We can guess that the biological clock is also not immune to the effects of aging. It may be that one reason our sleep isn't even worse than it is as we age is that the two opposing sleep processes—sleep debt and clock-dependent alerting—are both declining in parallel.

It's one of the cruel ironies of life that just as we are entering retirement and finally have more time to sleep, nature plays a nasty trick on us and offers us less sleep and poorer-quality sleep. If we live long enough, we all seem to go through a reverse development. Like babies, we grow more and more dependent on others, have less control over our bowels and bladder, and have more trouble eating solid foods. Sleep is also part of this bemusing pattern: As we grow older our sleep becomes less consolidated. We wake up more often at night and nod off more often during the day. In very old age, the fragmented sleep pattern spreads throughout the day and night; researcher Sonia Ancoli-Israel found in a study of elderly nursing-home patients that there was not a single hour during any 24-hour period in which they were not both asleep and awake. Ultimately we tend to die in our sleep.

I have reached the age of 70. It's only now, looking back over the span of my own life and my changing sleep patterns, that I can see the true arc of my circadian rhythms and how they've periodically collided with the demands of career and family. Not surprisingly, I've come to realize that I work best and enjoy life most when I adopt a sleep schedule that is appropriate to my age.

When I was younger, against all advice I give now, I stayed up late and very often didn't get enough sleep. That was in part due to the ridiculous traditions of medical schools, which require students to fatigue themselves to the breaking point. Much later, when I began to understand sleep debt, I became much more careful to monitor my own sleep needs and turn in early if I was pushing myself too far. But one unavoidable problem with sleep research is that it has to be done at night. I basically had the sleep pattern of a shift worker: up at night doing work, then awake during some of the day. My clock was always a little out of sync, and I often woke up in the middle of the night, my racing mind not letting me go back to sleep. On the other hand, in these early years my circadian clock tended to keep a night-owl schedule anyway, so staying up late worked fairly well.

As the decades passed, I tried to keep my late-work schedule, even though it was becoming nearly impossible. But 11 years ago my middle daughter was struck by a car and suffered severe brain damage. My wife and I went through a terrible year. Our daughter required 24-hour care. I had to get up very early every day to relieve my wife and was exhausted every night. I was still trying to run the Stanford Sleep Center, and I found that the only way I could get the necessary work done was to start extremely early. Soon I found that this routine fit very well with my changing circadian clock. My daughter no longer requires the same level of care, but the early-morning hours, from about 3:00 or 4:00 until 9:00 or 10:00, remain my most productive. The positive side of my late-life early-morning hours is that by lunchtime I've already put in a full day's work.

I think what I fear most as I get older is a real failure of the sleep process. I'm hopeful that very soon we will have safe medications that mimic the action of the biological clock, granting us the fully alert wakefulness and deeply satisfying sleep of our preteen years. Reclaiming healthy sleep late in life would not only relieve some of the problems of aging but it also might help lengthen life and grant us more years of physical and mental vigor.

PART TWO

When Sleep Fails

ON A MAP, the border between the United States and Canada is a distinct line across 3,000 miles of grasslands, mountains, and rivers. Along the actual borderline, you can stand in one place and be in the United States and take one step and be in Canada. There are places where this borderline is clearly delineated, such as at crossings and along the Saint Lawrence Seaway. But in other spots there is no obvious dividing line between countries: no river, no fence. In these borderlands, people can pass back and forth easily, and there is a mixture of cultures. The laws of either nation are sometimes difficult to enforce, and communities quickly learn to live with a certain element of lawlessness, where people enforce their own rules.

Just as nations have borders, sleep and wakefulness are like two great states with a common boundary. In their struggle with each other for supremacy over the brain, they have come to a power-sharing arrangement in most of us; as the biological clock plays referee, we step across the border twice each day, entering the land of sleep at night and crossing back into wakeful consciousness in the morning. And because it is a crossing we have made thousands of times during our lives, we have become fairly adept at making the twice-daily transit between the two very different countries of wakefulness and sleep.

But when sleep fails, this border can become a war zone. Wakefulness refuses to surrender to sleep, and sleep invades our waking moments. The neural border guards may refuse to let us cross into the land of sleep. Sleep fails as the result of any of a number of malfunctioning sleep processes. Sleep disorders can arise from problems in any component of the body machinery—from the biological clock; from injury, toxicity, physical illness, mental illness; from work and schedule problems. Sleep disorders can last one night, a few weeks, or be lifelong. They can arise at any age, from birth to death, affecting male and female alike. Some sleep disorders are completely invisible until they cause a catastrophe, and others could not be more visible.

But whatever the cause of sleep disorders, when sleep fails the borderline between waking consciousness and sleeping stops functioning as it should; stops being the well-defined, well-controlled line we expect. We are forced to fend for ourselves in the lawless borderlands between the two.

Chapter 6

Insomnia

IN 1977 I was a member of an advisory panel of psychiatrists, pharmacologists, and epidemiologists convened by the Institute of Medicine of the National Academy of Sciences to evaluate the state of research and medical practice on insomnia and sleeping pills. The other two sleep researchers and I were not surprised but the other members of the panel were shocked to find that there were really very few good scientific studies on insomnia and almost no sleep laboratory studies of the effectiveness of treatments for the problem. Our review led to modest improvements in research and clinical trials of sleep medications, which have since continued to improve. However, when I started writing this book I began closely surveying the field once again—and found myself somewhat daunted. What I came to realize is this: There are so many different types of insomnia, attributable to so many different causes, that it is nearly impossible to make generalizations that will describe all cases of insomnia in a meaningful way. I believe that we sleep specialists, in a laudable effort to communicate, have inadvertently imposed an awkward and rigid organization on the topic. The problem is that this organization, in my opinion, tends to obscure as much as it enlightens.

For instance, in almost every book on the subject you will read that insomnia can be divided into those types that last one to several nights and are "transient" and those that last weeks, months, or years and are therefore "chronic." But when you look at large numbers of individual cases, the distinction is less clear-cut. I've come to believe that "chronic" insomniacs defined as people who have trouble sleeping every night without exception for months or years are fairly rare. In most cases, people have trouble sleeping for a few nights, and then sleep well for some nights before the trouble returns. This type of sleep disturbance is better labeled "chronic-intermittent" insomnia. Likewise, stress is usually described as one of the prime causes of transient insomnia, but if a stress continues for a long period, then the insomnia may well continue beyond the two-week cutoff.

So what is insomnia? In the first place, there is no such sleep disorder. Insomnia is not a disease—it is a symptom. Insomnia is simply some sort of difficulty sleeping. Like a pain in the stomach, which can be a sign of many possible ailments—appendicitis, gallstones, food poisoning, peptic ulcer, and so on—each of which has its own requirements for treatment, difficulty sleeping has many different causes.

Most people, including most doctors, have trouble grasping this basic and important point. Over and over again I see insomnia being regarded as a specific illness rather than a symptom. Even my colleagues and I will occasionally fall into the habit of referring to insomnia as if it were a single disorder, because it's handy to talk about it that way. But that habit can obscure the true nature of the problem.

The fact that insomnia is regarded as a single disorder rather than a symptom goes to the heart of why it's so poorly diagnosed. In the practice of medicine, a doctor deals with symptoms and signs that in many cases will lead to the identification or diagnosis of a specific disease. A "symptom" is defined as something a patient feels and communicates verbally to a doctor. A "sign" is what a doctor observes directly. Since insomnia is never observed directly by a doctor (unless he or she is a sleep specialist in a laboratory setting), it should always be dealt with as a symptom, and doctors should search for the cause of the symptom. They seldom do.

Therefore, what most people mean when they say "I have insomnia" is that they are having trouble falling asleep or sleeping as long as they wish or when they wish. The task of any sleep specialist is to diagnose the cause of the insomnia and to initiate proper treatment.

In my mind, insomnia is also somewhat different from other sleep problems in that victims are always certain they have difficulty sleeping. I don't think I have ever heard of anyone saying "I may have insomnia or I may not. I really don't know." Also, when severe insomnia is associated with daytime fatigue, irritability, anxiety, im-

paired concentration, waves of drowsiness, and a host of other difficulties, the sufferers are always certain about the cause-and-effect
relationship. People who suffer from severe insomnia will never say
"I don't know why I am so tired all the time." So in this sense, while
some sleep problems can be hidden from the victims, insomnia is
usually not.

Unlike the self-imposed sleep deprivation of a demanding job, a
crying baby, final exams, or some other situation that carries the
prospect of relief—the knowledge that at some point you will decide
you have reached your limit and you will partake of the blessed act of
going to sleep—insomnia denies you any relief from the crucible of
sleep deprivation. You are trapped, seemingly unable to escape,
knowing that you'll have a much harder time functioning the following day.

The Fragility of Sleep

Although it is difficult to get really accurate information on how
many people have insomnia, the causes and their severity (in large
part because the term is so misunderstood), at least half of all humans
acknowledge that they sometimes have trouble sleeping. The prevalence of insomnia raises the question of why human sleep can be so
fragile and prone to malfunction. After all, cats and dogs don't seem
to have any trouble falling asleep.

I believe a vital evolutionary reason for insomnia may exist. Most
animals sleep and wake almost wholly according to their circadian
rhythms. As their sleep debt waxes and their clock-dependent alerting wanes, they get tired and go to sleep. In humans, other parts of
the brain can play a role in staving off sleepiness when the alerting
mechanism of the biological clock has turned off its juice. During
crises, we have the life-saving benefit of being able to push the limits
of our bedtime, replacing clock-dependent alerting with the psychological drive to keep the mind alert and ready to react.

But the price we pay for this evolutionary advantage may be insomnia. Our much-needed ability to transcend, when necessary, the
limits of clock-dependent alerting can assert itself when there's no
threat keeping us awake. For example, doctors' sleep has been studied on normal nights at home vs. on-call nights when they can
expect to be awakened to attend to patients. During on-call nights,

doctors have disrupted sleep even when they are not called to perform their duties.

If someone has a small sleep debt, a relatively small amount of stress or vigilance, such as being on call, will disturb sleep. For most people, though, disturbed sleep leads to an accumulation of sleep debt. This increased sleep pressure overcomes alerting and lets the person sleep through the night once again. The previously vigilant house physician will sleep through the phone call, the stressed worker will eventually sleep through an alarm clock. When stress is truly severe, and goes on interminably, there will be a persistent difficulty sleeping, and presumably a very sleep-deprived equilibrium finally is established.

It may be that there is an optimum level of predisposition to insomnia—a particular point on the sleepiness-alertness continuum where we have maximum daytime alertness most of the time and insomnia just a few nights a year. But even if you're not an on-call doctor or police officer, you probably have more stress than you can easily compartmentalize into the part of your life on the "awake" side of the border. If you frequently have trouble sleeping because of an overaroused mind, one reason is our stressful, overstimulating environment. Part of the cost of our fast-paced 24-hour modern lifestyle is that our psychological alerting is in overdrive, keeping us "on call" when we most need to be asleep.

How Serious a Problem?

My goal in writing this chapter is to be as clear as possible in guiding the reader to a helpful understanding of insomnia. I think the best way to accomplish this is to take you step by step through the various causes I consider when I am presented with a case of insomnia and the implications of each cause. I have not included several disorders that are extremely rare.

The very first dividing line in addressing any problem of insomnia is whether it really bothers you. The problem may be very severe: trouble sleeping every night with only a very small and fitful amount of sleep. Or it may be merely a little troublesome: an hour awake in a strange bedroom before falling asleep, and no insomnia the next night.

Occasional trouble sleeping is surely part of the human condition and should not necessarily cause concern. Last summer I woke up at about 1:00 A.M. scratching a mosquito bite. I rolled over, ignored the mild itching, and expected to return to sleep. Then I heard that superannoying, high-pitched buzz in my ear. I slapped at it and once more tried to go back to sleep. Again, the high-pitched mosquito sound. After a few more rounds between me and the mosquito, I jumped up, turned on the bedroom light, and began to look around the room for the pesky bug. After a futile search I applied repellent liberally and returned to bed. By this time it was nearly 2:00 and I had gotten myself wide awake. After about 15 minutes of not feeling sleepy, I said, "Oh, hell," got up and had some coffee, and started working on this manuscript. I knew I would pay the price of some sleepiness and impaired motivation later in the day, but I did not want to waste time lying awake in bed. Since I recognized the cause of my problem and solved it by resolving never to leave screen doors open, the insomnia itself caused me no worry or concern whatsoever. Nor should such an episode bother anyone.

On the other hand, if I woke up in the middle of the night for no apparent reason and could not go back to sleep for a long time, I would be annoyed. If, in spite of my fatigue, the same thing happened the next night and my fatigue the next day was worse, I would definitely be concerned. If I had insomnia on the third night, I would be galvanized into action. I would begin to really worry and aggressively seek an explanation. Very severe difficulty sleeping even for only several nights can not only be debilitating but very dangerous.

Here is one of the many horror stories that I have collected about the dangers of insomnia: In August 1991 an extended family was vacationing at a California beach—two sisters, Helen and Rose, their husbands, and their children. The summer idyll was interrupted by the news that the armies of Saddam Hussein had swept into the neighboring emirate of Kuwait. Two days later Helen's husband, a reserve officer, was called to active duty. Literally overnight, he boarded a transport plane bound for the Persian Gulf.

No one knew what lay ahead, and Helen worried that her husband could be in combat within a matter of days. In the midst of all of this, Rose's husband suffered a sudden pulmonary embollism while jogging on the beach. In critical condition, he was evacuated to a nearby large city hospital via helicopter, and Rose went with him, leaving her three children in the care of her very anxious sister.

Alone with four children and worried sick about both her husband and her brother-in-law, Helen was so consumed by stress and anxiety that she couldn't sleep at all. Who could blame her? After three nights of lying awake imagining worst-case scenarios in the Persian Gulf and in the city hospital, Helen was so exhausted she could not take it anymore. Wisely, she made an appointment at a local clinic and asked the doctor for something to help her sleep. In spite of her extremely stressful circumstances, unwisely this doctor would not prescribe a sleeping pill, suggesting instead a glass of warm milk, a hot bath, and soothing music.

After another sleepless night, Helen was simply too exhausted to care for the children in her charge. She called her mother, who lived about 200 miles away, and asked if she could bring the kids there for a few days. Helen packed up all their belongings and set out for her mother's house. Although she was still a nervous wreck, Helen started to feel some relief at the prospect of her mother's help. But with the relief came the first dangerous hint of drowsiness. No longer masked by all the stress and anxiety, the sleep debt that had been accumulating over the previous four nights began to assert itself.

In midafternoon, as Helen was driving through a small town, the unthinkable happened. Without slowing the car in the slightest, she drove through a red light. Helen still does not remember approaching the town or seeing the red light, but she does remember the piercing, nightmarish squeal of brakes as a pickup truck smashed into the side of her car. She and her child in the front seat sustained negligible injuries. Her sister's three children in the backseat however, were more seriously injured, but fortunately survived.

Another story, closer to home:

When I was just getting started at Stanford University, a couple I knew quite well left for a driving tour of France. Two weeks later my wife and I were shocked and dismayed to get a postcard from the husband tersely announcing that his wife had been killed in an automobile crash. When he returned, he told us between barely stifled sobs that he had fallen asleep at the wheel while driving in the French Alps. The car went off the road and crashed into a ravine. His young wife sustained fatal head injuries while he walked away with only minor cuts and bruises. He attributed his horrible lapse to severe jet lag. After a 12-hour red-eye flight from San Francisco to Paris, they had rented a car at the airport and immediately begun their tour, giving his body no time to adjust to the nine-hour time shift. For five nights leading up to the accident he had experienced great difficulty in falling asleep; his sleep debt was enormous by what tragically proved to be the last day of his wife's life.

If you remember nothing else from this book, you must remember these stories and the extremely important principle they are intended to illustrate. When a normal sleeper experiences severe difficulty sleeping, whether from stress, jet lag, or pain, the episode is no different from experimental sleep deprivation in the sense that the individual's sleep debt is mounting rapidly and the tendency to fall asleep will become very strong. If you lie awake most of the night worried, anxious, and unable to sleep, it would never occur to you that you would fall asleep driving or while doing some other potentially dangerous activity. But during the day you are like a tightrope walker carrying a huge load—one slip, one distraction, one letdown, and sleep is upon you like an epileptic seizure.

In summary, you should definitely be concerned about trouble sleeping when the problem persists more than a night or two, when the cause of the problem is not clear or is not easily resolved, and, most important, when there is a negative impact on your daytime function, mood, or performance. Finally, it may well be that your level of concern should be the highest when difficulty sleeping is a secondary consequence of stress, travel, pain, and so on. You are in harm's way, and whatever the cause of your insomnia, it could be horribly compounded by an unintended sleep episode.

What Causes "Transient" Insomnia?

As I mentioned at the beginning of this chapter, sleep specialists like to divide insomnia into two categories: "transient" cases lasting only one night to a week or two, and "chronic" cases lasting weeks, months, or years. These are useful categories, but sometimes they are a little too rigid. People often have a few nights of trouble sleeping, then a few nights of good sleep, then more nights of insomnia. In fact, once an individual has more than a single episode of transient insomnia, the possible patterns of insomnia are almost infinite. The two stories I just provided illustrate two of the three main circumstances that can temporarily disturb sleep: hyperarousal, rapid time zone or schedule change, and environmental disturbance. As the stories demonstrate, the fact that these sleep disturbances are temporary in no way mitigates the need to deal with them.

Hyperarousal

In a number of surveys, and in my own personal experience, hyperarousal caused by stress and worry is the most frequently mentioned cause of temporary sleeping difficulties, and is reported by about half of all those who have experienced insomnia. The degree to which sleep is disturbed is generally a function of the severity and duration of the stressful circumstances. I should note that hyperarousal also may be caused by happy circumstances: Excitement about a lucky windfall or something wonderful that will happen the next day can cause sleep problems the night before.

Time Zone and Schedule Changes

When our circadian rhythms are disrupted by jet lag, shift work and other major schedule changes, insomnia often results. An individual's clock-dependent alerting is thrown out of synchrony with new light and dark cycles, arousing the body when the "alarm" should be turned off. When people move quickly from one time zone to another, their bodies don't have time to catch up. Although some people may feel better in a day or two, others don't and their body's biological rhythms take a full week or more to catch up to the new time.

Sleep Environment

This should be obvious. Noises from traffic, plumbing, or neighbors are often blamed for insomnia. On the other hand, people soon habituate to repeated meaningless noise and tend not to wake up. When my wife and I first moved to New York in the late 1950s, our apartment was right next to the elevated railway. The screeching brakes of the trains entering the station kept me up much of the first night. In the morning I was incensed. "Why didn't the landlord tell me about this?" I fumed. "Now we'll have to move!" But by the next night I was both seriously sleep deprived and somewhat habituated to the sound of the brakes. I slept much better that night and

just fine most nights thereafter, although the trains kept on screeching. Personally, I'm somewhat skeptical that environmental factors
are of overriding importance as direct causes of insomnia. However,
I think sensitivity to the environment can be magnified by other
factors, such as stress or anger. As I suggested, being disturbed by
noise is usually transient, but if you feel that the noise is being made
maliciously and deliberately to annoy you, it is likely that your sleep
will be very disturbed.

Bouts of transient insomnia account for three-quarters of all cases
of insomnia. The causes are usually temporary, and, when the cause
recedes, so does the insomnia. People resolve their personal problems, leave the hotel, or rotate back to the day shift. When resolved,
transient insomnia is usually forgotten or dismissed as a minor incon-
venience. I want to make it eminently clear, however, that transient
insomnia is still a health and safety issue that demands serious attention and effective treatment. Even after a single night of bad sleep,
you can feel awful the next day and find your performance severely
impaired. Being extremely tired can make even minor difficulties
seem hopeless. A few nights of little or no sleep can make you unsafe
to yourself and others: People with insomnia are many times more
likely to have automobile accidents, not to mention the large-scale
disasters potentially caused by sleep-deprived airline pilots and train
engineers.

When people complain of extreme daytime fatigue resulting from
insomnia, it is always tempting to say: "Why don't you just take a
nap?" In the first place, it is likely that they cannot nap. If the
insomnia is caused by stress and anxiety, those feelings will come to
the forefront with greatly increased intensity as soon as the sufferer is
lying alone with nothing to distract him or her from them. The
reasons people can't sleep at night will be the same reasons they can't
nap during the day. Individuals in the vise of anxiety and stress fall
asleep only if they are caught off guard, such as while driving, working, or carrying out some other sedentary but distracting activity.
Accordingly, when physicians casually suggest that napping is the
easy solution to the problem, it must seem callous and unsympathetic
to the patient.

Late to Bed or Early to Rise?

Once it is clear that someone's insomnia is persistent, that is, recurring frequently or nearly every night, one of the first things I do is determine if the difficulty is with falling asleep or waking up too early. If you think you have an insomnia problem and it is confined to being unable to fall asleep, it is likely that the insomnia is the result of a circadian rhythm problem. You now know from what I have told you about the biological clock that strong clock-dependent alerting occurs typically in the evening. When the biological clock is alerting the brain at a time that you want to schedule your bedtime, you will have sleep-onset insomnia. When evening alerting keeps people up late and it is then difficult for them to get up in the morning, we call the problem delayed sleep-phase syndrome, or DSPS. To the unenlightened, it is sleep-onset insomnia.

In 1970–71, I was the resident fellow in a Stanford student dormitory that housed 90 students. We actually set up a sleep laboratory in the basement. I trained a small group of very bright students to attach electrodes and prepare volunteers for sleep recordings. At the time we had just opened our sleep disorders clinic and I was interested in sleep-onset insomnia. I was interested in how long it would take students to fall asleep. Thirty-six students volunteered to go to bed in the sleep laboratory at 10:00 P.M. on various nights. Thirty-one took longer than 30 minutes to fall asleep, which conformed to the then-conventional definition of insomnia. Four fell asleep within 5 to 10 minutes, and one required about 20. We then had the 31 "insomniacs" go to bed at midnight and still 18 required 30 or more minutes to fall asleep. The other 13 fell asleep within 10 minutes. I don't think any of the students considered themselves insomniacs, but they had as much trouble getting to sleep as patients whose complaint is difficulty falling asleep. Of course, we now know that the inability of the students to fall asleep was completely due to late-night clock-dependent alerting.

The other problem, waking up too early, is often considered to be a hallmark symptom of depression. But the biological clock can run too early as well as too late. If someone has consistent difficulty staying asleep in the morning, we always ask, "Are you sleepy or tired in the evening, and do you fall asleep in front of the TV?" If the answer is yes, this is the mirror image of delayed sleep-phase syndrome, designated formally as advanced sleep-phase syndrome (ASPS).

For some years now the treatment has been bright light in the morning for DSPS and bright light in the evening for ASPS. The usual prescription is sitting in front of a bank of fluorescent lights for a couple of hours. Sitting in front of a bright light box is not always the easiest thing to schedule into one's day, but a new device on the horizon should make it easier. It is a pair of glasses that delivers bright light to the periphery of the retina through fiber optic guides. The device is portable and so unobtrusive that it hardly disturbs the wearer.

Other Major Causes of Persistent Insomnia

For those who have persistent insomnia that is not due to biological clock problems, a large percentage will find that their insomnia is caused by one of three physical causes—restless legs syndrome, gastroesophageal reflux, or fibromyalgia.

In 1998 the Omnibus Sleep Poll, carried out by the National Sleep Foundation as part of National Sleep Awareness Week, found a large number of those who experienced difficulty sleeping on a frequent basis reported creepy, crawly feelings in their legs that went away when they moved about. The symptom is always associated with a disorder called restless legs syndrome. The hallmark of this syndrome, uncomfortable and sometimes painful feelings in the legs which create a desire to move them, causes difficulty sleeping. When symptoms occur, victims vigorously flex, stretch, and cross their legs to ease their discomfort. Usually patients prefer to walk about if possible. The feelings are relieved briefly, but return shortly thereafter.

Although the disorder is called restless legs syndrome, or RLS, the restlessness occasionally includes the arms and other muscles. There is a clear tendency for the prevalence to increase with age, but the syndrome may occur in children. There does not appear to be a gender difference. The basic cause of RLS is unknown, but it is somewhat more common in patients suffering from iron deficiency/anemia and kidney failure with dialysis.

This very important sleep disorder could not be easier to spot. We simply ask, "Do you have creepy, crawly feelings in your legs when you are sitting or lying that go away when you walk about and that are worse at night?" If the answer is yes, the diagnosis will almost be RLS. Unfortunately, few doctors or patients know enough to make the correct identification, and the vast majority of restless leg victims suffer for years without a diagnosis. As I have said, there is a major knowledge gap in the medical care system. What could be more grotesque than the fact that 15 to 20 million Americans with RLS have fallen into that gap?

I consider the restless legs syndrome a sleep disorder for four reasons. First, since it is extremely difficult for restless legs syndrome victims to lie still, they have great difficulty obtaining adequate sleep. Two, RLS symptoms are typically worse at night. Three, restless legs syndrome has a high association with an independent sleep disorder, periodic limb movement during sleep. And four, only sleep specialists can be depended on always to identify such patients and give them the relief they need. Restless legs syndrome was first described by Karl Eckbaum in the 1940s. It is thus the second major sleep disorder, after narcolepsy, to be identified and characterized. However, it was not identified as a sleep disorder, nor was it solidly linked with insomnia and with periodic leg movement during sleep, until our work at Stanford.

A retired dentist who had very severe restless legs syndrome and didn't know it was finally diagnosed by doctors in our Walla Walla/ Moscow primary care project. He thought his agitation and discomfort were a by-product of getting older. "I didn't know what the problem was," he said. "All I knew was I couldn't sleep." This bedeviled man could not even sit in a chair to read. His restlessness at night was overwhelming, and he became very severely, chronically sleep deprived. After more than 15 years of unremitting misery, the dentist mentioned his problem to newly educated primary sleep physician Dr. John Grauke in Moscow, Idaho. Of course, Dr. Grauke recognized the true problem instantly and prescribed an effective medication. Literally overnight, the dentist experienced miraculous relief.

Many others are not so fortunate. The National Commission on Sleep Disorders Research received a letter from the spouse of a suicide victim who had apparently given up hope after years of trying to find out what was wrong with her. The husband was very bitter. "Once I learned about restless legs," he wrote, "I was absolutely certain that was her problem." About a year ago, a woman in Milwaukee who had severe restless legs syndrome was undergoing angioplasty. During the operation, first one and finally three physicians struggled to hold her legs. While they were doing this, the woman died. The Restless Legs Syndrome Foundation has, in its files, numerous other horror stories of victims being restrained inappropriately. People who know they suffer from restless legs syndrome must be sure to notify all involved health professionals during any type of medical or dental procedure. More mundane precautions involve always obtaining an aisle seat on airplanes and in theaters.

What people say to explain their bizarre restlessness would fill a book. Explanations include: "I guess this is because I stand on my feet all day." "I guess that I'm neurotic." "I was a hyperactive child and it has persisted into my adult years." Since the prevalence of the syndrome is high, yet it is often undiagnosed, frequent problems and tragedies have resulted.

One of the Stanford Clinic's most grateful patients is a San Mateo veterinarian who had a very severe problem with restless legs syndrome. It had progressed to the point where he was getting very little sleep at night so that he was drowsy nearly all the time. He was a dedicated Rotarian, but at this point in his life, during meetings, he would sit down, immediately fall asleep for a couple of minutes, and then abruptly stand up and begin to pace and kick and flex his legs. After a time he would sit down again, and this bizarre behavior would be repeated. He quickly realized he could no longer participate in these social activities. He finally saw a neurologist who referred him to Stanford, and the relief he obtained with treatment basically, he said, "miraculously [gave] me back my life." Before coming to the clinic he had contemplated giving up his practice, since he could not remain in one position long enough to carry out the required activities of a veterinarian.

Since many physicians are unaware of restless legs syndrome, such complaints lead them in the wrong direction. Two summers ago I was attending the summer meeting of the house of delegates of the American Medical Association. During a policy meeting of about 150 physicians, I made some brief remarks about the danger of restraints if someone had restless legs syndrome. When several doctors asked what I was talking about, I asked how many people in the audience were familiar with restless legs syndrome. Not one physician's hand went up.

In the early days of the Stanford Clinic, patients with this problem were relatively rare. Thus, even I was guilty of underestimating the true extent of this disorder. In fact, it is now clear that the prevalence of restless legs syndrome is quite high. However, properly designed studies to carry out an accurate assessment of population prevalence have yet to be done. A large sample in Quebec, Canada, yielded a figure of 14 percent; several other nonrepresentative samples have suggested at least 10 percent, and the Restless Legs Syndrome Foundation, in order to maintain credibility, supports a very conservative figure of 5 percent. Even this lowest figure would comprise more than 10 million people in the United States, and it is likely that these percentages are the same in other countries.

We are sure that only the tiniest fraction know what is wrong with them. As with other sleep disorders, the millions of victims are not the only ones who lose sleep. Spouses, if they are in the same bed or even in the same room, will almost by definition be chronically sleep deprived.

Astoundingly, in our primary care project in Moscow, Idaho, nearly 30 percent of the clinical population reported unambiguous symptoms of the syndrome. As with every other sleep disorder, none of the patients had been given a diagnosis of restless legs syndrome before coming to us. Something has to be done about this terrible disorder. Restless legs syndrome has got to be the biggest completely unaddressed health care priority in America.

The first step is education. As I have said, no other condition is more easy to recognize. Furthermore, dramatically effective new treatments are available. There is absolutely no reason on earth why millions of people should continue to suffer this torment. For these reasons, health care professionals should be taught much more about this syndrome. If the National Institutes of Health does nothing else, it must carry out a population study to document the prevalence as well as the health and quality-of-life impact of restless legs syndrome. As the syndrome is so common, there should be a high research priority to find a cure or learn how it might be prevented.

Gastroesophageal Reflux

Sometimes the flow of stomach acid back into the lower esophagus (gastroesophageal reflux) causes sleep to be disturbed. If the acid makes it all the way to our throat and larynx, the sleeper will awaken coughing and choking. However, if the acid flows back only into our lower esophagus, the sleeper will wake up but won't know why. This was demonstrated in experiments in which a drop or two of acid was passed through a tube into the esophagus near the stomach. Even this small amount of acid caused the sleeping subject to wake up even though he did not report feeling heartburn or other sensations.

When frequent difficulty sleeping, particularly frequent arousals, is not diagnosed and resolved, very few if any physicians would suspect gastroesophageal reflux and have a patient sleep with a device in the esophagus to measure acid. Even sleep disorders clinics rarely do this as part of their routine sleep tests. Accordingly, we do not have a clear idea of the prevalence of gastroesophageal reflux as a cause of insomnia.

Heartburn is a very common disorder of waking patients. Gastroesophageal reflux is potentially a much more common cause of insomnia than heretofore assumed, and should always be considered. Medications that block acid secretion are now available without a prescription, and the simple step of not eating a full meal before going to bed will also help. In patients who complain of difficulty sleeping with no apparent reason and occasionally awaken with heartburn, gastroesophageal reflux should definitely be considered as a cause.

Fibrositis Syndrome (Fibromyalgia)

Fibrositis is a disorder associated with pain in muscles and tendons, characteristically with points of tenderness in certain typical locations. There is always daytime fatigue and very commonly difficulty falling asleep and staying asleep. When someone with fibrositis syndrome is finally referred to a sleep disorders clinic, a sleep test will usually record an abnormal EEG pattern called alpha–delta sleep, in which regular rhythms in the alpha frequency range are seen riding on large, slow delta waves.

It is seldom obvious why patients have difficulty sleeping. Of course, pain will disturb sleep. When patients with fibrositis syndrome are given the Multiple Sleep Latency Test, their results rarely suggest severe sleep deprivation. Thus, a large sleep debt is not likely to be the main cause of the daytime fatigue. It is my impression that this problem is highly prevalent. The society patient groups estimate that there are over 10 million sufferers in the United States.

One extremely interesting discovery about this disorder is that when patients are experimentally sleep-deprived, there is a significant increase in pain. For ethical reasons, not many of these experiments have been carried out. In my mind, this issue deserves much more research. Is there a sleep pathology or disturbance? Is there some sort of sleep pathology that is causing the pain, is the pain disturbing the sleep, or is it a combination of both? This raises a general question: will sleep deprivation make pain worse in general?

Insomnia Associated with Psychological, Emotional, and Psychiatric Problems

Frequent or persistent problems sleeping are very commonly associated with depression and other psychiatric problems. When these problems—phobias, anxieties, neuroses, and so on—are not obvious, spotting the true cause of the insomnia becomes more difficult.

The question of treatment is a little tricky. Generally, these cases are handled by psychiatrists. Although many sleep specialists are psychiatrists, psychiatrists in general outnumber sleep specialists by somewhere between 20 or 50 to one, and most of them have no expertise in sleep disorders. The insomnia problem, therefore, may very well not be treated directly, and not enough outcome data exist to indicate how frequently an insomnia problem clears up if the underlying psychiatric condition is effectively treated.

Disorders Requiring a Sleep Test for Diagnosis

Once all of the aforementioned causes of every night or frequently recurring insomnia are ruled out, there still exist several possible causes that can be identified with certainty only by polysomnographic testing (although sometimes careful questioning can elicit clues). Perhaps the most common of these is periodic limb movement disorder (PLMD), which, as mentioned earlier, is very frequently, although occasionally not, associated with restless legs syndrome. In periodic limb movement disorder, the sleep test will show recurring episodes of repetitive and highly stereotyped limb movements during sleep. The movements always involve the legs, rarely the arms, and consist of extension of the big toe, partial flexion of the ankle, knee, and sometimes the hip. They are frequently sufficiently vigorous to cause an awakening. Victims will complain of insomnia and unrefreshing sleep. Self-awareness of the leg movements is rare, but a bed partner may report being kicked and disturbed. The severity of the problem depends upon how frequently the movements occur, but what is most impressive is their clocklike regularity. I have often stared almost in awe as the polysomnograph machine records a burst of electrical activity in the anterior tibialis muscle exactly every 30 seconds (flexing every half-minute is common, but the period may vary). Studies have shown a very strong relationship between age and PLMD with prevalence figures as high as 40 percent in individuals over the age of 65.

The second cause is central sleep apnea, in which breathing simply stops during sleep and is resumed only when a patient awakens. The severity of central sleep apnea is related to the number of times the victim stops breathing during sleep. Snoring can occur but is usually not prominent. Sometimes central and obstructive sleep apnea can occur together (mixed apnea), but in central sleep apnea itself there is no obstruction. There is no truly effective treatment for this condition. Happily, central sleep apnea is rare.

A third diagnosis that can be made only by carrying out a sleep test is called sleep state misperception. From the viewpoint of a sleep specialist, this is a very interesting and perplexing condition. It is diagnosed in about 5 percent of cases where patients who complain of persistent insomnia, when tested, show completely normal sleep. In my opinion, this is consistent with the slogan "The brain never sleeps," which is to say that the brain actively induces and maintains sleep. In some people, brain activity may be at a higher level that in some way makes victims feel they were awake even though they were unquestionably asleep. Most of these people do not say they have had no sleep whatsoever, but their estimate is a lot less than what actually occurs. Insomnia in these instances should not be associated with increasing sleep debt or an abnormal MSLT.

The problem of sleep state misperception can sometimes be resolved by persuading people that their sleep is normal no matter what they think. Once, a young woman flew out from the East Coast to see me without an appointment. She came to my office and told the receptionist she would wait until I showed up. I saw right away that she looked awful and was obviously desperate. She had resigned from a Peace Corps assignment overseas because her insomnia was so bad. I tested her daytime sleepiness with the MSLT and her nighttime sleep in the sleep laboratory over two nights. Right away I noticed that the MSLT showed her to be less sleepy in the daytime than the average person off the street. When the nighttime testing began, she fell asleep fairly quickly and slept well the whole night. The same thing happened the second night. Yet after both nights, the patient was sure she had slept hardly at all. When it came time to discuss the results of the tests, I sat down with her and went over the EEG recordings from both nights page by page. In my most comforting and reassuring, yet authoritative, manner I said, "I have been doing these sleep recordings almost all of my adult life, and your tests show absolutely perfect, normal sleep. These are just beautiful sleep spindles, and this is wonderful slow-wave sleep." I explained to her that the brain is not inactive during sleep, and I reassured her with great firmness that she didn't need to worry ever again about the quality of her sleep. I would like to add that I taped our discussion. When we were done, I gave her the tape and said, "If at any time during the years ahead you begin to worry, please listen to this tape." The patient flew back East and had no further problems with insomnia.

Interestingly, if people who suffer from sleep state misperception are given sleeping pills, they often say that they slept more than usual, even though the all-night recording has shown that their sleep time didn't really increase at all. In these cases, the sleep medication doesn't so much improve sleep, but rather decreases the feeling of having been awake.

Primary Insomnia

At last we are left with two distinct diagnoses that are often lumped together as "primary insomnias." The first, and by far the most common, is psychophysiological insomnia, also called learned insomnia or conditioned insomnia. This disorder is one of the most frequently diagnosed in sleep clinics. The diagnosis is considered when the patient interview suggests a great deal of anxiety and tension around getting ready for bed and getting ready to go to sleep.

Often patients describe getting enough sleep as the greatest struggle in their life. When patients give a history of sleeping better in a strange environment than in their own bedroom, this is usually a positive sign—in the foreign environment, the cues and conditioned signals that create tension are either absent or else greatly reduced. These individuals maintain a focused absorption on their sleep problem. Most sleep specialists have a collection of dramatic examples. Terrible insomnia but sound sleep when forced to spend the night on the floor at O'Hare Airport during a storm. Can't sleep at home but slept hanging from the side of a mountain. Much more commonly, this characteristic or feature is not sufficiently clear.

A clinical diagnosis of psychophysiological insomnia must also include a daytime consequence, usually irritability, anxiety, and depressed mood. Finally, the polysomnogram must show disturbed sleep in terms of a prolonged sleep latency—20 minutes or more—and an abnormal amount of wakefulness during the night.

The second diagnosis is idiopathic insomnia, which was originally called childhood-onset insomnia, and refers to a lifelong inability to obtain adequate sleep. It is presumably due to an abnormality in the brain mechanisms that control the sleep-wake system. The disorder is definitely not common and the exact prevalence is unknown. The crucial feature is the onset at an early age. The presence of daytime symptoms and certain mild neurological signs differentiate this diagnosis from the findings in a normal short sleeper.

In spite of these general criteria for insomnia, there has long been some confusion about how to classify patients who seemed to sleep a lot more than they thought. For example, as the reader now knows, it is the fundamental belief of the sleep professionals that the loss of an hour or two of sleep every night add to cumulative sleep debt such that the sleep tendency during the day should steadily increase. In a few more days the sleep loss ought to be producing strong feelings that should be difficult to ignore, such as waves of drowsiness and burning eyes. Finally, behavioral changes should be apparent to others: falling asleep while watching television, nodding off whenever one is sedentary. If the nightly sleep loss was more substantial, say four hours, it would be impossible for this to happen every night because the homeostatic sleep drive would simply become so strong that sleep is inevitable.

Considering all this, the insomnia that many sleep clinic patients complain about is questionable. In one of our earliest scientific publications in the 1960s, we analyzed laboratory sleep questionnaires, the patients' test results, and the severity of their complaints. The overall result was a very sizable discrepancy between the severity of the complaint and the severity of the objective sleep disturbance, as measured in sleep laboratory recordings.

In one striking research example, a patient complaining of severe insomnia was recorded on ten consecutive nights in the sleep lab. He stated on his questionnaire each morning that it took between one and four hours to fall asleep, with an average of about an hour and a half. The objective test, however, showed that it never took more than 30 minutes for him to fall asleep, and he averaged about 15 minutes. Another chronic insomniac in this research project wrote on her questionnaire each morning that she never slept more than $5^{1}/_{2}$ hours, and her ten estimates of her own sleep time averaged about four hours. Her actual average sleep time derived from the polysomnographic testing was six hours and twenty minutes.

At that point in time, there was no widely accepted definition of insomnia in terms of the objective sleep parameters, but in order to do a clinical trial, a cutoff had to be set. So in the 1970s in order to qualify as an insomniac, an individual had to take at least 30 minutes to fall asleep, to sleep fewer than 6 hours, and/or to have multiple awakenings during the night. Patients who actually had a diagnostic polysomnogram at a sleep clinic generally met these criteria or worse, but large numbers of volunteers for clinical trials of sleeping pills who were first screened to be sure they qualified did not meet these criteria. As time passed, we sleep specialists began, in clinical practice, to rely less on the objective sleep parameters and more on the complaint of the patient. If someone is miserable and they say it is because they have insomnia, then they have insomnia.

When the multiple sleep latency test was validated and began to enjoy widespread use, three groups of sleep researchers, including ours, reported that large numbers of chronic insomniacs were fully alert in the daytime, scoring at or near the ceiling of the MSLT. To give an example, we compared two matched groups (matched for age, sex, etc.) of normal sleepers and chronic insomniacs. The insomnia complainers were significantly more alert than the normal controls, and fully 14% were at the ceiling of the MSLT, never falling asleep in the daytime. I hasten to add that the several hundred chronic insomniacs involved did exhibit about every level of daytime sleep tendency. I have mentioned that many individuals who complain of severe insomnia over a long period of time deny ever feeling sleepy in the daytime and these results were certainly consistent with this. The easiest but not very satisfactory explanation would simply be that these people just have too much anxiety in the lab to allow themselves to fall asleep, even though they may be very sleepy. However, the sleep loss they describe should overwhelm this anxiety. An answer to this conundrum has been supplied by the outstanding research of Mike Bonnet and Donna Arand.

Bonnet and Arand first used sleep recordings from 10 primary insomniacs to produce identical sleep disturbances in a group of matched normal sleepers for 7 nights. They were doing this in order to determine if specific sleep patterns were responsible for the secondary insomnia symptoms reported by the insomniacs. Specifically, these symptoms were increased tension and confusion, decreased vigor, personality disturbance, subjective overestimation of poor sleep, increased body temperature, and increased 24-hour whole body metabolic rate. They also had increased multiple sleep latency test (MSLT) values. On the other hand, normal sleepers with the sleep patterns of insomniacs displayed symptoms more akin to mild partial sleep deprivation than the symptoms of primary insomnia. Bonnet and Arand concluded that the secondary symptoms reported by patients with primary insomnia are probably not related to their poor sleep per se. Data from this study and others support the contention that the indirect symptoms of insomnia, including poor sleep, are secondary to central nervous system hyperarousal.

Treating Primary Insomnias

The primary insomnias are usually difficult to treat. Because these disorders are chronic, there have been exhaustive efforts to develop nondrug treatments for them. Most physicians will not prescribe effective sleep medication for only a few days, let alone chronically. I do believe that a dedicated, caring, and, above all, knowledgable physician can ease insomnia in almost every case, but doing so may require a great deal of time. One of the problems I have with most of the lay-level books published on insomnia is that they promise that people will "sleep well in five days" or find the "miracle sleep cure." People with chronic insomnia should know a cure is never this easy, and it's foolish and counterproductive to tell them so.

There are a variety of general techniques that can be tried to alleviate primary insomnia. These approaches include improving sleep hygiene (which is a good idea for everyone), relaxation techniques, stimulus control, cognitive techniques, and sleep state restriction. I will discuss each in turn.

Improving Sleep Hygiene

The simple goal of good sleep hygiene is to do everything possible to foster good sleep at night. Sleep hygiene includes nonpsychological elements, such as avoiding caffeine before bedtime, but many of the elements are behavioral. Keeping a regular schedule is one of the most important behaviors for healthy sleep. A regular schedule helps train your sleep cycle in the same way that running at the same time every morning conditions you to prepare for exercise at that time. Sticking to a regular sleep schedule seven days a week is a sacrifice worth making if it helps you maintain peak condition throughout the week. Consider it "doctor's orders." I have had to excuse myself early from many a dinner party because I needed to be in bed. Better sleep hygiene is much more extensively discussed in Chapter 19.

Relaxation Techniques

Relaxation has long been used to fight the body's sleep disruptive physiological arousal. The most widely known technique is called progressive relaxation training. With this method, insomniacs learn to relax systematically, first by tensing and relaxing the feet, then the legs, then the hands, then the arms, and so on. They also concentrate on controlling breathing and think about the pleasant sensations. When people practice this technique during the day and before bedtime, it can be very effective in removing anxiety that interferes with sleep both at the beginning and in the middle of the night.

Stimulus Control

One important part of improving our chance to fall asleep is to abolish as much as possible stimulating activities or thoughts as bedtime approaches. Keeping away from things that are disturbing before you try to go to sleep may sound obvious, but it is amazing how often people will get themselves excited, upset, anxious, or angry before going to bed. For example, they watch the late news, seeing stories on rape, murder, fatal accidents, and corruption, and then wonder why they can't sleep. Other pitfalls include doing homework, paying bills, or checking e-mail right before going to bed. People have the misguided belief that they are making good use of their time by getting a jump on tomorrow's headaches. But focusing on things that cause psychological arousal right before bed is more likely to disturb sleep and undermine productivity the next day.

One of my colleagues had a patient, Ron, who was a classic case of an insomniac who couldn't leave his work at the office. Ron started his own electronics company and developed chronic insomnia that persisted for years. He typically spent the hours before bed worrying and obsessing about the next day and all things that might go wrong. After a session of this late-night work, he wasn't ready for sleep, he was ready to do battle! Ron was living through tomorrow's crises today. My colleague required him to designate a specific half hour immediately after dinner as "worry time," when he could make a list of all the things that caused him anxiety and think about how to address them. He was absolutely forbidden to spend even a minute worrying after those 30 minutes. Ron spent the remainder of the evening doing things that were calming and relaxing, such as reading a good book. These techniques played a key part in eventually breaking the cycle of his psychophysiological insomnia.

Cognitive Techniques

Techniques that engage the mind with some simple, repetitive problem are longtime favorites for battling sleeplessness. The mental attention that these tasks require offers a distraction from thoughts that interfere with sleep. Counting sheep is the classic example. Some people use repeated calculations, such as starting with a number (say, 1000) and subtracting another number (say, 17) again and again.

Another method that sometimes works to get the mind off the subject of sleep is, paradoxically, to make staying awake a goal. Trying to stay awake for as long as possible often counteracts the fear of not being able to sleep. Doing so, patients relax enough to let their (usually substantial) sleep debt take over, and they drift off to sleep.

Sleep State Restriction

One of the techniques that I like to use to fight insomnia is a more formal version of the cognitive technique just mentioned. It is called sleep state restriction. The idea is to order a patient *not* to sleep. I favor this technique for patients who are exaggerating their symptoms or have honest misperceptions about their sleep but cannot accept the possibility that they might be able to sleep normally. I don't want them to feel I am accusing them of lying, and it allows me to avoid a confrontation on this point. If someone comes to me and says, "Doctor, I sleep only four hours a night," I say, "Okay, I want you to go to bed at 3:00 A.M. and get up at 7:00 A.M." After sleeping only four hours, the patient usually has built up a lot of sleep debt and feels pretty sleepy. Then we add half an hour of sleep every night, until a week later the patient is up to a solid seven and a half hours a night. This technique requires a high degree of commitment by the patient and is not suitable for everyone.

Alternative Therapies

The following "alternative" therapies sometimes are used to treat insomnia. None have been truly tested. Nonetheless, at public lectures, etc., I often encounter someone who swears by one of them. I'm happy for that person, but I have no way of knowing if anyone else might benefit.

Hypnosis

Hypnosis has limited effectiveness in promoting relaxation and fighting insomnia. For one thing, true hypnosis demands the presence of a hypnotist, so it's usually not something you can try at home. Second, the hypnotic trance is very different from sleep; it is more of a highly suggestible state of relaxation, so a trance doesn't naturally lead directly into sleep. (In cases of psychophysiological insomnia, however, hypnosis may be useful in relieving people of undue anxieties.) The third difficulty with hypnosis is that some people are resistant to it.

Self-hypnosis may be another matter. What is called self-hypnosis is really a voluntary relaxation technique that is similar to meditation. Self-hypnosis, meditation, and yoga can put the body and mind at ease and ready for sleep. In one study patients were instructed to lie still with eyes closed and focus on their breathing, thinking the words "in" and "out" as they inhaled and exhaled. This technique proved to be just as effective as the progressive relaxation technique in fighting insomnia.

Biofeedback

Biofeedback is a technique whereby patients learn how to monitor and control physiological responses. Patients are hooked up to machines that monitor electrical resistance in the skin or brain waves. Through feedback from the machine, they can learn consciously to control physiological tension and relaxation. Some research has shown that biofeedback can be effective, but biofeedback's use is limited by the need for regular access to the right equipment.

Acupuncture

There have been no good studies of the benefits of treating insomnia with acupuncture or acupressure, although some practitioners claim they can treat insomnia successfully 90 percent of the time. I have to confess to being dubious about these claims, because the studies I've read don't conform to accepted scientific protocol.

Massage

Massage helps people relax physically and mentally, and as a result masseurs report that people often fall asleep on the massage table. Of course, to be most effective the massage would have to be given right at bedtime, in your own bed. Like biofeedback and acupuncture, this is impractical for most people, unless you live with someone who is proficient at massage.

Herbs and Home Remedies

People regularly ask me about herbal treatments for insomnia, or home remedies, and want to know if they work or if there have been scientific studies of their efficacy. Generally I find that valerian, herbal teas, warm milk, and the like have not been well tested scientifically. The few studies usually are small or very limited, and don't represent even the beginning of a true clinical trial. If sleep research were as well funded as cancer research, I'm sure we would have time and money to find these answers. Right now we don't. When asked if these treatments work, my response is: We don't know. If you try them and they help you, that's fine, especially if you have transient insomnia and don't want to take prescription sleeping pills. But for chronic insomnia, my advice is that if you really want to get answers, talk to a sleep specialist.

Melatonin

In the early 1990s, some of my colleagues began investigating the use of the hormone melatonin as a sleep medication, testing it on laboratory animals to determine toxicity or side effects. The substance appeared very promising, and in the mid-1990s, researchers applied to the drug-regulating arm of the Food and Drug Administration to test melatonin's safety in humans. The FDA denied the request, requiring more animal trials first. In a classic instance of bureaucracy's left hand not knowing what the right hand is doing, the food-regulating arm of the FDA soon afterward approved the sale of melatonin as a food additive. As a "natural substance," melatonin became available without any testing whatsoever. An onslaught of very positive coverage in books for the layman and other media encouraged people to take melatonin not only to help them sleep but also to improve their general health, happiness, longevity, and virility—claims that have never been scientifically substantiated and that some of us feel are patently ridiculous. Thus began one of the largest uncontrolled and unregulated clinical trials in medical history.

What we do know about melatonin is that it is a hormone secreted by the pineal gland in the brain that lets the body know that it is dark outside. For humans, melatonin directs the body to prepare for sleep; for nocturnal animals like rats, its release is a sign to start waking up. Long winter nights lead to higher melatonin levels in the body, and short summer nights lead to lower levels. Among nonhuman mammals, changes in melatonin levels regulate hibernation, sexual activity, and sex hormone production. Since humans tend to be sexually active year round, melatonin does not seem to affect these cycles, although changing melatonin levels do play a role in initiating sexual development at puberty.

The sleep-inducing effect of melatonin works in counterpoint to the alerting effect of light. In very low doses (up to 0.5 milligrams for the average adult), melatonin can shift the phase of the biological clock. Melatonin rises naturally right before falling asleep, and ingested melatonin can produce the same sort of surge. Melatonin is most likely to affect the phase of the biological clock when it's synchronized with changing light levels. For example, if you usually can't get to sleep before 1:00 A.M., you may be able to get to sleep earlier by ingesting melatonin shortly after the sun sets. In other words, taking melatonin at night causes a phase-advance (earlier to bed and earlier to rise), whereas melatonin in the morning induces a phase-delay (later to rise and later to bed).

Since melatonin can constrict blood vessels, there is some concern that it may pose a danger for people with cardiovascular disease. Biologists also have observed some effects on human sperm and egg cells. Melatonin may have effects on human reproductive cycles analogous to its effects on reproduction in other mammals.

When patients ask me if they should be experimenting with melatonin, I first remind them that the hormone is less carefully regulated for purity and dosage than are prescription medications, and that much more research into its actions remains to be conducted. Nevertheless, melatonin does seem to help some people, so I don't discourage interested patients from trying it in small doses as a remedy for transient insomnia and jet lag. It may help night workers sleep better during the day, and totally blind people may be able to synchronize their clocks to melatonin instead of light.

Relationship Between Temporary and Persistent Insomnia

Unfortunately, sleep specialists know very little about how an initially transient insomnia becomes a chronic insomnia. Sometimes insomnia persists because the initial cause, such as shift work or posttraumatic stress disorder is severe and long-lasting. In other cases, the sleeping difficulties persist long after the initial problems have gone away. Most commonly, we are completely uncertain about how a normal sleeper becomes an insomniac, whose frequent nights of poor sleep definitely undermine quality of life and daytime function. Most insomnia experts speculate that occasional, limited bouts of insomnia cause the victim to begin worrying about being able to sleep. This creates an ongoing tension that interferes with sleep and reinforces the worry. Some people are probably more vulnerable to this than others.

One important fact that we have learned is that the lower someone's sleep debt, the more vulnerable they will be to a bout of stress-related or other types of transient insomnia. One of my teaching assistants, who always fell asleep about five minutes after going to bed, was enthusiastically lowering his sleep debt by sleeping an extra hour or two each night. Suddenly, to his great surprise and dismay, he began having trouble falling asleep at night. He had lowered his sleep debt beyond some critical point and the routine worries of student life were sufficient to prevent sleep. Had he not completely understood the reasons for his "insomnia," he might have started worrying and obsessing about it, and causing his sleep problems to persist.

I know that if people take intelligent action early in the course of insomnia, they can nip it in the bud, before it grows into a frequent or persistent problem. Any normal sleeper who has a bout of difficulty sleeping should, first of all, be able to identify the cause. This is true almost without exception. Everyone should know enough to understand and actively manage their sleep. Even if you cannot remember your last bout of difficulty sleeping, be ready when sleep problems do strike. Unlike those whose chronic insomnia rises out of a prolonged case of temporary insomnia, the victims of the kind of heightened physiological arousal or hyperarousal described by Mike Bonnet and Donna Arand may just have insomnia as a result of an individual constitutional characteristic. On the other hand, I have come to suspect that there is a lot more posttraumatic stress disorder among these patients than we now realize. Early childhood experiences of physical or sexual abuse are often either repressed or not mentioned out of shame. At the risk of repeating myself, here again it is necessary to call for much more research on insomnia.

I also feel that this is the time to make a very strong pitch to everyone—normal sleeper, good sleeper, poor sleeper, whatever—to improve their sleep hygiene, as described in Chapter 19, as much as possible. Sleep hygiene principles are not laws, they are principles to follow as much as possible within the bounds of common sense. Remember, we want to keep sleep debt down for optimal performance—but when sleep debt is low, people are much more vulnerable to bouts of insomnia, and the principles of sleep hygiene become much more important.

Treating Insomnia: The Case for Sleeping Pills
The biggest challenge to treating insomnia is persuading doctors and even the people who have insomnia that it is a serious problem. In

our uninformed society, most doctors and lay people consider insomnia a nuisance condition even less important than the common cold or flu. We now know that insomnia can be a deadly problem that we fail to treat at risk to our lives and the lives of those we love.

As a lifelong sleep specialist, I believe that the two sleep issues that are most misunderstood and mythologized by doctors and the general public are, first, the problem of insomnia and, second, the use of sleeping pills to treat it. The reasons are various, but the results are depressingly familiar. Ignorance yields bad medicine and dangerous behavior.

In a survey administered in my most recent undergraduate course, "Sleep and Dreams," an astounding 94 percent of the students agreed or strongly agreed with the statement "Sleeping pills are addictive." However, there is no evidence that currently marketed prescription sleep medications are addicting. How in the world did nearly all of these young students from widely diverse backgrounds develop such a belief?

Just as puzzling is the fact that three-fourths of the students agreed or strongly agreed with the statement "Sleeping pills should not be taken unless you have had difficulty sleeping for more than a month." This belief runs completely counter to the conclusions reached by a special consensus panel and numerous sleep experts at a 1983 special conference under the auspices of the National Institutes of Health, where all agreed that safe and effective sleep medication is the treatment of choice for transient insomnia. Again, how did these students arrive at this belief?

Compounding the problem of a misinformed public is the outdated attitude of most physicians toward sleep medications. In a study of approximately 500 primary care physicians scattered across the country, about 90 percent stated their belief that sleep medications are addicting and that they have serious side effects. Not long ago I was serving as a consulting sleep expert at an FDA hearing involving the sleep medication Halcion (triazolam). One of the physician witnesses began his remarks with the provocative statement: "Using a sleeping pill is like swatting a mosquito with a sledgehammer."

Many people believe that insomnia is one of the most common problems in primary care medical practice. They think doctors are inundated by patients asking for sleeping pills and, as concerned citizens they worry that such pills are dangerously overprescribed. Nothing could be further from the truth. Insomnia is very common, but it just is not diagnosed or treated in medical practices. For example, consider the stereotypical image of a doctor immediately reaching for the prescription pad when a patient complains about trouble sleeping. Extensive national surveys carried out in the early 1980s showed that only about 10 percent of patients with insomnia were given a prescription for sleeping pills, and those patients almost never used them for more than a few nights. People who occasionally take sleeping pills report consistently that these medications effectively relieve their symptoms and that, should the insomnia recur, they would like to use them again. Critics who assert that sleeping pills are overprescribed invariably point to patients who take sleeping pills every night for years. These patients are a very small minority. For the vast majority of insomnia sufferers, many recent studies show that sleeping pills are in fact underprescribed.

The reality, confirmed by my own extensive observations of primary care medical practice in recent years, is that patients almost never seek help specifically for insomnia problems and that doctors resist prescribing sleeping pills on the rare occasions when patients do complain about trouble sleeping.

Erroneous beliefs have led to a state of affairs that defies rational analysis. In those very rare instances when doctors do prescribe something for insomnia, they favor medications that have not been carefully tested for safety and efficacy in treating sleep—such as antidepressants and antianxiety drugs—over the most recent generations of sleeping pills that have been specifically developed for and have been proven useful in treating insomnia. Some health professionals deride sleeping pills as merely symptomatic relief that doesn't address the underlying problem. But from the patients' point of view, symptomatic relief is exactly what is needed. This is particularly true when the insomnia problem is stress-related and temporary.

Insomnia patients find themselves in a classic catch-22 situation: They don't report insomnia because they believe the only thing a doctor can do for their insomnia is give them a sleeping pill, which they irrationally fear. But to many patients, the only thing worse than taking a sleeping pill—which leads inevitably to addiction, they believe—is being denied sleeping pills by a disapproving primary care physician. Rather than risk addiction or the scorn of their doctor, patients may believe it is far better to suffer on their own or resort to folk remedies—which may or may not work.

I have personally experienced another doctor's disdain when she was asked to prescribe sleeping pills. Every year I give a lecture to undergraduates at Cornell University, and on my most recent trip I noticed a student who looked terribly sleepy. It turned out that she had recently endured a serious personal crisis that left her severely sleep deprived. Unable to sleep at night or to skip classes for a daytime nap, she appeared desperate. Knowing what bad things can happen when someone is that sleep deprived, and fearing she might suffer some terrible accident, I placed a call to the student health service. I told the doctor who I was, and that this student needed sleeping pills for a few nights. The doctor seemed resistant, so the Cornell professor who was my host got on the phone and said I was one of the foremost experts in the world on this subject. Our pleading only strengthened the student health doctor's resolve: "I'm not going to be a pill pusher for you or anyone else," she said to me. It did no good to argue that no one was going to get addicted from a three or four day supply of sleep medication. By the scorn and indignation in her voice, you would have thought I was Joe Sleaze, the local drug dealer. All I could do was tell the student to try to find a doctor who would help her get the sleep she desperately needed.

A Brief History of Sleep Medications

At the root of the unfortunate discrepancy between perceptions of the danger of sleeping pills and the reality of their safety and effectiveness is the sometimes tainted history of earlier sleep medications. Sleeping pills are haunted by an inglorious past, even though today's medications are far safer and more sophisticated. To truly appreciate the widespread prejudice against sleep medications, and to understand why these concerns are no longer valid, it is helpful to have a historical perspective.

The problem with many older medications traditionally used to induce sleep is that they depress the central nervous system enough to cause unconsciousness and, at higher doses, death. The history of drug development for insomnia has been a quest to develop sleep-inducing medications that are safe at higher doses, are not addictive, wear off quickly, so that the user doesn't feel sleepy the next day, and don't have side effects. Sleep-inducing medications of the past generally failed on all of these counts. Part of the problem is that most of those medications were developed for other purposes, and their sleep-inducing quality actually was a side effect itself—usually one of many.

Drug treatments for insomnia probably have been around for as long as people have suffered from sleeplessness. From ancient times until the nineteenth century, the most common sleeping potions contained alcohol, opium, or a dilute solution of the active ingredient in the opium poppy, morphine. Morphine, of course, was and still is used mostly as a painkiller. It also affects the digestive system, and a tincture of morphine called laudanum was long used as a treatment for stomach problems. The trouble with morphine derivatives is that they induce virtually every side effect that we wish to avoid in a sleeping pill. Morphine is addictive, it affects mood, it lasts for many hours, and at high doses it can cause coma and death. At low doses it can make people excitable. But without synthetic alternatives, morphine and alcohol were the sedatives of choice.

The first synthetic sleep drug was chloral hydrate, introduced in 1869. This drug and its cousins were chemically classified as bromide salts and became known as bromides. (Shortly thereafter, people started using the term "bromide" to mean an unexciting platitude or truism.) These medications were no great improvement over existing ones because they also could be addictive, and an overdose could kill. Chloral hydrate became notorious in the popular mind as the active ingredient in "knockout drops."

It wasn't until 1903 that barbital was developed, which gave rise to a large class of sleep-inducing compounds called barbiturates. Although developed for anesthesia, barbiturates were widely prescribed as sleeping pills well into the 1970s. The most common types were secobarbital (most commonly known by the trade name Seconal), amobarbital (Amytal), and pentobarbital (Nembutal). Barbiturates depress the central nervous system enough to induce deep unconsciousness in high doses. At lower doses, they can release inhibitions; Amytal became popularly known as "truth serum" after psychiatrists started using it to lower patients' inhibitions during therapy sessions.

The drawbacks of barbiturates as sleep aids soon became apparent.

They were very addictive and caused a "high," increasing their potential for abuse. Tolerance progressed rapidly—after taking a steady dose for only a week or so, the body adapted to the drug by reacting less to it, necessitating ever higher doses. As the dosage increased, there was also the ever-present danger of accidental overdose, because the difference between a therapeutic dose and a lethal dose is relatively small. Sometimes the overdose was not accidental. In the 1950s and 1960s many Hollywood celebrities and ordinary citizens alike attempted suicide by taking a handful of barbiturate sleeping pills, often in combination with alcohol. I believe that the intentional and unintentional abuse of barbiturates has prejudiced doctors and patients against all sleeping pills.

In the 1970s doctors started prescribing a completely new and much safer type of medication: benzodiazepines. The first of these was chlordiazepoxide (Librium), followed shortly thereafter by diazepam (Valium). These early benzodiazepines actually were created and certified to treat anxiety. Doctors in the United States could prescribe them for sleep, but the FDA never certified that they were safe and effective for that purpose. Consistent with the history of all sleep medications, the sleep-inducing properties of Librium and Valium were useful side effects rather than their primary indication. After a spate of highly publicized deaths from barbiturates in the 1950s and early 1960s, the benzodiazepines offered important improvements in safety; they were largely ineffectual in suicide attempts, and since they didn't create tolerance, dosages didn't need to be increased. Yet the early antianxiety medications still could be addictive, as was most widely publicized with Valium.

Sleeping Pills Today
The first benzodiazepine drug approved by the FDA as a hypnotic—a certified sleeping pill—was flurazepam (trade name Dalmane), developed in the early 1970s. Halcion was the next FDA-certified sleeping pill, but it has had some troubles. Since 1982 the FDA has been investigating extremely rare cases in which people taking Halcion allegedly became violent or suicidal. Since the FDA found the drug to be entirely safe when used properly, it lowered the recommended dosage and added warnings to the label to watch for anxiety, abnormal thinking, and behavioral changes.

A new class of hypnotic medications has been developed that is safer and more effective than any that have come before: the imidazopyridines. One sleep medication in this class that currently is available in the United States is zolpidem (trade name Ambien). More compounds in this class are under development. Ambien is a short-acting hypnotic that does not induce tolerance and has little or no potential to become addictive. Marketed in Europe since 1987, it was approved for use in the United States in 1992. Ambien's duration of action in the bloodstream is short. By the time the night is over, the drug has been metabolized to the point where the patient no longer feels its effects. This means that Ambien doesn't cause residual drowsiness the next day, unlike long-acting benzodiazepines such as Dalmane, for example, which has a much longer half-life. Ambien is also an improvement over the benzodiazepines because it is much more selective in how it interacts with nerve cells.

To be approved as a medication specifically recommended for insomnia, a candidate "hypnotic" (the name used for sleep inducing drugs) must pass an incredible array of tests involving many normal volunteers and patients with insomnia. Such tests are very expensive, and it would cost more than $100 million to evaluate just one compound. These days Ambien is the most-prescribed hypnotic in the United States and except for Halcion and an older compound, temazepam (Restorial), doctors hardly prescribe anything else. Today Ambien is by far the best-evaluated sleeping pill and the most effective and safest. Its increased safety and effectiveness is largely due to its increased specificity.

The barbiturates, benzodiazepines, and imidazopyridines all work through the same process. They activate the brain's governor, a brake that holds back nerve activity and keeps the nervous system from burning itself out. The lever that turns this brake on is called the GABA receptor, and it is actually a multiplex of docking stations for a variety of regulatory molecules. Barbiturates attach themselves to one part of the GABA complex and act very broadly to depress all nerve activity. Benzodiazepines attach themselves to another part of the receptor and act in a more targeted way; generally, they relieve anxiety, relax muscles, and induce sleep. Ambien and other nonbenzodiazepine medications in development are more specific yet: They attach themselves to only one subtype of the benzodiazepine receptor. Among the benzodiazepines and Ambien, each individual medication has its own strengths and weaknesses, and every patient reacts slightly differently to any particular medication. But most sleep specialists believe that Ambien is currently our best available drug treatment for insomnia: It induces sleep with the fewest side effects in the most people.

Sleep medications have improved a great deal over the years, and as we come to understand more about sleep, they should get better still. But social attitudes about sleeping pills haven't caught up with the scientific work on these substances. A colleague of mine surveyed attitudes toward sleeping pills in 1990 and found that the number-one reason people avoided these medications was that they considered them "sinful." Yet it seems to me that taking sleeping pills to get good sleep—even for extended periods—is inherently no more sinful than taking daily doses of heart medication or an antidepressant, such as Prozac. If a nonaddictive sleeping pill that does not induce tolerance and has very few side effects is the only way that someone can get good sleep and feel fully awake during the day, there is nothing "sinful" in taking it. These medications can save lives and are justifiable if their benefits outweigh their risks.

Over-the-Counter Medications

To me, the millions of sleep sufferers who are driven to self-medication are the most eloquent testimony to the underuse of prescription hypnotics. Most over-the-counter "sleep aids" have no proven efficacy. The primary ingredient in such sleep medications is usually an antihistamine, which was developed originally as an allergy medication that affects the immune system. Since histamines also act as neurotransmitters, histamine neurons are related to general alertness, firing more frequently when we are most active. Antihistamines may induce sleepiness by damping down the activity of these nerve cells, but antihistamine activity is fairly general and has many other effects such as agitation, dehydration, and constipation. The body also starts to become tolerant of the medications the longer they are taken, leaving users vulnerable to "rebound" insomnia—insomnia that occurs after they stop taking the medication. Antihistamines also stay in the system much longer than hypnotics do, another reason they are a poor substitute for sleep medications that act with more precision.

For all of these reasons, sleep specialists generally recommend against taking over-the-counter sleeping pills for insomnia.

Successful Treatment: Integrating the Whole

The following example nicely illustrates the fact that in cases of chronic insomnia, the road to healthy sleep is often not straight or easy. Instead, I work with the patient to find the cause of the insomnia by carefully ruling out possible causes in the step-by-step approach I described earlier in this chapter. Finding the source of the insomnia is more than half the battle. This case is also a good example of how working hard with the advice of a specialist eventually can lead to relief.

In this example, a Stanford professor came to me because she was having trouble sleeping. Again, what I asked first was how long the insomnia had been going on, what was the pattern of sleep troubles over many nights, and how serious a problem she felt it was. Then I looked for the typical factors associated with pure circadian insomnia. I felt she had a mild DSPS, but that it was not the major problem. With a few more questions, I satisfied myself that restless legs syndrome, fibromyalgia, and SER were unlikely. Then I carefully reviewed the stresses in her life. She was a very ambitious woman who put a lot of pressure on herself. She regularly worked hard and stayed up late, and then had trouble sleeping. The problem became worse over time, until she became concerned enough to come to me.

Her research projects were very exciting, but she was under a great deal of pressure to produce results. She didn't have tenure yet and was working hard to prove her worth. I asked about her sleep habits and environment. She tended to work right up until bedtime, an obvious no-no. There was also a problem with the bedroom environment, or rather, her bedmate. Her husband was a lark and was therefore already long asleep by the time she went to bed. Lying awake in the dark while her husband slept soundly beside her often caused her to feel resentment, an emotion that further interfered with sleep.

At this point, her insomnia seemed to be rooted in stress and I decided to hold a nighttime sleep test in reserve. She felt ambivalent about taking sleeping pills even for a short time, so I told her some easy things to try. I instructed her to stay away from caffeine and keep alcohol ingestion low. Before bed she was to take warm baths.

Lastly, when she turned off the light and closed her eyes, she was to focus on a pleasant memory, perhaps a favorite movie or a past vacation, walking through each part of it until she fell asleep. I also asked her to keep a sleep diary. She seemed relieved and eager to try my suggestions.

When the professor returned a few days later, she had tried all of these things and her sleep was a little better, but the insomnia was still a problem. Next I wanted to know whether we were dealing with persistent psychophysiological insomnia or just persistent stress. "Look," I told her, "you've made a little progress. Let's work on reducing your stress at bedtime and try that for a couple weeks to see if we can make things a lot better." We decided that she would set aside an early-evening "worry time" to list her worries, then not think about them again before going to bed. She also agreed to try additional relaxation techniques.

When she came back two weeks later she was dispirited and reported that her insomnia had not improved. Now I was afraid that her sleeping problem was not just due to stress but was the beginning of a psychophysiological insomnia, in which her fear of sleeplessness was itself getting in the way of falling asleep. I made arrangements for all night clinical polysomnographic testing. The results ruled out periodic limb movement disorder, central sleep apnea, and for sure, sleep state misperception. She really had disturbed sleep. Because the disturbance was somewhat worse early in the night with a long sleep latency that later in the night, I began to suspect that she had a delayed sleep phase that was worse than I initially thought. I recommended that she try using bright lights in the morning to try to shift her sleep phase and make her wake up earlier in the day and get sleepy earlier in the evening. I also suggested she try a low-dose sleeping pill for one week. Some people start to feel anxious and desperate because they fear they will never sleep well again. I wanted her to know that if she was really desperate, she could get to sleep. At this point she was willing to try anything, so I prescribed a low dose of Ambien. I also asked her to call me every morning to let me know how things had gone the night before.

Using both bright light in the morning and sleeping pills at bedtime, she began sleeping better right away. She felt much better during the day, and she didn't dread going to bed anymore. After a week she was very much relieved, and she no longer needed the morning light exposure. Now the trick was to show her that she could have this sleep even without the pills, so I proposed the following: I would give her one sleeping pill every day for the next week, but sometime during the week I would switch from a sleeping pill to a placebo. If the root of her insomnia was mostly anxiety about sleeping, then taking a pill, even a placebo, should help her. She would also continue to call me every morning to let me know how she had slept the previous night, so I would know right away if things weren't working out as planned. She continued to sleep well through the week. "Well," I said after the week was over, "you've been taking the placebo for four days now. I think you are cured." She was overjoyed, and continued to sleep well after that.

Making Use of What We Know

In the past quarter century we have learned an enormous amount about all the insomnias, but relatively few scientists have been involved directly in insomnia research and little money has been directed at the problem. So, while I lament that we have much yet to learn, we have learned a great deal that can be very helpful to insomnia sufferers. I know that the vast majority of people who are concerned about difficulty sleeping are not receiving the benefits of the knowledge we have worked so hard to accumulate.

It is maddening that insomnia is always oversimplified. In fact, each case is different. As my experience with the professor shows, success comes from recognizing the differences and crafting individual treatments. People have to take the responsibility for educating themselves about sleep. People must find a professional who is knowledgeable on the subject, intelligent about applying that expertise to their individual case, and able to spend the necessary time working with them. Whether insomnia is transient or chronic, it should be treated aggressively as the serious and potentially life-threatening health problem that it is.

Chapter 7

Snoring and Sleep Apnea:
The Midnight Stranglers

THE FOLLOWING CASE is typical: I had a patient who was a corporate executive with a salary in the high six figures. About 10 years prior to seeing me, he began to suffer from fatigue. His initial effort to obtain medical help resulted in a diagnosis of depression. Various antidepressant medications were prescribed, but his fatigue only worsened. Shortly thereafter, he began to have an increasingly difficult problem with high blood pressure, which did not respond to very aggressive treatment. His fatigue finally reached a point where he was unable to meet the demands of his high-level position. He could not get things organized; his thinking was impaired. He frequently canceled meetings because he was too tired. Finally, he was asked to leave his company.

When I saw him he was at the end of his rope and had been unemployed for three years. His marriage was on the rocks because of his irritability and apathy. He said he had been downright miserable for at least five years and was beginning to wonder what the point of staying alive was. Although he had endured 10 years of suffering and countless visits to various medical specialists, I was quite certain of his diagnosis after looking at him and asking three or four questions. A laboratory sleep test confirmed absolutely that his problem was not depression, not chronic fatigue syndrome, but a hidden killer called apnea. Treatment was quick and easy, and his physical and mental problems subsided dramatically.

Apnea is an unrecognized killer, but it is hiding in plain sight. Every night more than 50 million Americans stop breathing. In a stunning evolutionary failure, nature endowed us with throats that tend to collapse during sleep and stop air flow but did not endow our sleeping brains with the ability to start breathing again calmly. At this breathless moment, the immediate future holds only two possibilities: death or waking up to breathe. In the worst cases, no air enters the lungs for 40, 50, 60 seconds, or longer. The muscles of the diaphragm struggle harder and harder against the blocked throat, without success. Carbon dioxide builds up in the bloodstream and the level of life-giving oxygen falls precipitously. After a minute or more the brain is panicking, suffocating, screaming out for oxygen. The skin and lips turn blue. Just when death seems imminent, the sleeper suddenly struggles awake and the tongue and throat muscles tighten, allowing oxygen to flood into the lungs in a series of gasping, snorting breaths. Oxygen is restored to the blood, and the fatal course is reversed. Instead of being alarmed and staying awake, the victim is immediately asleep again. After a few seconds snoring begins—and the cycle starts again, repeating hundreds and hundreds a time a night.

That is what sleep apnea looks and sounds like to an objective observer—but apnea victims have no memory of their all-night life-and-death struggle for breath. It never ceases to amaze me that sleep apnea victims can awaken hundreds of times in a single night and remember nothing of that torment. It's hard to measure how much real sleep such patients lose, but it is at least a third of their time in bed. And when sleep is interrupted this many times, it has little value in reducing sleep debt. Victims of this midnight strangler may be aware that they have lost their energy and are tired all day, but they never know the reason unless someone they believe (but who?) tells them what is going on at night and how it is affecting them.

The severe consequences of this sleep disorder and its very high prevalence make it one of the most serious general health problems in America. I have heard people who should know better contend that any phenomenon that is this common can't be abnormal. Nothing could be further from the truth.

Apnea—a Greek word for absence of breath—remains the most underdiagnosed deadly problem in medicine. In its 1992 report to the U.S. Congress, the National Commission on Sleep Disorders Research estimated that 38,000 fatal heart attacks and strokes in the United States each year are due to apnea. I would call it the silent killer, a phrase also used for high blood pressure generally, except that obstructive sleep apnea is far from silent. People with apnea usually snore so loudly that their snoring is compared to jackhammers, sounding loud even through doors, through walls, and down halls. And yet the true significance of this loud warning remains unappreciated by people and their doctors.

The warning isn't always ignored by those who must hear the snorers, though. A few years ago a woman was actually arrested and subsequently charged with disturbing the peace because her neighbors complained that her snoring was so loud. A patient of mine told me that when he was in the army he would go to bed inside his barracks, and in the morning he would wake up to find himself outside on the parade grounds, where other soldiers had carried him, bed and all. The wife of another patient told me that her next-door neighbor had pounded on her door one day and demanded to know what kind of animal she was keeping in her house. "That's no animal," the patient's wife replied, "that's my husband." Recently several students petitioned me to do something about a student who slept in the dormitory room next to them. His loud snoring greatly disturbed their sleep and even caused the wall to rattle, they said. I quickly arranged a sleep test for the student, and was not surprised to learn that he had very severe obstructive sleep apnea. More alarming was the associated finding of high blood pressure, although the student was only 20 years old.

Nearly 40 percent of the population has some sleep apnea, and half of those cases are clinically significant. That means that at least 20 percent of the people walking in to see their family physician have a dangerous level of apnea. The number of doctor visits attributable to apnea is probably much higher, because apnea causes a wide range of health problems that force people to see their doctors. One of the most common problems is extreme fatigue, since apnea sufferers' actual quantity and quality of sleep is very low. Yet these people are not properly diagnosed. I conclude that family practitioners catch fewer than 1 or 2 percent of their patients with apnea. Even those with the most flagrant symptoms are rarely identified.

Who are these unlucky people? They're all around you; you may be one too. People who are overweight or obese are more likely to have apnea, but thin people can have it as well, depending on the width of their throats or the shape of their jaws. Obvious cases of obstructive apnea tend to start appearing in both men and women in their 30s, 40s, and 50s, but it can strike even children. The overall prevalence of apnea in men is about one in four. The prevalence of apnea in women lags behind that in men until after menopause, when it increases to a similar level.

In all of medicine, I can't think of a single other serious condition that is so common, life-threatening, treatable, and yet so unrecognized. It's as if diabetes were well known to laboratory researchers, and effective insulin had been developed, but physicians were completely unaware that diabetes existed. As with sleep apnea, doctors unable to recognize diabetes would notice their patients becoming inexplicably ill, and could run lots of tests on them without finding the cause. Undiagnosed, diabetic patients would slowly get worse, succumbing to kidney damage, blindness, peripheral neuropathy, blood vessel blockage, and gangrene. As their patients began to die, the doctors still wouldn't know why because they had never learned about the disease. The doctors would try to treat the consequences of diabetes, but their efforts would stand little chance of success because they wouldn't be addressing the root cause of the problems. The unnecessary misery and loss of life would continue.

The tragedy of undiagnosed sleep apnea is especially striking because there are very effective treatments and often the condition can be completely cured. As a compassionate person, when I think of all the deaths that could have been prevented, all the lives in jeopardy every night and so little being done about it, I am so shocked that I have become something of a zealot on this issue. About five years ago, I found myself extremely frustrated that primary care physicians at the Stanford Medical Center (even here!) did not seem to be interested in our sleep disorders clinic. I walked into our internal medicine clinic and offered the five people sitting in the waiting room a free sleep test. I further enticed them by mentioning that the test normally would cost $1,000. Four of the five people wanted the "free test." Of those four, two had severe apnea. They had spent years going from doctor to doctor, trying to find the cause of their health problems, which were due almost totally to apnea.

Sometimes my zeal to save people can lead to embarrassing situations. I was recently on a plane flying back from a speaking engagement when I noticed that the passenger across the aisle from me would fall asleep and stop breathing for long periods every couple of minutes. I knew from experience that he had severe, perhaps life-threatening sleep apnea. I thought about saying something when he awoke, but during the entire trip I never found a way to broach the subject gracefully. It's hard to just start talking with a stranger about his health problems. Once I left the plane, however, I began to have second thoughts. I had the chance to save this man's life, and yet I said nothing. Then fate intervened—I got a second chance. Along with a number of others, I headed for the rest room in the airport terminal, and as I was standing at the urinals I realized my sleep apnea victim was standing next to me. This time I didn't hesitate, blurting out "You have a serious problem that needs attention immediately!" Before I had a chance to say more, he gave me a withering look, quickly zipped his pants, and scurried out of the bathroom.

In a few instances like this my efforts came to naught, but on the whole I feel very good about what I have accomplished: By now I and my colleagues at Stanford have saved thousands of lives. If we count patients treated by all our medical disciples, the number must total hundreds of thousands of lives saved in the United States and perhaps a million people worldwide. And yet we have barely started to address the tens of millions of apnea victims right here in the world's most medically sophisticated nation who continue to suffer without diagnosis or treatment.

Snoring

A colleague once suggested a little educational exercise that I use frequently when I am talking to a lay audience. "How many of you," I say to them, "have a sleep disorder?" Generally, not more than one or two hands are raised, often none. "How many of you snore?" I then ask. About half of those in the audience raise their hands. I wait while they look around at one another, some smiling and laughing because snoring seems funny and there are so many hands in the air. After a suitably dramatic pause I tell them, "Every one of you with a hand in the air has a sleep disorder." I then go on to explain why: Snoring is a sign that your breathing is impaired while you sleep. If you snore, you need to know how badly your breathing is impaired, and what the consequences are.

We snore because our throats represent one of nature's biggest compromises. The throat is a tube that must serve multiple functions: breathing, talking, eating, and drinking. But the engineering requirements for these activities are different. The tongue and upper airway must be very flexible for the exquisite task of creating all the different sounds we use in speaking. This is equally true for swallowing food and fluids. For breathing we should have a stiff tube that could not collapse while we suck air into the lungs.

The throat's rigidity for breathing is accomplished partly with the help of muscular tension, but when we go to sleep, the muscles in the throat tend to relax. As we inhale during sleep, suction and air passing through the throat cause its soft sides to pull inward. As the throat is pulled inward, rebounds, and pulls inward again it sets up a rapid vibration, like a flag rippling on a windy day. That vibrating flesh creates a loud rumble: snoring. Loud snoring is a sign that breathing is strained, that the throat is almost closing down. The narrower the throat becomes during inhalation, the harder the diaphragm has to pull to get enough air. The result is a vicious cycle in which increasing suction from the lungs and increasing air flow through the throat pull the throat closed even more, making the vibration stronger, the snoring louder.

In healthy sleepers, relaxing the throat and tongue muscles is not enough to cause apnea or even loud snoring, not enough for what engineers call "structural failure" to occur. Yet the differences between sleepers without apnea and those with apnea are very small: If the throat is already a little narrow, or if it is narrowed by extra fatty tissue, the suction on the sides of the throat is increased. Accordingly, the risk factors for apnea include enlarged tonsils or lymph nodes, obesity, and a naturally small airway. The first sign of impending failure, like sagging beams on an old bridge, is snoring.

When Snoring Becomes Sleep Apnea

Not everyone who snores has sleep apnea, but in general, the louder the snoring, the more likely that the sleeper has apnea. There are really two types of apnea: central sleep apnea and obstructive sleep apnea. Central apnea occurs when the diaphragm, the brain, or the nerve connection between the two makes little or no effort to pull air into the lungs. At present, there is no effective treatment for central sleep apnea. Fortunately, this variant of sleep disordered breathing appears to be rare.

Obstructive sleep apnea is by far the more common type, and when I use the phrase "sleep apnea" I will always mean obstructive sleep apnea.

In obstructive sleep apnea, as with snoring, the walls of the throat are pulled together by the suction created during inspiration (breathing in). But in obstructive sleep apnea, the throat stays closed. To get an idea why, imagine a beautiful day at home, a gentle breeze wafting in through your windows and out the open front door. If the door is wide open, the air circulates freely. But if the door is open only a foot or so, the breeze pulls on it a little; as the door starts to move it narrows the gap more, increasing the speed of air passing through and the pressure on the door, until it slams shut. The danger results from the "door" remaining shut—because even though the diaphragm relaxes at the end of the breath, the throat remains closed. Remember that the throat closes at the beginning of inspiration, after most of the air in the lungs has been exhaled. This is why blood-oxygen levels fall faster than they would if you were holding your breath, which most people do after taking a big breath. To make things worse, the respiratory cycle continues for the diaphragm. The diaphragm makes a tremendous and futile increasing effort to pull air in, and then relaxes and lets a little air out—in effect, ratcheting out all the remaining air in the lungs.

I used to explain snoring and apnea to my students by saying that the throat in sleep is like a soggy paper straw. When using those old paper straws on a thick milkshake, the harder you sucked, the more likely you were to collapse the straw. This is analogous to how the throat collapses in apnea. Most students today have never seen a paper straw, but I hope the analogy is helpful to some of you.

When air does not get into the lungs, the oxygen levels in the bloodstream begin to fall. In many cases the level of oxygen in the blood falls to dangerous levels. Apnea victims sometimes reach the kind of blood-oxygen level you would experience if you were suddenly transported from sea level to the top of Mount Everest. Air Force experiments in low-pressure chambers have shown that someone who has not been conditioned to operate at that altitude will become unconscious within minutes and die shortly afterward. Brain damage is another possible result of such low oxygen levels.

Once the apnea victim rouses and begins to breathe, oxygen levels rise—but another kind of stress is initiated. The heart starts pumping madly and blood pressure rises rapidly to alarmingly high levels. In some cases sleep specialists have measured transient systolic pressures at this moment as high as 300 mm Hp. Most people who get their blood pressure checked know that this is unbelievably high. Normal systolic pressure is about 110 or 120. Such pressures night after night can eventually cause damage to organs and small strokes in the brain. If the cardiac arteries are already partially blocked, this sort of hard work can also cause heart failure.

In 1973 Christian Guilleminault and I proposed the measure that is still used for the clinical definition of sleep apnea and for rating its severity. We called it the Apnea/Hypopnea Index (AHI). Hypopnea is the term we use when the throat doesn't quite close entirely, but air flow is reduced sufficiently to lower oxygen and cause an arousal. The AHI score represents the average number of apnea and hypopnea episodes that a patient has during an hour of sleep. We decided that an AHI of 5 should be the lower limit for making a diagnosis of apnea, so a score of less than 5 (breathing stops fewer than 5 times per hour) is considered too low for clinical diagnosis and doesn't require treatment. However, treatment may be necessary if a patient has an AHI of 5 to 10 with other signs or symptoms of apnea, such as daytime fatigue or high blood pressure. Although not all my colleagues agree, I feel strongly that people with an AHI of 10 to 20 should definitely consider treatment, even if they are not feeling sleepy during the day. In my opinion, anyone with a score over 20 should always be treated—they have or will soon have a serious, life-threatening problem.

The Stanford team led by Christian Guilleminault recently has identified patients whose loud snoring and excessive daytime sleepiness aren't associated with apnea—their breathing doesn't actually stop. It seems that the increased effort of breathing, sometimes associated with flailing movements, wakes the sleeper for a few moments. Christian named this variant of sleep disordered breathing upper airway resistance syndrome. A spouse might notice that snoring is interrupted as the sleeper coughs, clears the throat, or mumbles something, perhaps turning over afterward. The snoring stops only for a moment or two, then resumes. This is the same kind of arousal that occurs in patients with obstructive sleep apnea, and it also needs to be evaluated carefully.

The Discovery of Sleep Apnea

Obstructive sleep apnea was the third major sleep disorder to be discovered and characterized; the first was narcolepsy, which I will tell you about later, and the second was restless legs syndrome. Nearly a century passed between the first and the third discovery. In 1956 a group of American pulmonary physicians identified patients who were extremely obese and extremely sleepy during the day. They named the condition "Pickwickian syndrome" because the patients resembled "Joe, the fat boy," a character in Charles Dickens's *Pickwick Papers,* who was so drowsy he would fall asleep standing up. Unfortunately, the American researcher studied the patients only in the daytime and attempted to explain their severe drowsiness by attributing it to high levels of carbon dioxide in their blood. Had the doctors understood that they should have studied the patients while asleep as well, they might not have missed a great discovery.

Nine years later, in 1965, two separate research groups in Europe reported that Pickwickian patients periodically stopped breathing in their sleep, and the researchers realized that this was the more likely cause of the patients' daytime sleepiness. The European findings went entirely unnoticed in the United States, partly because they were published in obscure journals, but mostly, I think, because no one was very interested in anything that had to do with sleep.

In 1970, shortly after we had launched our sleep clinic, I was asked by a Stanford pulmonary specialist to do sleep recordings on several Pickwickian patients whom he had hospitalized at the Palo Alto Veterans Administration Hospital. Our findings dramatically confirmed the finding of obstructive sleep apnea that the Europeans had made five years earlier. At the time I attributed the patients' breathing problems to their massive obesity, but our perspective changed greatly after we were joined by Christian Guilleminault in January of 1972. Christian insisted that we make the recording of respiratory parameters a routine part of our all-night clinical sleep evaluations. After we started monitoring each patient's breathing, it seemed as if nearly everyone who came to our clinic seeking help was suffering from severe obstructive sleep apnea.

I should explain that what little renown we had achieved up to that time was the result of my previous studies of patients with narcolepsy. I had opened a narcolepsy clinic with the late Dr. Steven Mitchell in 1964. At the time, anyone noticed to be excessively sleepy in the daytime was suspected of having narcolepsy. Since we were the only such clinic in the world, sleepy patients were sent to us from all over. When we became aware of the connection between apnea and excessive daytime sleepiness, we realized that many of these patients weren't suffering from narcolepsy, as others thought, but from obstructive sleep apnea.

Although most of our patients were overweight, they were far from being "Pickwickian," and we decided to rename the disorder sleep apnea to serve as a more general classification. By November 29, 1972, we had learned enough to give the world's first continuing medical education (CME) course on the diagnosis and treatment of sleep disorders. Because a discipline does not exist unless it can be taught, I have suggested that the date this course began might be recognized as the official birthday of the clinical, scientific discipline of sleep disorders medicine.

By this time we were aware that even thin people could have obstructive sleep apnea and that far-advanced sleep apnea was definitely dangerous. I remember one incident that occurred in 1973 as vividly as if it had happened last night. I was monitoring the sleep recording of a patient when the tracing of the patient's heartbeat, or electrocardiagram (EKG), went totally flat. My first assumption was that the amplifier had malfunctioned, or else that the EKG electrode had come loose. After fiddling with the equipment for a few seconds, I literally jumped out of my skin as I realized that the patient's heart had stopped beating. In a total panic, I rushed into his bedroom, ready to perform emergency cardiopulmonary resuscitation. By the time I got to his bed, he was snoring and gasping, and obviously alive. When I returned to the control room and examined the EKG record, I found his heart had stopped beating for 11 seconds. I was told by a cardiologist that if your heart stops for 20 seconds or more, it's likely to be the end of the game because at that point the cardiac muscle has real trouble resuming beating again on its own. You can imagine how closely we watched the patients' recordings from that point on. Our ultimate nightmare would be to have a patient die while under our care.

The danger of apnea stems not only from heart problems and high blood pressure, but also from the incredible sleep debt that apnea sufferers carry around with them since they get almost no continuous sleep at night. People with severe apnea typically carry so much sleep debt that they fall asleep while driving, eating, or talking. As I mentioned earlier, before apnea was discovered we assumed that most of these patients had narcolepsy—we had no idea that sleep apnea was so common or occurred in people who weren't obese. Like Dickens's "fat boy," people with severe apnea can fall asleep at almost any time of the day. Without knowing it, many experience frequent recurring microsleeps, brief periods when EEG activity representing sleep intrudes into the waking state. They tend to have the same health, performance, and mood problems common to all severely sleep-deprived people, making them a danger not only to themselves but to others.

The most common danger is falling asleep while driving. People with apnea are much more likely to be involved in auto accidents. Some studies suggest that such people have an accident rate 10 times that of the general population. Usually these people have no idea why they are falling asleep behind the wheel. As recently as 1991, during a visit to a college in another city to inspect their research facilities, a staff member who showed me around said, "I should come to your meeting. I fall asleep all the time." I questioned her and found out that she was a loud snorer and had high blood pressure. A year before I met her, she had fallen asleep at the wheel and collided head-on with another car. She was hospitalized in intensive care, where she received full neurological workups and was seen by about 20 different doctors. None of the physicians asked her about her sleep or her pattern of chronic sleepiness. After recuperating she was released, but she still tended to fall asleep all the time. No one in her family would drive with her anymore. I referred her to the local sleep disorders center, where my sleep apnea diagnosis was confirmed and she was successfully treated. Her sleepiness disappeared in a week, despite the fact that she had been tired and sleepy in the daytime for about 10 years.

Although daytime fatigue and tiredness—or outright drowsiness—are usually one of the most troublesome, easily detectable symptoms for apnea patients, they are not the only ones. A variety of other difficulties are common, including esophageal reflux, frequent nocturnal urination, heavy sweating at night, morning headaches, raspy throat, personality changes, and loss of hearing—even male impotence and the reduction of sex drive in both men and women. And yet, when patients go to doctors with these apnea-induced symptoms, their physicians nearly always miss the true cause. Even the by-products of excessive daytime sleepiness—diminished performance, diminished mental acuity, forgetfulness, poor concentration, disorientation—frequently are ascribed to some other problem, like Alzheimer's disease. The fact that sleep apnea and marked obesity often go hand in hand means that many of the health problems caused by apnea are erroneously attributed to the patient's weight.

Even if people with advanced sleep apnea don't kill or maim themselves in an accident, they will have significant health problems for years. The high blood pressure that damages blood vessels in the heart, kidneys, brain, and other organs can lead to a long, slow decline in their physical well-being. These patients eventually find that they can't exert themselves physically at all without being out of breath, their biochemistry gets out of whack, and they suffer multiple heart attacks or strokes, one of which eventually kills them.

In the early days of the Stanford Sleep Disorders Clinic, we tried to learn as much as possible, as fast as possible, about the cardiovascular side of the problem. Accurately monitoring blood pressure during sleep without disturbing patients was not easy, since we had to place pressure transducers in the heart or major arteries. After Italian sleep researcher Elio Lugaresi reported nocturnal hypertension associated with snoring and apnea in 1975, Christian Guilleminault persuaded Stanford cardiologists John Schroeder and Ara Tilkian to spend nights in the hospital's clinical research center monitoring systemic and pulmonary arterial blood pressure in as many patients as possible. They consistently observed huge rises in blood pressure, as if the patient were lifting heavy weights. Typically such observations are carried out for only a few nights. However, it is not difficult to imagine the damage to blood vessels that can build up under this hypertensive pounding all night, every night, year after year.

Our cardiology colleagues also introduced us to the technique of using a 24-hour EKG recorder that patients could take home or use in the sleep laboratory, with the results then analyzed by computer. Until such an analysis was possible, no one could afford to regularly spend hours and hours scanning a continuous paper tape recording. The computer would quickly locate the episodes where the most severe and serious abnormal heartbeats occurred, and we could make a paper copy of these episodes for inspection. They were spectacular!

During apneas, the heartbeat always slowed, often so much that it appeared to stop. Indeed, as I had already discovered, the heart often *did* stop. Most of the problems that would alarm cardiologists if they were seen in a daytime EKG, we observed in our patients at night. The heart was struggling under a double burden; in addition to the autonomic problems caused by the struggle to breathe, the heart muscle itself was being starved of oxygen and was beginning to fail. Like a car engine that is just beginning to sputter as it runs out of gas, the failing heart begins having serious rhythm problems. The most serious of these is a wild, uncoordinated, rapid heartbeat, called ventricular tachycardia, which, if it continues, is fatal.

Christian Guilleminault published some papers showing dramatic improvements when severe apnea patients were treated with tracheostomies. Prior to treatment there were dramatic cardiac abnormalities during sleep; a completely normal heartbeat returned when the tracheostomy tube was opened. When the tube was closed again during sleep, the abnormalities returned. When a severely ill sleep apnea patient dies during sleep, the direct cause is likely to be a fatal cardiac arrhythmia.

Our studies did not attract serious attention from either academic or practicing cardiologists in the 1970s, a sad state of affairs that pretty much continues to this day. A few cardiologists are now beginning to act on this information. I sometimes think that even though Christian's results are two decades old, they should be published again. I simply cannot understand how the cardiology community can continue to ignore them.

When patients suffer from severe obstructive sleep apnea, some degree of cardiovascular disease (high blood pressure, coronary artery disease, heart attack, or stroke) is almost always present. The big problem is that such patients often have other risk factors for cardiovascular disease—most notably obesity—to which cardiologists tend to attribute the problem. I am happy to report that a few groups of cardiologists—a tiny band among the thousands around the world—are reporting stunningly beneficial results of treating obstructive sleep apnea in patients with congestive heart failure. These results may someday turn the tide.

I mentioned one such case from Walla Walla, Washington, in the beginning of the book, but I will give a little more detail here. The story was reported to me early in 1998 by Dick Simon. The local cardiologist referred a patient to Dick who was in far-advanced congestive heart failure. The cardiologist referred the patient, by the way, not because Dick is a sleep specialist, but because he is an excellent internist, and the cardiologist thought Dick might be able to think of something that could prolong the patient's life. The patient, an overweight 60-year-old, could walk only one block without getting short of breath. The slow failure of the heart muscle caused massive tissue bloating (edema) of his lower limbs. He could not lie down because the pressure of tissue and body fluids on the heart and lungs also made him very short of breath. His activities were confined largely to sitting around his house all day long, frequently dozing in his chair. The congestive heart failure was assumed to be secondary to high blood pressure, neither of which was responding to the 10 different medications he was taking.

While in Dick's waiting room, the patient fell asleep, and Dick immediately diagnosed a previously unidentified, severe obstructive sleep apnea. After several weeks of treatment, this patient became a new man. He could breathe when lying down, he could walk up a flight of stairs, his edema was gone, and he felt, and continues to feel great. Of the 10 medications he was taking for his heart, blood pressure, and fluid retention, he now takes only two.

I would like to go on record as saying that I am absolutely convinced that obstructive sleep apnea plays a major role in causing high blood pressure, heart disease, and stroke. This is a controversial issue, but for now I urge everyone who has high blood pressure, heart disease, or concern about a stroke to ask themselves two questions: Am I tired in the daytime? And have I been told that I snore? If the answers to both questions are yes, my unalterable position is that checking for the presence of apnea is mandatory, even if the sleep test is nothing more than putting a tape recorder next to the bed at night. I expect that this warning will be largely ignored, just as early warnings about the health risks of tobacco were ignored. All I will say at this point is that I expect to live long enough to enjoy a full vindication as this position gains mainstream acceptance. The evidence supporting a causal role for obstructive sleep apnea at night in the development of cardiovascular disease throughout the day continues to accumulate, albeit not as rapidly as we would wish. I am not the only one who has arrived at this conclusion—only the most vocal.

I recently took an informal poll of a number of my seasoned sleep specialist colleagues to see how many felt that obstructive sleep apnea was a cause of high blood pressure, heart attack, and stroke. I can't say that I was surprised when they all reported that they believe that apnea is a cause for all three potentially fatal disorders. Almost certainly the nonspecialist skeptics have never monitored the polysomnographic tests of obstructive sleep apnea patients. When apnea has progressed to a severe level, chronic cardiovascular problems are always present.

Again, a supremely important question of this complexity can be answered with absolute certainty only by mounting a very well-financed research program, one that will be possible only if sleep research is better funded than it currently is. Ultimately, it is a matter of devoting sufficient resources and accumulating enough scientific data to convince even the most diehard skeptics.

Apnea in Older People

The prevalence of apnea rises as humans get older, probably because all tissue, including tissue in the airway, becomes less firm as we age. This flabbiness makes it easier for the throat to pull closed and stay closed. Hormonal changes probably also increase the risk of apnea. Therefore, apnea should be one of the first things doctors consider when elderly patients have problems with sleepiness, high blood pressure, or cognitive problems—but doctors almost never do this.

Patients who are sleep deprived due to apnea are likely to get confused more easily. They might become forgetful or have difficulty balancing a checkbook. Often doctors and relatives assume that these problems are early signs of Alzheimer's disease or other senile dementias. Or doctors might think that daytime fatigue and irritability are the results of depression. I think that apnea is not recognized most of the time in the elderly because people often assume that the elderly are always sleepy, absentminded, and confused. People tend to say, "Well, he's old. What do you expect?"

I know of one patient who went to a doctor after he nodded off while driving with his 12-year-old grandson and hit a concrete guard rail. Luckily, both were okay. The doctor guessed that his loss of consciousness might be due to epilepsy and gave him drugs to treat it. When things did not improve, the patient saw a psychiatrist, who diagnosed depression and prescribed an antidepressant. Still, his condition worsened, and he began to lose interest in everything around him. His psychiatrists increased the dose of the antidepressant, to no effect, then switched him to a high dose of another drug. When that didn't work, the doctor gave him still another antidepressant, which also failed to make him feel better. He was then subjected to a number of expensive brain scans to look for a tumor or ministroke that might explain the problem, but nothing was found.

Two years later his wife saw a *Reader's Digest* article that described apnea's characteristic loud, intermittent snoring. She thought, "That's my husband." She took the article to their doctor, who dismissed it. Not someone to be put off easily, she called the local sleep center and arranged for her husband to be examined. At the sleep center, the husband fell asleep in the waiting room and his apnea was immediately apparent. One week after treatment began he said he "felt reborn"; he continued to feel fine after discontinuing all his other medications.

I wish I could report many more such success stories, but unfortunately we are not seeing nearly as many older patients as we should. Although the prevalence of apnea increases with age, the percentage of people with apnea seems to start falling again after about age 70. This is not because we are treating older patients more successfully. Rather, it is probably because people with apnea tend to die sooner than their cohorts and never make it to old age.

Apnea in Children

I became concerned about the dangers of obstructive sleep apnea in children very soon after we launched the Stanford sleep clinic. Among our first patients in 1972 were an 11-year-old boy and a 13-year-old girl. The boy, Raymond M., had developed high blood pressure over the previous six months. Raymond's family had a history of high blood pressure, but never so early in life. He first came to the pediatrics department at Stanford, where doctors performed an array of tests, trying in vain to discover the cause of the hypertension. A pediatrician noticed that the boy was very sleepy during the day and recommended that he see our Dr. Guilleminault for this seemingly unrelated symptom.

Christian reviewed Raymond's case with the boy's mother and found that Raymond had been abnormally sleepy most of his life. During the past two to three years it had become worse. His teachers complained that he fell asleep in class and that he had "behavioral problems"—inattention, hyperactivity, and aggression. His mother also confirmed that Raymond had been a loud snorer since he was very young.

An overnight test confirmed what we had immediately surmised, Raymond had severe apnea. The boy stopped breathing an average of 55 times every hour, and his throat stayed closed for at least 30 seconds, and sometimes 65 seconds, each time. Because he stopped breathing for an average of 45 seconds out of almost every minute of the night, Raymond was getting very little actual sleep. With each episode of apnea, the available oxygen in his bloodstream fell sharply, often to less than half of what it should be.

Christian notified Raymond's pediatricians that his sleep problem was serious and probably also the cause of his high blood pressure. "What's the treatment?" they asked. Christian replied that the treatment was a tracheostomy—putting a breathing hole in the throat. (By this time, several had been done in Europe.) "Have you ever done this before?" When Christian replied in the negative, the shocked pediatricians preferred to find another reason for the high blood pressure and to continue searching for an alternate treatment.

Six months later the blood pressure problem was worse in spite of aggressive medical treatment. With high blood pressure now threatening his life, Raymond finally had his tracheostomy, which allowed him to breathe normally when he slept.

Within ten days of surgery his blood pressure was miraculously down to normal. Furthermore, he was no longer sleepy during the day. We followed Raymond for the next five years, and he continued to develop normally. But we had to keep fighting with his local pediatricians, who wanted to close the tracheostomy because he seemed to have recovered. They just didn't understand that the problem was still there and that his high blood pressure and sleepiness would return if the treatment was reversed.

After our success with Raymond, the pediatricians were more willing to try a tracheostomy with a sleepy 13-year-old girl who had extremely high blood pressure that did not respond to the most potent medication. Again a seemingly hopeless hypertension miraculously disappeared after putting the breathing hole in her throat. Unfortunately, years of oxygen deprivation appeared to have caused some brain damage. Her IQ was then measured at 75, although she had been, we were told, of normal intelligence as a young child.

We have seen many children in our clinic since our group published the first description of obstructive sleep apnea in children in 1976. Obstructive sleep apnea can occur in children of any age, from infants to teenagers. Even though the various treatments now available for apnea are less invasive than a tracheostomy, the vast majority of pediatricians ignore the problem. I know there are huge numbers of children out there who are undiagnosed, who are being robbed of their health and intelligence before they get much of a chance in life. In a research project we're conducting in Moscow, Idaho, we have found that 40 percent of the children have noisy breathing and 10 percent had outright sleep apnea. Usually cases like this are resolved by taking out the tonsils and adenoids, so there is no excuse for compromising a child's health and mental development by missing a completely curable problem.

Parents should frequently listen to their children breathe during sleep. When bending over a sleeping child in a quiet room, parents should find the sound of breathing to be barely audible. The breathing should appear effortless, in the same way it is very easy to blow air through a short, wide tube as opposed to a very thin straw. And the breathing should be through the nose. Of course, the child should not have a cold when parents attempt this type of observation.

Breathing that seems to require effort, or produces any sort of noise, such as snoring or wheezing, demands further investigation. Snoring is not normal and should always be cause for concern, no matter what anyone thinks. Many parents have listened to their children sleep and heard noisy breathing, but have come to think that this is normal.

When I was a boy, tonsils were known mainly as the home of germs. Children who often had strep throat had their tonsils removed. With the advent of penicillin and other antibiotics, our concern about tonsils and adenoids has virtually disappeared. Yet this lymphoid tissue in their airway may be the single worst culprit in children's obstructive sleep apnea. Parents should not allow the specter of surgery to deter them from giving their children the healthiest possible sleep. Furthermore, simple, painless, and safe methods to shrink tonsils and adenoids with microwaves may soon be widely available.

On a related topic, I believe that every pregnant woman and her husband should receive information about sleep and breathing, particularly during the first pregnancy. It is not uncommon for previously nonapneic women to develop obstructive sleep apnea during pregnancy, or for mild apnea to become very severe.

Sudden Infant Death Syndrome

Almost every time I speak to the lay public about sleep apnea, someone raises a hand and says, "What about sudden infant death?" wondering if apnea could be the cause. Sudden infant death syndrome

(SIDS) was first recognized as an entity in 1963. Amazingly, a high school classmate, friend, and near neighbor of mine in Walla Walla, Washington, whose first child died suddenly and inexplicably, played a major role in bringing this problem to light. SIDS is classified as a sleep disorder because death always occurs during sleep. Seemingly healthy and happy babies are put down for sleep and later found dead in their cribs. Every year more than 7,000 American babies, about 1 baby out of 500, die of SIDS, which is far too high a number. Starting in 1973, there were a few reports of sleep apnea in siblings of SIDS cases, and occasionally an infant was found in time to be resuscitated.

In the intervening years, enough studies have accumulated to rule out obstructive sleep apnea as the major cause of SIDS. In the United States and several other countries, the number of deaths due to SIDS has been reduced significantly by the recent "back-to-sleep" campaign, which persuades parents to always place their infants on their back, never on their stomach, when they are being put to sleep.

As I have already indicated, many infants do have obstructive sleep apnea, and a few pediatric sleep specialists are beginning to address the issues involved in treatment when the cause is not large tonsils or adenoids or a correctable airway malformation. It appears that the problem does not come instantly out of the blue; noisy breathing and restless sleep are strong clues.

Treating Sleep Apnea

If the bad news about sleep apnea is that it's widespread, life-threatening, and underdiagnosed, the good news is that it can be safely and effectively treated. Doctors can treat severe apnea in one of two ways: by enlarging the air passage or by holding that air passage open mechanically during sleep. There are a variety of surgical and non-surgical treatments for apnea, some of which work very well and others that are more questionable. These treatments include continuous positive airway pressure, surgery, and a new microwave technology.

Continuous Positive Airway Pressure

In the last decade and a half, continuous positive airway pressure (CPAP) machines have been the most effective way of treating obstructive sleep apnea. To use the machine, a small, comfortable mask is fitted over the nose, leaving the mouth uncovered. Patients must sleep with their mouth closed, aided by a chin strap, while the machine gently blows air into the nose at a pressure slightly higher than the surrounding air pressure. Although this sounds odd, most people get used to it quickly.

The first CPAP machine was developed by the Australian pulmonologist Colin Sullivan in 1981. Sullivan found, as we did, that many people could not be persuaded to have a tracheostomy, even when they clearly needed it to save their lives. Some patients would refuse a tracheostomy even if I told them that they could very well die that night. Desperate to do something for these patients, Sullivan finally found an alternative to tracheostomy. His brilliant concept was blowing air into the nose to keep the throat open. His first machine was his home vacuum cleaner—he attached the hose to the other end so that air blew out, and then attached a mask to the patient's nose. As with today's much more refined versions, the positive air pressure provided by the machine prevents the airway from collapsing.

Literally within minutes of achieving the correct CPAP pressure to maintain an open airway, patients with obstructive sleep apnea start sleeping like people who have gone without sleep for many days. For the first week or so after starting to use the machine, patients will spend a great deal of time in deep sleep, while there is a marked decrease in the lighter sleep stages. Patients often report that there is a dramatic increase of daytime alertness and energy after just a few nights on CPAP. As one witness testified before the National Commission, "My mind was so sharp and clear that I felt like I had a brain transplant."

Although the theory of nasal CPAP is simple, using it is not so simple because everything has to be adjusted properly. The air pressure must be high enough to maintain an open airway during all stages of sleep and in all body positions, but not so high that the pressure is bothersome. This requires careful monitoring and adjustment by a qualified sleep professional. The mask and machine itself also can be disturbing. While most patients have no problem with the treatment, a few patients feel that sleeping with a CPAP machine is like sleeping with a vacuum cleaner running in your ear and a diving mask on your face. For these patients, using the device consistently requires commitment and understanding.

Recent studies have shown that some people tend to use the machine less often than they say they do. I believe that people tend to lose sight of the benefits of CPAP because eventually they forget how awful they used to feel without it, while they are reminded every night of the machine's drawbacks. Nevertheless, CPAP works wonders for those who have no problem using it all the time, which is the case for about half of all apnea patients. CPAP is a very well-established treatment, and most insurance companies will cover the cost of the machine.

Another approach to treating obstructive sleep apnea is to keep the airway open by moving the lower jaw forward. This is accomplished by a variety of dental appliances that are inserted in the mouth at night. While these devices may sometimes be a little less expensive than other treatments, I am skeptical of their effectiveness in reducing severe apnea sufficiently. Relatively few well-designed studies have been done to show that these appliances work well, nor has patient compliance been carefully evaluated.

Surgery

In 1981, the same year that nasal CPAP was introduced, a surgical procedure developed by doctors in Japan to alleviate snoring was introduced to the United States as a treatment for obstructive sleep apnea. The surgical procedure is called uvulopalatopharyngoplasty— a mouthful of a name, which is why almost everyone uses its acronym, UPPP. This surgical treatment for apnea consisted of cutting away excess tissue at the back of the throat, including the uvula, the tonsils, and parts of the soft palate. The UPPP procedure was widely used until follow-up studies by sleep specialists found that it completely eliminated apnea or reduced AHI levels to below 5 in only about 10 percent of all cases. UPPP does reduce snoring, however, but this outcome can create a new danger, because snoring is the warning that something is wrong. It would be like taking the battery out of a smoke alarm rather than preventing a fire. Often when people claim to sleep better after the UPPP surgery, an objective test in the sleep lab shows that the apnea is just as bad as before. In a few cases, apnea actually becomes worse, probably as a result of scarring at the back of the throat.

Several years ago there was a huge marketing push to do UPPP with a laser instead of the scalpel. Using a laser offers almost no benefit, except that there is less bleeding during surgery. Also, while claims are made that laser surgery is painless, patients undergoing this approach generally report severe postoperative pain.

The Stanford Surgical Approach

For more than a decade and a half, the Stanford Sleep Disorders Clinic has teamed up with two outstanding ear, nose, and throat (ENT) surgeons, Drs. Nelson Powell and Robert Riley, both of whom also have degrees from dental school and have training in maxillofacial surgery. They are members of a very tiny group of surgeons who qualify as sleep specialists and have worked consistently to develop new and better surgical treatments for obstructive sleep apnea. Their procedures provide a cure of obstructive sleep apnea in a majority of cases, and with rare exception, all their patients improve substantially. Their approach combines the standard UPPP with ingenious procedures to pull the large tongue muscle forward and away from the back of the throat. This is accomplished by cutting out a small rectangle of bone in the front of the jaw, to which the tongue muscle is attached. They then pull this piece of bone out, rotate it 90 degrees, so it cannot fall back, and trim and fix it permanently. This maneuver pulls the tongue forward and adds more than a centimeter to the airway diameter, without any visible external changes.

Whenever any sleep apnea patient receives a treatment, the efficacy of this treatment must always be carefully evaluated. Unfortunately, most surgeons and dentists around the country do not carry out polysomnographic follow-ups. Well over 1,000 patients have undergone this surgical procedure at Stanford, and postoperative sleep tests show that 60 to 70 percent are entirely cured.

New Technology

Some patients with obstructive sleep apnea absolutely cannot tolerate the CPAP treatment. Other people who tolerate the treatment well for a few years, and who fully understand the improvement in their lives, nonetheless begin to wish that they could be cured and dispense with the machine. As I have said, surgery is another option, but the results have generally been very poor except at Stanford and a few other places.

A very promising new treatment has been developed by Nelson Powell. In recent years medical specialists have used radio-frequency energy to shrink the prostate gland and certain other targets. After sitting next to a urologist on the plane and talking about radio-frequency tissue reduction, Nelson had the inspiration to use the technique for shrinking tissue in the upper airway. To make a long story short, he hooked up with medical entrepreneurs and convinced them that this could be a very successful technique for treating apnea. Together they developed safe and effective equipment and conducted a very careful series of trials, first in animals and then in humans.

The procedure is basically quite simple. After a local anesthetic is administered, small needles are inserted into the tissue that needs shrinking. A very precise and controlled dose of radio frequency waves is delivered to the target tissue only at the needle tips. The area around the needle tips is coagulated and absorbed, leaving only a tiny internal scar. This treatment results in an overall reduction in tissue volume. The Food and Drug Administration approved the technique for treating snoring a few years ago. Recent clinical trials show that it works on the base of the tongue, which is the primary culprit in most cases of obstructive apnea. After reviewing these data, the FDA has approved the technique for treating obstructive sleep apnea.

This approach has numerous advantages over conventional surgery. It does not require an operating room or hospitalization. It is easily done as an outpatient procedure. The treatment itself takes only a few minutes and is bloodless and painless. Although there is some swelling immediately after the procedure, posttreatment pain is much less severe than that from ordinary surgery, and what little pain there is can be controlled easily with over-the-counter painkillers. Because there is so little discomfort, patients are willing to come back for successive treatments. This is in contrast to laser surgery, after which pain can inhibit the desire to return for further treatment. There also is no wound on the tongue or sutures that can come undone. To date there has been not a single untoward incident in our surgeons' hands. And for the first time, there is a possibility of comfortable and convenient treatment that can cure many sufferers, even those individuals whose obstructive sleep apnea is currently mild—meaning we can stop the disorder before it gets much worse.

Nelson Powell and his colleagues Bob Riley, Rob Troell, and Kasey Li are among the finest physicians on the face of the earth, and I have followed their work with great admiration at their care and ingenuity. I am certain that their technique will continue to improve and have wider applications. Such an approach may become the procedure of choice for tonsillectomy and adenoidectomy in children, and pediatricians may also become much less reluctant to refer children to surgeons for treatment of obstructive sleep apnea. It is important that those who use the technique are well trained and, above all, understand sleep mechanisms and sleep disorders. With such a promising treatment right at hand it is all the more important to insist that medical students receive adequate education about the diagnosis and treatment of obstructive sleep apnea and other sleep disorders.

Light at the End of the Tunnel?

Along with a steadily increasing band of colleagues, I have been diagnosing and treating obstructive sleep apnea for more than a quarter of a century. Every physician today who has practiced sleep medicine for any length of time has seen one miraculous recovery after another. Even so, every patient who has been treated successfully is probably matched by one whose treatment is less than satisfactory, and these are both vastly outnumbered by those who are unidentified. The advent of managed care hasn't made things any easier; to get to a sleep specialist, most people now have to be referred by a primary care physician who most likely won't recognize the patient's sleep problem. Of course, for managed care to pay for treatment, it must be fully effective—and of course, no treatment is fully effective for every patient. Thus, every effort must be made to increase the effectiveness of treatments and to achieve ways to provide a lasting cure. I believe that radio-frequency technology holds the greatest promise for a highly accessible and successful treatment.

Meanwhile, for every sleep apnea victim who has been restored to normal functioning and health, there are several hundred who are going downhill without knowing why. For anyone who cares about their fellow human beings, this is totally unacceptable.

I got a taste of this anger when I questioned one of the patients whom we rescued from the Stanford Internal Medicine Clinic waiting room. Remember, these patients were not coming in for sleep problems, had no idea they had sleep problems, and came to the sleep clinic simply because we walked into the waiting room that day and offered them a free exam. I interviewed this patient about three weeks after he was diagnosed and put on nasal CPAP treatment.

"How are things going on the CPAP?" I asked.

"Absolutely terrific," he replied. "I mean, the difference in the quality of my life is amazing. I don't know how I can possibly measure it. I really just thought that I was getting older, and that's the way life was going to be. But now it's really not."

"Look back at the quality of your life before treatment," I continued. "How impaired do you think you were?"

"Really a lot. I would say 50 percent, sometimes nearly 100 percent. The quality of my life before this treatment was really awful. How can I describe it? It was just so difficult to make decisions and to get things done. I just didn't have the power or the energy to deal with my life. Now my blood pressure is controlled with about a quarter of the medication I was on previously, with no diuretic at all. It's just terrific. I used to spend a lot of time watching TV and dozing off. Now I have the energy to pursue other interests. I just bought my first computer, and I'm reading again now that I can stay awake to enjoy it. It's really terrific."

"Your diagnosis of sleep apnea was made completely by chance," I reminded him. "You may have had this condition for eight to ten years. And every one of your doctors has failed to recognize the symptoms. How do you feel about that?"

"Really angry," he immediately replied. "Bitter. I mean, it's inexcusable and gross incompetence. I'm mad as hell. I really just don't understand how a doctor couldn't diagnose this. It's easier to diagnose than a broken arm, for heaven's sake. You ask a few simple questions and you don't need an X ray. The thought that I spent so many years with such a low and deteriorating quality of life, and feeling really miserable, really, really aggravates me. And to think how many other people are walking around right now seeing their physician for these symptoms and not being recognized is inexcusable. If I had to have mortgaged my house to pay for this treatment, I would have done it in a second. It would have been an easy decision. The quality of my life in the past was really terrible, and now it's really terrific."

I'd like to add one of my favorite successful treatment stories, told to me by an anonymous sleep specialist. He was treating a man and wife, both of whom were very overweight and had severe obstructive sleep apnea. In addition to having all the typical symptoms, they emphasized that they had lost all interest in having sex. When they came back after several weeks of being on nasal CPAP, they commented, "Those hoses may make us look like elephants, but hallelujah, we're making out like rabbits."

Chapter 8

Ambushed by Sleep: Narcolepsy and Other Sleep Disorders

IT IS NIGHT in a small village. A young woman puts out the light and goes to bed. She lies on her back for a few minutes, quietly looking at the ceiling. She notices a strange brightness at the window, a glow that slowly fills the room with an eerie light. She is frightened, feeling that something horrible is about to happen. She tries to get up but finds that she is completely paralyzed. She cannot move her arms or legs; she cannot sit up or roll over. Suddenly a strange and frightening being appears at her window and begins to drift toward her. She wants to scream, to run, but her muscles won't respond. She can't utter a sound, can't even look away. Then the creature reaches out with an alien finger and probes her body, molesting her sexually. After a seeming eternity, the intruder stops his torture and floats away. The glow slowly fades from the room. A few minutes later the young woman can move again, and she runs to the door trying to escape the horrible memory.

A scene from the *X-Files*? Testimony of an alien abduction from the supermarket tabloids? On the contrary, the year is 1432, and the young woman has been visited by an incubus, a demon believed to come at night to assault women, often sexually. In the folklore of the time, the spawn of such nocturnal encounters were witches, goblins, and deformed babies. In some legends, King Arthur's magician,

Merlin, is the product of such a visit. Sometimes men were assaulted by a female demon, called a succubus.

It is interesting to note how much stories of medieval incubi and succubi have in common with modern stories of alien abduction. People who feel they have been abducted by aliens often say that such visitations start at night while they are in bed. Many times the "victims" are unable to move, paralyzed. Sometimes a strange light shines on them and they are transported to an alien spaceship. There they are often probed with needles and strange medical instruments. They feel indescribable terror. Later they are returned to their home, with no physical marks but a vivid memory of everything that happened.

These stories may have a common root. They all may be products of very vivid "hypnagogic" (associated with sleep onset) hallucinations. Vivid hallucinations, behaviors, and terror are all fascinating symptoms of some of the sleep disorders that blur the line between sleep and wakefulness. People with narcolepsy, sleepwalking, night terrors, sleeptalking, and REM behavior disorder can get stranded in sleep's borderlands, where everyday rules of thought and behavior don't seem to apply.

Most people have experienced simple hypnagogic images or sensations upon falling asleep. The most common are isolated images or feelings that float through our consciousness, like having our skin lightly touched, or a feeling of floating. A common and unpleasant feeling is one of falling suddenly, leading to a startle and an abrupt jerk of the limbs. More frightening, but completely normal, are hypnagogic images like a bright flash of light, or sounds such as a loud bang that seems to come from inside the head. These images and sensations are almost always very fleeting, and because the sleeper is not yet deeply asleep, they often cause a return to full wakefulness. Indeed, they are remembered only if the sleeper wakes up.

Narcolepsy
Truly vivid hypnagogic hallucinations occur when someone falls immediately or very rapidly into REM sleep without going through the intervening non-REM sleep stages. When REM sleep occurs so quickly, the dream story often begins exactly where wakefulness

ended and is a seamless stream of consciousness from the real world to the dream world. Occasionally this can happen to normal individuals if they are extremely sleep deprived, or after waking up later in the sleep cycle, when REM is favored. However, hypnagogic hallucinations are frequent and are a true torment in patients who have a sleep disorder called narcolepsy.

What we don't know is why the content of these vivid hypnagogic hallucinations is so often very unpleasant or downright terrifying. People report being fully awake and aware but completely paralyzed. Sometimes they see a strange light. Most often there is pervasive fear, sometimes so strong that people are sure they are about to die. Other parts of their hallucination, which may include people, animals, parts of objects, or just shapes, have a mysteriously nightmarish quality. Personally, I have never had a patient who reported experiencing an alien abduction, but many people have told me that they saw intruders in their bedroom, that they saw someone coming in the window, or that they heard footsteps getting closer and closer and knew they would be murdered in their bed. One patient of mine was sure she saw a frightening stranger walk in and out of her bedroom every night for a year before her narcolepsy was diagnosed. Only after diagnosis did she finally believe that no one else was there. Prior to that she had kept silent for fear of being thought insane.

I became interested in narcolepsy when I first read about it as a sophomore in medical school before I ever saw a case. Six years later in 1958, I met my first narcoleptic patient. He went to bed in my New York sleep laboratory and passed directly into unambiguous REM sleep in less than a minute, a phenomenon I had never seen in several hundred all-night sleep recordings on adults. I knew instantly that this could be an important discovery, and I begged him to come back the next night. He returned several times, and each night he went from wakefulness immediately into REM sleep. It finally occurred to me to study him during daytime naps. Again he passed directly from wakefulness into REM sleep, a sequence that we later found, as I have mentioned before, in normal newborn infants—but only in very special circumstances in adults. Otherwise, people always proceed predictably through non-REM sleep stages 1 through 4 before entering REM sleep. I was very excited to find in narcolepsy a pattern of sleep so different from the norm.

The scientific importance of narcolepsy is that it is a sleep disorder caused by malfunctions in the primary brain mechanisms that induce normal sleep. Understanding and curing this disorder will inevitably advance our understanding of the processes of normal sleep and wakefulness. For people with narcolepsy, the most important and debilitating effect of the disorder is that they are unbearably sleepy all the time. Their struggle to stay awake is relentless, and whenever they let down their guard, sleep immediately overcomes them. Even when they are on guard, they are often overtaken by sleep—in the middle of a sentence, while eating, or even during sex. Such unintended sleep "attacks" may last up to 10 or 20 minutes, and then victims wake up feeling somewhat refreshed. Soon afterward, they become sleepy again.

The most dramatic component of the narcolepsy syndrome is "cataplexy"—attacks of muscle weakness or near-total paralysis that occur suddenly, last for a few seconds or minutes, and vanish. People who have cataplexy might collapse into a chair or onto the floor, conscious of everything around them—able to see and hear, but unable to move. Just as in REM sleep, the heart and breathing muscles operate normally, as do the muscles in the eyes. However, the muscles of the arms and legs remain completely limp. If the cataplectic attack lasts a bit, one can pick up the victim's arm and shake it like a rag doll's, then let it flop back to the person's side. When the episode is over, voluntary muscular control returns and is completely normal.

Before I discovered that muscle paralysis is normally associated with human REM sleep, it was impossible to explain cataplexy. Others had erroneously assumed the attacks to be epileptic seizures not related to the sufferer's pervasive sleepiness. Contributing to the strangeness of cataplexy is the fact that an attack typically is precipitated by strong emotion—anger, laughter, or just getting excited. For this reason, cataplexy was often interpreted as a psychological defense in people who were assumed to be deeply afraid of being too emotional.

For a few patients, only highly specific situations or emotions will trigger an attack. For example, one patient who was a hunter had cataplectic attacks at the moment of the kill as he tried to pull the trigger of his hunting rifle, and when trying to slice rare roast beef.

Other patients have their attacks when becoming angry at a spouse; or when laughing at a joke. Many narcoleptics learn which emotions are most likely to trigger attacks, and condition themselves to push those emotions out of their minds or avoid situations where they might arise. In those with very severe cataplexy, any strong emotion will trigger an attack.

Once I was sure that narcoleptic patients consistently fell immediately into REM sleep from wakefulness, I wanted to establish that cataplexy is the same paralytic process that occurs normally in the rest of us for about two hours every night during REM sleep. It certainly appeared to be, but I wanted to be sure. People don't recognize that REM sleep is the only time they are completely paralyzed. During REM sleep, tendon reflexes like the knee jerk completely disappear; at any joint both the flexor muscles and the extensor muscles are paralyzed and completely limp. Voluntary muscle control vanishes, but breathing continues and the eye muscles are not paralyzed. I decided to induce cataplexy by getting patients to laugh and then looking for these same patterns of paralysis.

One thing I learned while trying to do this experiment is that humor is extremely fragile in a laboratory setting. Telling patients jokes that might have been hilariously funny at a cocktail party simply did not work in the lab. We spent a fair amount of time collecting surefire funny stories, which also failed. We floundered like bombing stand-up comics, until we found that allowing subjects to view the television show *I Love Lucy* worked. They reliably laughed and collapsed. Sure enough, during a cataplectic attack, the patients could move their eyes in response to commands, they could breathe more or less normally and inhale and exhale in response to commands. As in REM sleep, during the paralysis they were completely flaccid; tendon reflexes were completely gone and their arms and legs were completely limp.

We also found that if patients remained undisturbed and were comfortable, a complete cataplectic attack would often lead them into a full-blown REM sleep period with a dream. Many of the dreams were smoothly continuous with the waking experience and then might take off into some bizarre convolution, such as one where I summoned 20 medical students into the room to make fun of the patient. Since this sort of hallucination is common, it is easy to understand the speculations at the beginning of this chapter: If one can image someone with narcolepsy living in medieval times, all of the symptomatology would seem supernatural. Even in today's world, the sleep-onset REM period dreams are often confused with reality. I had a patient who came to work on Saturday several times because she had dreamed that her boss had requested it. Occasionally people with narcolepsy are neither clearly awake nor clearly asleep; they may be existing simultaneously in two entirely different states of mind. While we were examining one patient in the laboratory, he reported that as he listened to us he was aware that he was in the laboratory, but he felt that he was also lying paralyzed in the street outside and was terrified that he would be struck by a car.

We also found that it was hard to elicit cataplexy in front of the camera. Years ago, a young Morley Safer and his *60 Minutes* crew came to Stanford to get film for a segment on sleep disorders. The only way to share the full impact of narcolepsy with the public was to make sure Safer got to film at least one full-blown cataplectic attack. We asked our most cataplectically gifted patient what was the surest trigger for an attack and he said, "shooting pool." Since developing narcolepsy he stopped playing pool because he would repeatedly fall to the floor. We found a neighbor with a billiards table and set the whole thing up. Morley Safer and the patient played pool; the lights were on, the camera rolled, and I stood by ready to enlighten the audience when the dramatic event took place. But it didn't take place. The camera rolled. Finally one of the crew said, "I think we've exposed about $10,000 worth of film; we don't have much more. [This was before videocameras were widely used.] Should we keep going?" Morley Safer said, "Well, don't worry, we'll edit out every-thing except my one or two good shots and we'll show that," at which point the patient began to laugh and melted to the floor. It was a great segment. Some years later I was surprised and delighted to encounter Safer on a train in Italy, entirely by chance. We had a nice chat during which he commented that he remembered the cataplectic attack as vividly as anything in his entire career as a re-porter.

Despite being sleepy all day, people with narcolepsy don't sleep well at night. In fact, their sleep resembles that of people with little or no sleep debt, compared with that of normal sleepers. Narcoleptic patients typically spend much more of their night in light sleep and less time in the deepest stages of non-REM sleep. This is exactly the opposite of what is seen during the nighttime sleep that normally follows sleep deprivation.

It is nearly impossible for people with narcolepsy to lead normal lives. Relationships are often damaged irreversibly when patients fall asleep during a conversation—or even during sex. We always encourage patients' spouses to accompany them to the sleep clinic so that we can explain that it is the disease, not boredom, that causes their mate to fall asleep at these emotionally charged moments. But if private life is difficult, social situations are strewn with potential land mines. One of my patients suffered a severe cataplectic attack at a party. Overhearing a funny remark, she collapsed to the floor while the trayful of champagne glasses she was carrying smashed all around her. Even though she tended to have attacks very infrequently, after this single traumatically embarrassing moment she withdrew completely from an active social life.

Narcolepsy can strike people at almost any age—it has been identified in children as young as three and has first emerged as late as 50 in a few adults—but the peak time of onset is during adolescence, suggesting that the sexual maturation of the brain may play a role. It's particularly harmful when narcolepsy occurs in children and isn't recognized; I knew of one case in which parents beat their narcoleptic child repeatedly for being uncooperative, lazy, and a liar until finally her illness was diagnosed.

But anytime the disorder strikes, it can be perplexing and highly disturbing. When the cataplectic attacks are the first problem to appear, it is obvious to victims that something is terribly wrong, but they cannot find a reason. In most cases, however, the first symptom of narcolepsy is excessive daytime sleepiness, which may develop insidiously over several years or come on quite rapidly. The onset of cataplectic attacks may occur almost at the same time as excessive sleepiness; but the development of cataplexy is more commonly delayed two or three years. Occasionally the first manifestation of narcolepsy is hypnogogic hallucinations. One of my patients experienced her first symptom when she got into bed one night and found a rattlesnake beside her. It is impossible to imagine how terrifying this must have been. She called the police, who came and searched her apartment from top to bottom. Since she'd been up all night, she lay down on her couch the next afternoon for a nap and again there was the rattlesnake. Hysterical with fear and confusion, she was hospitalized in a psychiatric ward. It will not be difficult to believe she was a basket case by the time I saw her.

People who aren't knowledgeable about narcolepsy may shun someone with the disorder or decide not to marry them or have children. Although there is a genetic component to the disorder, narcoleptics are only slightly more likely than the general population to have children who also develop the disorder. Given our ability to treat narcolepsy very effectively, the very slim chance of passing it to another generation should not influence such decisions.

Surveys conducted to evaluate quality of life for people with narcolepsy have found that patients often suffer from double vision, memory problems, balance disturbances, and personality changes. About two thirds of respondents say that narcolepsy was responsible for their frequent rear-end automobile accidents. People also report experiencing paralysis at dangerous moments and as a result, burning themselves, nearly drowning in the bathtub, or having accidents or close calls while driving, to name just a few mishaps.

Narcolepsy affects about .05 percent of the population, or 1 in 2,000 people. This figure is fairly constant worldwide. Although it has a lower prevalence than insomnia, sleep apnea, or restless legs syndrome, narcolepsy is still a relatively common disorder: Half as many women develop narcolepsy as develop breast cancer, and the disorder is five times more common than leukemia.

After studying my first narcoleptic patient in New York, I very much wanted to locate more patients to see if they would also show sleep-onset REM periods. At the time, I was working with a psychoanalyst, Charles Fisher, who was trying to find the unconscious motivation behind my first narcolepsy patient's constant daytime fatigue and sudden attacks of paralysis. At any rate, Fisher and I polled doctors and hospitals all over New York City and managed to find four other people with narcolepsy, all of whom exhibited the same sleep pattern.

When I moved to Stanford University in 1963, I intended to continue studying narcolepsy, but none of the local physicians had ever seen such a patient and my efforts netted a big fat zero. Convinced that there must be at least a few people with narcolepsy in the area, I did something I had never done before: I placed a small want ad in the *San Francisco Chronicle*: "If you are sleepy all the time and have attacks of muscular weakness when you laugh or get angry, please write Stanford professor at this address." The ad ran only a few days, but over 100 people responded, at least half of whom definitely had the disorder. If memory serves, none of these individuals knew what was the matter with them. In one fell swoop, I learned that narcolepsy was far more common than I had previously thought and that doctors apparently didn't know it existed. I soon had more experience with this disorder than almost anyone else in the world. I was dismayed to find that patients had been suffering for an average of 15 years before they came to me, and that they had seen an average of five different doctors without receiving a correct diagnosis. It was also my first indication of how little medical students were still taught about sleep disorders.

Because I and one junior colleague, Dr. Stephen Mitchell, were at the time the only doctors in the area knowledgeable about treating narcolepsy, we began to assume the responsibility for the care of these patients. In 1964 Dr. Mitchell and I opened the very first clinic in the world devoted exclusively to treating sleep disorders. This service was supposed to pay for itself by billing patients. Unfortunately, most of the patients either didn't have jobs or were poorly paid, probably resulting from their history of falling asleep on the job. The clinic went broke within a year. Nevertheless, the seed was sown.

My involvement in taking care of patients with narcolepsy and in allowing them to volunteer for research studies led to my desire to develop a full-fledged clinical service to help such patients. Although the clinic failed to produce an income, I continued to take care of many of these patients, while at the same time they contributed to our scientific observations.

Letting Sleepy Dogs Lie

One problem with narcolepsy research in the 1960s was a lack of methods to find a clue to the underlying brain abnormality in humans. We made several attempts to collect and analyze spinal fluid from narcoleptic patients, but we had no control group and it was understandably difficult to recruit volunteers. What we really needed to find was an animal model for narcolepsy.

By 1972 our consistent efforts to make movies of cataplectic attacks had yielded some pretty good film clips. That year I showed a couple of them in a presentation at the annual convention of the American Medical Association. Afterward a neurologist approached me and told me that he knew about a dog that had similar attacks. When I contacted the dog's veterinarian, he offered both bad news and good news. The bad news was that he had put the dog to sleep because he mistakenly assumed the animal had intractable epilepsy. The good news was that he had made a movie of the dog having several attacks. I viewed a copy of the film and decided that the attacks certainly looked a lot like cataplexy—but only by observing the dog directly and doing some tests could I have been certain.

The next year at the annual meeting of the American Academy of Neurology, I showed both my human film and the dog film. Another neurologist approached me and told me about a female French poodle in Saskatoon, Canada, that had identical behavior. This time I managed to get in touch with the owner, and I convinced him to donate the poodle, whose name was Monique, to Stanford for tests. Monique did indeed have narcolepsy, and her cataplexy was severe.

In order to try to breed more such dogs, we agreed that the next time Monique came into heat, we would get her back to Saskatoon to mate with her brother. Since both dogs were genetically similar, breeding the two would increase the chances that they would pass on the narcolepsy trait to their offspring. When Monique finally did come into heat, I excitedly called a major airline and told them that I had a narcoleptic dog that I had to ship to Saskatoon as part of a scientific experiment. "No sick dogs on the airplane, sir," I was told. I tried to explain that the dog was not actually sick, that it had a genetic disorder. "I'm very sorry," the airline employee said, as if speaking to a child, "regulations do not allow sick animals on the airplane." I was desperate and incredibly frustrated. Here we had the chance to make a breakthrough in the study of narcolepsy and I couldn't get the poodle back home because of a regulation that didn't even apply. I would have chauffeured Monique the 3,000 plus miles to Saskatoon myself, but the event coincided with the memorable 1974 gasoline shortage.

As a last, desperate act I called my congressman's office and explained the situation to an aide. "I'll see what we can do," he said. A few minutes later the phone rang. It was the president of the airline: "We'd like to help you in any way we can, Professor." Monique flew to Saskatoon but, alas, the union did not produce any pups.

My determination to find more narcoleptic dogs and breed them was undiminished by this setback. Monique and I toured veterinary schools around the country, exhibited the unique attacks of cataplexy, and asked those in the audience to keep an eye out for any animal that seemed to exhibit such abnormalities. During the next few years veterinarians from around the country sent us about a dozen dogs that we diagnosed with narcolepsy. In 1977 we successfully bred a litter of Doberman pups all of which developed narcolepsy and in later years we collected other breeds with the disorder. We still have the original Dobermans' descendants residing at Stanford's sleep center. As with humans, canine narcolepsy doesn't involve pain. The dogs simply collapse, albeit dramatically when they get excited, for example when we give them a new toy or a favorite snack. A minute or two later they are back up again as if nothing had happened. As far as I can tell, our narcoleptic dogs are all healthy and happy and have no idea they are different from normal dogs.

Through selective breeding and genetic analyses of blood samples from the dogs, my colleague at Stanford, Emmanuel Mignot, is very close to finding the gene for narcolepsy in dogs, called *canarc-1* (from canus—Latin for "dog"—and "narcolepsy"). This gene is particularly interesting because its location on the chromosome is associated with a group of natural immune system genes, raising the possibility that narcolepsy is partly an autoimmune disorder or that the sleep mechanism is closely related to immune function. The genetics of narcolepsy are more complicated in humans than in dogs: In dogs one gene is enough to pass on the trait, whereas in humans it is not. For example, in identical human twins (who by definition have identical genes) if one twin has narcolepsy, there is only a 30 percent chance that the other will have the disorder. Other genes, or environmental and developmental factors, must play a part in precipitating narcolepsy in humans.

In 1977 a little item in *Sports Illustrated* magazine mentioned that the bullfighting industry in Spain was in trouble. The bulls would enter the arena and suddenly fall down. They would recover and fall again. The Spaniards considered such a bullfight a joke, a serious cultural problem. *Sports Illustrated* reported that a group in Madrid was offering a reward of several million pesetas to anyone who could solve the problem. I was dazzled by the possibility that I could be the one with the answer and possibly fund my research for the rest of my career. I was therefore very disappointed when I found that this seemingly huge sum of money was only about U.S. $25,000. Nevertheless, I was convinced that the falling bulls had cataplexy fostered by excessive inbreeding, and my professional curiosity was greatly aroused.

I sent a close friend who had previously lived in Spain on a mission to obtain movies. Videocameras did not exist at this time, and since the longest rolls of Super-8 movie film available were three minutes the camera could not be run continuously. There was no way to predict exactly when a bull would fall, so my friend was always two or three seconds too late. He attended countless bullfights and had lots of movie footage of bulls on the ground, but he never actually captured the cataplectic attack itself. Although the Spanish veterinarians never identified the cause, the problem was finally solved by eliminating the bovine strains in which the falling tendency occurred. My friend did manage to turn the escapade into a hilarious magazine article entitled "El Toro Tanglefoot, or Sitting Bull Revisited."

Later we confirmed that narcolepsy could exist in species other than dogs and humans when we found several ponies that had cataplexy. I imagine that wild animals with narcolepsy would not survive very long, since any tendency to collapse when frightened would quickly lead to the animal becoming dinner for a predator.

Treating Narcolepsy
There is currently no cure for narcolepsy. We treat the disorder by providing stimulants to counter patients' pervasive daytime sleepiness. Cataplexy, hypnagogic hallucinations, and sleep paralysis are pure manifestations of REM sleep and must be treated with different medications. Most often antidepressants are used because they block REM paralysis (the source of cataplectic paralysis).

For many years the treatment for narcolepsy has been limited to amphetamines and the amphetaminelike Ritalin. The latter is para-doxically—and controversially—used to calm hyperactive children. The main challenge in treating the abnormal sleepiness is adjusting the dosage to produce sufficient alertness without debilitating side effects, such as jitteriness, dry mouth, and, in rare cases, psychosis.

I believe that doctors' most common mistake in treating narcolepsy was and still is not using these drugs as aggressively as they should. Since amphetamines are widely abused, there is a moral taint to them, and physicians who know little about narcolepsy often feel uncomfortable prescribing them over a long period of time. Many patients also share this ambivalence, but such feelings are counter-productive. I always make a comparison to diabetes, where the pan-creas is not making insulin. Taking insulin prescribed by a physician is simply replacing what is lacking in the body to restore the health of the patient. In the same way, narcolepsy is a disease in which the daily periods of internal clock-dependent alerting appear to be miss-ing. The physician, then, is using drugs to replace this important internal function.

The best strategy for finding the optimal dose of stimulants is to let patients specify their own personal treatment goals, such as staying awake in the classroom or being able to drive a reasonable distance without falling asleep. Once these goals are set, stimulants are then provided in sufficient quantity to achieve these objectives. Overall, the goal of treatment should be for the patient to achieve as normal a life as possible. The main reason to establish individual goals is that the term "normal function" is too vague. Even if primary care phy-sicians never miss a case, they are likely to encounter only a few individuals with narcolepsy throughout their career; nevertheless, it should be no problem to work with the patient to get the very best results. A doctor should first prescribe a minimal dose of stimulant and then slowly raise the dose until the goal is met. Side effects should be tracked. If they become too bothersome, the medication can be changed.

One of the 10 appointed members of the National Commission on Sleep Disorders Research was a highly successful businessman who was also a victim of narcolepsy. Both his personal and professional lives began suffering as early as high school before his disorder was correctly identified. Once diagnosed and treated, however, he was able to fully exploit his exceptional talents. Recognizing his out-standing ability, I appointed him vice-chairman of the commission. I worked with him very closely for two years, and except for an occa-sional episode of partial cataplexy when excited, and a very occa-sional wave of drowsiness (both of which were trivial) he was as normal as anyone because he is adequately treated. His medication is a morning dose of 100 mg of metamphetamine every day, which has not changed for many years. He has a complete checkup of his heart, blood pressure and liver functions regularly, and has never had any problems or side effects.

As I write this at the end of 1998, the FDA has approved a promis-ing new treatment for narcolepsy. The narcolepsy medication, modafinil, marketed as Provigil, keeps people awake through mecha-nisms that are currently not fully understood. Modafinil is not an amphetamine, and its action does not resemble that of conventional stimulants, which broadly excite various nerve centers of the brain and cause a range of side effects from palpitations to an upset stom-ach. By contrast, modafinil causes few or no side effects. It may work at the nexus of the brain's sleep drive and clock-dependent alerting systems.

As with any drug, the biggest question will be the drug's long-term effects, although a six-month study of 61 patients revealed nothing that would raise concerns. During this study the patients experi-enced no effects on mood, blood pressure/heart rate, weight, or nocturnal sleep. A few patients complained of headache and dry mouth, but interestingly, those complaints were found almost as often in the group that received a placebo. All of the patients treated with modafinil reported a decrease in daytime sleepiness, and there was no evidence that patients had any tendency to increase the pre-scribed dose over time.

All of this is important because patients must use medications their whole lives, which typically means from age 15 on.

Sleep Disorders and Safety
For an adult in today's world, losing the right to drive an automobile can be catastrophic. Next to remaining undiagnosed, the fear of losing a driver's license is often cited as an important reason that victims of narcolepsy often do not avail themselves of treatment.

Since the 1960s, when I first became involved in taking care of patients with narcolepsy, I have been firmly convinced that the well-managed patient is no less safe than anyone else. Certainly, the effectively treated narcoleptic patient is safer than all the "normal" drivers who are severely sleep deprived. The answer to people's worries about traffic safety is not to deny narcoleptics driver's licenses but to greatly expand the identification and treatment of people with all sleep disorders. As I have always maintained, the vast majority of victims of sleep disorders remain unidentified. No drowsy driver should be allowed on the road. No one has a right to put not only him- or herself, but many others as well, at risk of injury, disability, and death.

Acting Out the Dream: REM Behavior Disorder

Many of us may think that being told that our dreams will come true sounds idyllic, but for people with REM behavior disorder, the dream is a nightmare. This disorder can be regarded as the opposite of narcolepsy. In narcolepsy, the muscle paralysis of REM sleep intrudes into waking life. In REM behavior disorder, muscles that should be paralyzed during REM sleep are not. REM paralysis fails, and the body acts out the brain's dream. Injuries to the dreamer and the dreamer's spouse are common.

REM behavior disorder was described for the first time as recently as 1985 by two sleep specialists at the University of Minnesota, Mark Mahowald and Carlos Schenck, and by Christian Guilleminault at Stanford. Now being identified frequently by sleep specialists, over 90 percent of REM behavior disorder patients are male. The disorder usually strikes after the age of 50, although we have seen patients as young as 9 at Stanford. REM behavior disorder seems to be progressive: Patients typically talk, twitch, and jerk during dreaming for years before they fully act out their REM dreams. In older patients a degenerative neurologic condition, often Parkinson's disease, usually accompanies REM behavior disorder. It is assumed that in these instances, the degenerative process may have affected the tiny area of the brain stem that controls REM paralysis.

As we have learned, the dreaming brain functions very similarly to the waking brain, processing thoughts and sending out messages to move limbs. Normally the instructions to move the eyes get through, but messages to move muscles in the rest of the body are blocked before they can leave the spinal cord. In REM behavior disorder, the messages are not halted, due to the pathology in the brain stem. People may just move their arms and legs in bed or talk in their sleep, or they may actually get out of bed and run around, without ever waking up or realizing that they are dreaming. The brain is blocking sensations from the environment and at the same time is replacing them with internally generated sensations from the dream world. As in every dream, the brain is directing the action—in effect, the body is just along for the ride.

To make matters worse, the dreams that are acted out are often violent or frightening. People dream of being chased or fighting for their life against enemies, demons, or wild animals. One man I talked to dreamed that he was playing football; he realized upon awakening that in attempts to avoid being tackled, he had collided with half the furniture in the room. Such nighttime behavior is dangerous. Patients often come in with bruises, cuts, and even broken bones they sustained during sleep. While they usually remember nothing of the episode, they may remember the dream itself.

It's difficult to say who suffers more when someone has REM behavior disorder, the terrorized and often battered bedmate, or the person who must cope with the eventual realization that he has harmed someone he loves, with no memory of the incident. Wives are often the ones who seek treatment because they cannot go on living with someone who punches, kicks, slaps, or chokes them in the middle of the night. One patient dreamed that he was choking a deer and woke up to find he was choking his wife. (She was shaken but all right.) Ironically men sometimes attack their wives while dreaming that they are fighting to protect them against an intruder. If some injury doesn't wake the dreamer, he usually is awakened by his wife's screams.

Several other characteristics make this disorder even more amazing. First, it can affect people who are almost never violent in daily life. One of Mahowald and Schenck's patients was a 77-year-old minister who had been acting out violently in his sleep for 20 years before he finally sought treatment after seriously injuring himself. Second, people who have had a violent outburst during the night usually wake up the next day feeling completely refreshed, as if they'd enjoyed a great night's sleep. The third strange feature of this disorder is that the autonomic nervous system, which governs heart rate, breathing, and other vital functions, seems to remain unaffected by these violent outbursts. Continuous recordings of patients' heart rate, breathing, and blood pressure show that they can thrash violently, swear, or jump around the room while the heartbeat remains at 60 beats a minute, the normal resting rate. The part of the body usually under voluntary control is running amok, while the part under automatic control continues as it would in normal REM sleep. In only a few cases, usually during the most extreme nightmares, do the heart rate, blood pressure, and rate of breathing increase.

Fortunately, the Minnesota sleep specialists have developed a fairly effective treatment for REM behavior disorder—clonazepam, a benzodiazapine that curtails or eliminates the disorder in about 9 out of 10 cases. People don't usually grow tolerant of clonazepam at the proper dosage, even when it is taken over a period of years. In the few cases in which clonazepam doesn't work, some antidepressants can reduce the violent behavior. Even when drug therapy seems to be working, it's still prudent to make the bedroom safe, eliminating all sharp and breakable objects. Some patients sleep in a bare room with only a mattress on the floor, covering the windows with heavy curtains. Many couples resort to separate bedrooms.

An animal model from long ago sheds light on the possible causes of REM behavior disorder. More than 35 years ago, the brilliant French sleep researcher Michel Jouvet observed that cats with damage in a tiny part of the brain stem will interrupt their non-REM sleep with episodes of hallucinatory behavior. They arch their backs, hiss, and bare their teeth at an unseen rival while their brain waves register normal REM sleep. When these areas are not damaged and become active during REM sleep or cataplexy, they trigger a sequence of nerve impulses from the brain stem to the spinal cord that instantly turn off the millions of spinal motor neurons that ordinarily command muscles to move.

It is possible that as we age, the brain atrophies or is damaged in this part of the brain stem in ways that aren't immediately apparent. Alternatively, it is also possible that the brain abnormalities that cause the disorder originate far earlier—perhaps in childhood or even in the womb—and then are revealed by the normal brain changes involved in aging. The fact that the vast majority of cases occur in men suggests that some hormonal element is probably involved.

Sleepwalking and Night Terrors

A sleep-deprived college freshman climbs out of bed in the middle of the night, silently opens the door of his dorm room, and walks down the hallway. His roommate wakes up, sees him, and asks where he's going, but the young man just keeps walking, seemingly unable to hear anything. If his roommate stands in front of him, the sleep-walker seems to look right through him. After five minutes or so the sleepwalker returns to bed and falls soundly asleep. In the morning he can't remember anything about his excursion.

A four-year-old girl sits up in the middle of the night and begins screaming. Her parents rush in and find her wide-eyed in terror. The parents ask what is wrong and try to soothe her. The child doesn't respond to their words and doesn't seem to see them. She keeps staring at something, terrified. Her parents keep saying "What's wrong, honey? What's wrong?" Soon they are equally frightened. After five seemingly interminable minutes, her crying and struggling subside, and without a word she lies down and slips back into a peaceful sleep. In the morning she can't remember what she was frightened about or even that she was frightened at all.

These are two examples of parasomnias (Latin for "near sleep"): sleepwalking and night terrors. Like people with REM behavior disorder, people afflicted with sleepwalking and night terrors will rise out of seemingly deep sleep and act as if they are awake; they typically don't respond to other people and have no memory of the incident the next day. Unlike REM behavior disorder, however, people are not dreaming when they sleepwalk and are not having nightmares during night terrors. In fact, neither sleepwalking nor night terrors occur during REM sleep. Sleepwalking often happens when people have become very sleep deprived, and both night terrors and sleepwalking are more likely to occur in the beginning of the night, when sleep debt is still high. Brain-wave recordings suggest that both sleepwalkers and night terror victims are passing back and forth rapidly between sleep and wakefulness. They wake up enough to get the most primitive parts of the brain working—the emotional brain and the basic motor centers—without engaging the brain's more reflective and self-aware functions. The sleep debt won't release its grip on the brain, so the sleeper never rises out of the blunted perception and amnesia that we all experience the first few moments after waking up. In true sleepwalking, there will be some perception but not high-level cognition: Sleepwalkers are able to recognize a door but do not know how to get a door open.

The absence of self-consciousness found in both sleepwalking and night terrors might be related to the global amnesia that people sometimes experience with extreme sleep deprivation. After all, perception is so intimately tied to memory that it is difficult to separate them. How conscious can you really be if you immediately forget what you are experiencing? Neuroscientist Gerald Edelman has proposed that consciousness is really a "remembered present," that self-awareness is an immediate memory of how we are feeling and what we are thinking. It is possible that sleepwalkers are not fully asleep, but that the part of the brain responsible for this remembering is not functioning as it normally would.

Most cases of sleepwalking and night terrors begin in early childhood, although they can continue into adulthood. Sleepwalking can begin as early as children are able to walk, but it mostly occurs between the ages of four and eight, then disappears spontaneously after adolescence. Sleepwalking seems to run in families (no pun intended), although many sufferers don't have a family history of the problem. It is interesting that it is at just around four years of age kids give up daytime napping, resulting in a maximum sleep debt at bedtime and a deep, consolidated sleep throughout the night.

Night terrors are most frightening not for the sleepers but for parents or others around them. Children with night terrors rise up out of a deep sleep seemingly truly terrified, often screaming with fright. Their eyes are open wide, as if seeing some horror that others cannot. Their hearts race, they may tremble, and they take short, shallow breaths. I can remember my own daughter terrified and whimpering in the night. Even though I was somewhat of an expert on night terrors, it was very difficult not to panic myself. "What's wrong? What's wrong?" my wife and I would ask her, but she just kept staring straight ahead, her eyes wide with fright.

Parents are understandably concerned when their children have night terrors. It is hard to see any child more scared than they have ever been before. Parents' inability to reach out and comfort their child is especially troubling. They often feel powerless, guilty, and somehow a failure as their child's protector.

I hope I can allay the anxiety and worry. A child in the middle of a night terror episode is in a sense still asleep. Such children are not having a bad dream and will almost never remember the episode. In fact, they may not be experiencing fear at all; it is their body that is expressing fright rather than their mind. Somehow it is not the conscious self that is terrified but some automatic process of the sleeping brain.

The best therapy is to focus on keeping children from harm. Speaking calmly and reassuringly to them—even though they don't respond—sometimes can slowly bring them out of their fright. Children usually calm down after 5 to 15 minutes and go back to sleep without ever really waking. If they do wake, they are confused and unable to say what was scaring them or even remember that they were scared. They'll probably forget the whole episode by morning.

About 3 percent of children experience night terrors, although many cases are probably not tabulated. Night terrors occur most often in children between two and five years of age and usually disappear completely by age seven. The disorder also may appear late in life, probably due to a form of epilepsy or organic changes in the brain. Like sleepwalking, night terrors tend to run in families. Episodes can be spurred by nothing at all, but may be more common when children have a fever, and are occasionally associated with taking medications. Sleep deprivation, which is more likely to occur in adolescents and adults, typically exacerbates these problems.

Sleepwalking or night terrors are less prevalent in adults. The attacks can have similar causes. When adults have persistent night terrors or sleepwalk, they should be evaluated by a sleep specialist. Anxiety or stress may prompt the brain to be awake. On the other hand, sleep deprivation and an overwhelming sleep debt keep the brain from fully awakening. Sleep-talking has similar causes. The brain is aroused enough to send commands to speak but not aroused enough to be conscious of the act.

Sleepwalking in adults is sometimes more akin to global amnesia. Some years ago I was scheduled to participate in a symposium on sleep disorders in Bologna, Italy, organized by my friend and pioneering sleep specialist Professor Elio Lugaresi. I was to take a polar flight to Paris and then catch a flight to Bologna. I boarded the flight in San Francisco and because I was sleep deprived, I went to sleep fairly quickly after the plane took off. My next memory was of being awakened by the flight attendant because we were landing. I looked out the window and saw buildings that I did not recognize. I was greatly puzzled because I am very familiar with the de Gaulle Airport and the appearance of the surrounding territory. To my utter amazement, we were landing at Bologna. I must have completely forgotten landing in Paris, getting off the plane, boarding a bus to another terminal, waiting for the next flight, and getting on it. In a sense I had been awake, but not conscious.

Sleepwalking also can be caused by excessive medication or by interactions between medications. The secret at the center of the very first mystery novel in the English language, Wilkie Collins's *The Moonstone,* is that the main character had sleepwalked under the influence of a sleeping potion and stolen a precious gem. Medication-induced sleepwalking is a particular problem for elderly patients who may have many prescriptions from different doctors. Too much alcohol also may initiate an episode of somnambulism.

Many people believe that stress can cause sleepwalking. The truth is that until stress produces a large sleep debt, a stressful situation will not be associated with sleepwalking. Nonetheless, this myth has persisted. An example of sleepwalking associated with stress appears in Shakespeare's *Macbeth,* a play that is full of sleep references. In this passage Lady Macbeth is feeling intense guilt about her role in goading her husband to murder the king and is observed sleepwalking by a lady-in-waiting and a doctor:

Gentlewoman: Since his majesty went into the field, I have seen her rise from her bed, throw her night-gown upon her, unlock her closet, take forth paper, fold it, write upon't, read it, afterwards seal it, and again return to bed; yet all this while in a most fast sleep.

Doctor: A great perturbation in nature, to receive at once the benefit of sleep, and do the effects of watching!

Gentlewoman: Lo you, here she comes! This is her very guise; and, upon my life, fast asleep. Observe her; stand close.

Doctor: You see, her eyes are open.

Gentlewoman: Ay, but their sense is shut. *The lady-in-waiting and the doctor observe Lady Macbeth speaking loudly and clearly as she tries to wash imagined blood from her hands.*

Doctor: Foul whisperings are abroad: unnatural deeds
   Do breed unnatural troubles: infected minds
   To their deaf pillows will discharge their secrets:
   More needs she the divine than the physician.
   God, God forgive us all! Look after her;
   Remove from her the means of all annoyance,
   And still keep eyes upon her.

Note how the doctor implies that Lady Macbeth's sleepwalking reveals problems of a psychological or spiritual rather than physical nature, and he dispenses the same advice doctors give today: Keep an eye on the patient and remove anything harmful from her way. In contrast to Shakespeare's doctor, modern sleep specialists no longer believe that people who sleepwalk or have night terrors tend to have some sort of very severe psychological problem—anxiety, fear, or guilt. A great deal of research convincingly shows that people who have any of the parasomnias—night terrors, sleepwalking, bruxism (tooth grinding), bedwetting, and the like—are no more likely to have psychological disorders than anyone else.

People tend to believe there are clear-cut distinctions between normal sleep and abnormal parasomnias, but I think it's often a difference in degree, not in kind. Few people sleepwalk in the stereotypical sense, but who hasn't turned off an alarm clock or taken a late-night phone call with no memory of doing it? Many doctors on call have had the experience of answering the phone in the middle of the night, talking to a nurse about a patient, then returning to bed and being unable to remember the call in the morning. "Boy," the nurse will say, "are you lucky I didn't do what you told me to do when I called last night." The doctor will be confused: "I don't remember your calling." We all experience episodes where the body is moving, but the mind isn't engaged. As University of Pennsylvania sleep researcher David Dinges describes it, "The starter is turning the engine over, but the engine's not catching."

Like the doctor in *Macbeth,* many people also find the blurred line between waking and sleeping unnatural and threatening. How can people be both awake and asleep, conscious but not conscious, aware of the outside world in some ways and unaware in others? If people act out, break things, or commit murder while they are sleepwalking or dreaming, should they be held responsible?

I know of at least one murder case where someone was acquitted on the grounds of sleepwalking, but I'm sure that in many more cases people have been convicted of perpetrating a crime while they were, in fact, asleep. I firmly believe any such conviction is unlawful. The sleeping self is like another person inside us, someone who is not subject to the same laws and norms as the waking world.

I admit that this idea raises some difficult questions about responsibility and accountability under the law. But we cannot hold sleeping people responsible for their actions for the same reason that we cannot hold insane people responsible; in order to do wrong in the eyes of the law, the accused has to be conscious and aware of his or her actions and their effects. If someone has an unforeseeable heart attack, passes out in the road, and causes a 10-car pileup, we can't hold that person responsible for the accident. The conscious self of the awakened state is, for all practical purposes, as different from the unconsciousness of sleep as one person is from another.

The truth of the matter is that the danger is most often to the sleepwalker himself. I know a woman whose husband and two sons were frequent sleepwalkers and night wanderers. Sadly, one son was sleepwalking on the highway one night and was killed when he was hit by a truck. Adding to her terrible emotional pain was the coroner's report, which indicated suicide as the cause of death. As a partial sublimation of her intense grief, she actively protested until, with the help of Mark Mahowald, who is a world-class expert in this area, she finally succeeded in getting the cause of death changed to a sleep disorder. She continues to work to increase awareness about these issues in the hope of avoiding more such tragedies.

Chapter 9

Our Chronically Fatigued Syndrome

A FEW YEARS AGO, I designed an experiment to find out if people are able to judge accurately how likely they are to fall asleep in a soporific situation. Forty-two student volunteers stayed up most of the night and then had a two-hour nap from 5:00 A.M. until 7:00 A.M. After this they were prepared for brain-wave recordings. They sat in front of a computer console, and at the end of every two-minute interval they were asked to judge their likelihood of falling asleep in the next two minutes (by clicking along a scale of 0 to 100 percent on the computer). In addition, throughout each two-minute interval they would click on icons that indicated they were aware of a yawn, drifting thoughts or hallucinations, heavy eyelids or eyes out of focus, head nodding, or actually falling asleep. Although the students were substantially sleep deprived, they were asked to try to stay awake during the hour of testing.

In general, the students were terrible at predicting how likely they were to fall asleep. They were videotaped continuously and brain waves were recorded, so we had extremely accurate, objective information on what happened. The students fell asleep many times in the intervals where they had predicted there was zero likelihood of falling asleep, and other times they predicted a 100 percent likelihood of falling asleep and did not.

The results are emblematic of how blind most people are to the role of the sleep drive in daily life. They accept readily that chronic sleep loss can be debilitating and dangerous, but they don't seem to recognize the urgent distress signals of fatigue, or appreciate their significance if they do, continuing to delude themselves that they know when they're at risk of falling asleep. All of the sleep episodes in our experiment lasted three seconds or longer, which is generally the time it takes an unresponsive driver to traverse a four-meter-wide highway shoulder at a speed of 60 miles per hour, at an angle of departure of only three degrees. In other words, three seconds of sleep is long enough to crash and die. If these student subjects had been trying to avoid sleep on the highway, and thought they could get off safely before sleep hit, they probably would not have made it.

In another study, I purposefully created a very boring lecture, which I gave at a senior citizens' center in the evening. Two assistants kept tabs on the small audience, each carefully watching half. Nearly all the seniors nodded off at least once. When questioned afterward, they all denied falling asleep.

The Cost of Sleep Deprivation

We are now in the midst of a pandemic of fatigue resulting from a long line of cultural, economic, health, and technological influences that can be traced back to long before Thomas Edison and his electric light bulb. Nonetheless, societal pressures to work more and at odd hours—evenings, weekends, the night shift, round-the-clock—have reduced our sleep time over the past century by about 20 percent. In the three decades since 1969, working Americans have added 158 hours annually—nearly a full month of work—to their workday (including the commute). Many of those extra hours are being carved out of sleep time, and more work has meant extending other responsibilities of daily life into nighttime hours. All major cities in the United States have 24-hour grocery stores, and other businesses are staying open later as well to accommodate people who work late and can run their errands only after getting off the job.

Add to the mix our own era's peculiar brand of "hedomasochism," the idea that we can and must do it all—work, family, sports, hobbies—and there is very little time left for sleep. The Puritan "hard-work" ethic of the nineteenth century has become the "work hard, play hard" ethic of the late twentieth century. Many of us are finding that we have run ourselves down so much that we have lost the ability to enjoy much of anything. We try to do top-notch work at the office, spend time with our spouse and kids, work out at the gym, cook and eat dinner, clean around the house, and stay up late to watch a movie. And before bed, we try to get a jump on the next day by reading reports or logging on to our e-mail.

The result of all this hard work and hard play is that we treat our sleep like a neglected child. We are resentful when the demands of sleep are inconvenient or too frequent. When we finally go to bed, we are frustrated when sleep doesn't come quickly. We express a longing for sleep while putting everything else ahead of it, spurning its cries for attention until it turns destructive.

What's the way out of this sleep-deprived time trap?

We can't very well turn back the clock and stop using modern technology. Nor do we want to celebrate the millennium by giving up all the conveniences and entertainments that prevent sleeping. Given the unending demands of our increasingly complex lives, getting more sleep is not a simple proposition.

I believe that the only solution is a radical rethinking of our relationship to sleep. We have no choice: The health threats of our modern antisleep culture are killing us. We have to face the fact that the freedom we have gained through the invention of electric lights and appliances, and more recently global communication and the Internet, requires that we make wise choices about how we use them. Unless these choices are based on knowledge about sleep deprivation and biological rhythms as well as what constitutes healthy, adequate sleep, we are likely to find ourselves sleepwalking into disaster.

In recent years some of my sleep colleagues around the world have looked outside the laboratory for data about the effects of sleepiness and sleep deprivation on performance in real-world situations. We joined forces with a prominent jewel in the federal crown, the National Transportation Safety Board. For those who understand sleep deprivation and sleep debt, there is definitely an increasing awareness that a large percentage of transportation accidents are linked to sleepiness or sleep-induced lapses in awareness. A huge proportion of assembly-line accidents also are attributed to the potent combination of sleepiness and monotonous tasks. Serious efforts to gauge the full impact of fatigue in critical industries such as aviation, medicine, trucking, and shipping, have made it clear (at least to those with a fundamental knowledge of sleep) that the problem is worse and more pervasive than anyone suspected.

The Not-So-Friendly Skies

Flying planes used to be a relatively straightforward task. Airplanes had a few basic controls, and flights were slow and short. But multiengined commercial aircraft have grown progressively more complicated. Automated aircraft controls, including autopilots and satellite navigation, make the pilot's job both easier and more complex, creating new possibilities for error. In fact, aircraft themselves are generally so well designed and thoroughly tested, and weather tracking so improved, that pilot error is now the most common cause of airplane accidents. This fact has increased the importance of learning much more about how humans perform when they are operating complex machinery, and how and why they make mistakes.

Now that airplanes fly faster and farther, sleep deprivation and circadian rhythms play a major role in how pilots perform in the cockpit. Any international flight crew can talk about the scheduling problems they have experienced and the burden of feeling sleepy in the cockpit on overseas flights.

An American Airlines flight to Cali, Colombia, in December 1995, illustrates the tragic consequences of human error caused by sleep deprivation. As the plane approached the airport in Cali, descending into a long, deep valley, the crew tried to program the plane's autopilot to lock on to a beacon called "Rozo." The copilot brought up a list of the navigation beacons starting with "R" by typing that letter into the computer. He selected the first beacon on the list, which is usually the closest. However, the sleep-deprived navigator overlooked the fact that the first was not "Rozo" but "Romeo"—a beacon more than a 100 miles away in Bogotá. The sleep-deprived human pilot didn't catch his navigator's mistake, and the plane's autopilot did what it was designed to do. It obeyed the command and, unbeknownst to the crew, made a slow turn to the left, toward Bogotá. Minutes later they realized something was wrong, but it was too late. The plane smashed into a mountain, killing 149 people.

The "black box" recording of that Cali flight is one of the most poignant narrations of pilot fatigue that I have read:

Captain: I called tracking one day and said, "Hey, this [expletive] international is doing me . . . I want you to spell out the legal rest." And that's where I got this from, and I wrote it down very explicitly. Ten hours crew rest.

First Officer: That's on international?

Captain: Yeah, if you fly less than 5¹/₂ hours.

First Officer: Which in this case . . .

Captain: That's our scenario. Ten hours crew rest, 30-minute debrief, and 1 hour sign-in. And you can't move that up at all, because it's an FAA thing. You roll those wheels before 11¹/₂ hours, you're [expletive].

[The captain mentions a pilot friend who had trouble flying international routes, then continues.]

Captain: He said he didn't mind it, he didn't mind driving back home at five o'clock in the morning. But to me, I'm like . . . it's torture.

First Officer: Yeah.

Captain: Torture in the [expletive] car, trying to keep awake and stay alive, uh-huh. I discussed this with my wife. I said, "Honey, I just don't want to do this, I hope you don't feel like I'm [unintelligible.] She said, "No way, forget it. You don't need to do that [expletive]. [Sound of yawning.]

It was a cruel irony that the pilot and first officer didn't hear the warnings in their own words. Their mistake is typical of those made by people who are too sleepy to pay attention to details that can spell the difference between life and death.

NASA—the National Aeronautics and Space Administration—conducted one of the most important programs in fatigue research to learn how pilots are affected by fatigue and to develop effective ways to recognize and counteract it. For many years the director of this

Fatigue Countermeasures Program was a former student and colleague of mine, Mark Rosekind. (I have fond memories of Mark entertaining kids at the Stanford Summer Sleep Camp with magic tricks. He also took this skill to NASA, where he taught a shuttle astronaut what became the first magic trick performed in space.) At NASA, Mark designed the first program to measure accurately exactly what happens to flight crews on long-haul and short-haul flights.

Mark and his colleagues boarded planes and wired up the pilots to portable EEGs. The pilots took skill and reaction tests on handheld computers at set intervals. After observing and testing pilots on commercial, transpacific flights between San Francisco, Japan, Hawaii, and Los Angeles, Mark came away with frightening results. The reaction times of pilots flying these routes during the night decreased by more than 25 percent, very similar to the blunted reactions found in people who have stayed up all night. Furthermore, the pilots frequently fell into brief episodes of sleep—episodes of falling asleep for 5 to 10 seconds. Fifteen percent of the episodes lasted more than 15 seconds. During these microsleeps, pilots were effectively out of touch with the world, unable to react to emergencies.

As Rosekind points out, these studies probably presented the rosiest possible picture, since the pilots knew they were wired to EEG machines and were being watched by an observer sitting in back of them, which should have created unusual motivation to stay awake. And yet, they fell asleep. Anecdotal evidence suggests that conditions are much worse in unmonitored situation. One pilot who testified before the National Commission on Sleep Disorders said that at times he was so sleepy that he was "nodding off as we got into take-off position."

Such impairment might not be so troublesome during the middle of the flight, when pilots are not likely to have many demands on their attention. But Rosekind's group also found that some pilots were conking out in the final 30 minutes of flight, during descent and landing of the airplane. Among the nine pilots in the study section, there were five episodes of microsleep during the last 10 minutes of flight. Think about that: They were falling asleep as they landed the plane.

Doctors Asleep on Their Feet

It's alarming, but somewhat understandable, that pilots crossing multiple time zones have fatigue problems. What's more disturbing to me directly is that the health care professionals in whose hands we literally place our lives—surgeons, anesthesiologists, and emergency room doctors and nurses—are themselves chronically and severely sleep deprived. It is not unusual for medical residents and interns—the foot soldiers of hospital and emergency room care—to work 100 hours during a week that includes two nights on call. After a few highly publicized malpractice cases due to sleepiness, doctors' shifts in New York are now regulated to last no more than 16 hours per day with at least one continuous 24-hour period off per week and a four-week average of 80 hours per week. Of course, if you do the math, you realize that someone working six 16-hour days in one week, for a total of 96 hours, would still be in compliance with these guidelines, as long as the person brought the average time down to 80 the following week. That leaves no more than four or five hours for sleep per day. But according to a recent exposé in *The New York Times,* these guidelines are routinely violated and emergency room doctors in hospitals throughout Manhattan continue to rack up 100-hour work weeks.

The scene inside operating rooms is frightening to contemplate. Surgeons, anesthesiologists, and nurses are all on call multiple nights a week. Doctors may be called into emergency surgery at 2:00 A.M., operate for five hours, and go straight into a previously scheduled 7:00 A.M. surgery. Patients have no idea that the surgeons preparing to cut into them are working on two or three hours' sleep or fatigued by a long operation the night before.

One story out of the scores that I have heard is particularly striking for the light it sheds on our not-so-benign neglect of sleep deprivation. In 1993 a team of Colorado doctors brought an eight-year-old boy into the operating room for what should have been a minor surgical operation. The anesthesiologist assigned to the case was notorious for working while extremely fatigued, and he admitted that he sometimes fell asleep during operations. But despite a seemingly universal awareness among other doctors and nurses of the anesthesiologist's frequent drowsiness at work, he was allowed to administer general anesthesia to the boy.

Surgeons avoid using general anesthesia whenever possible because sometimes there is only a small margin of error between a dose that produces deep unconsciousness and one that causes death. Everyone has a slightly different reaction to anesthetic medications, and a given dose has different effects on different people. These factors make anesthesiology the medical equivalent of flying an airplane. Both are highly complex, technological fields that follow a predictable routine most of the time. Usually anesthesiologists have little to do except monitor the instruments. When things go wrong, however, they can go wrong in a hurry. More than any other medical profession, anesthesiology consists of days or weeks of routine and somewhat tedious activity—and fleeting moments of sheer terror.

For the eight-year-old boy, things did go wrong. And in the critical moments that followed, the anesthesiologist failed to perform his duties properly. The boy died. In the resulting civil court trial, the doctor admitted he had made fatal errors during the operation but denied that he fell asleep. Nonetheless, the jury determined that the physician was guilty of "grossly negligent medical care."

This and similar tragedies highlight the enormity of the medical establishment's almost willful ignorance about the dangers of fatigue. If any physician was falling-down drunk when he arrived at the operating theater, he would never have been allowed to work. Being drunk impairs performance significantly, even if intoxication isn't so extreme that the drinker actually passes out. To say that someone can be held responsible for fatigue-induced errors only if they fall asleep is like saying that a drunk driver cannot be cited unless he actually passed out at the wheel. Yet trials and investigations of accidents caused by fatigued drivers, doctors, and pilots usually focus on whether or not the person actually fell asleep rather than on their state of mind in the moments before the accident.

Of course we must accept that doctors will occasionally make a mistake. No one is perfect. On the other hand, if a doctor makes a mistake because of fatigue, then that is unacceptable, in my opinion. Some years ago in an anonymous survey, 42 percent of the house staff of a San Francisco hospital, admitted killing at least one patient by making a fatigue-related mistake. Over the years, we have run the

Multiple Sleep Latency Test on nurses and resident physicians; I can remember only one who was not in the twilight zone of extreme sleepiness.

Unsafe at Any Speed

Even if we're not undergoing surgery or flying aloft at 30,000 feet, almost all of us engage in a daily game of Russian roulette where the stakes for competent performance are just as high. How? By driving a car. Given the enormous prevalence of sleep deprivation, it is surprising how little research has been done on exactly how sleep deprivation and circadian rhythms affect people's driving ability. But we do know that 33 percent of traffic accidents are traceable to sleepiness. And we know that fatigue is the number-one cause of fatal crashes in young drivers, ages 18 to 25. In a poll by the Gallup Organization, 31 percent of all adult respondents reported having dozed off at the wheel of an automobile, and 4 percent reported auto accidents due to sleepiness.

Fatigue likely plays a large role in most car accidents labeled "cause unknown." But one of the reasons fatigue is such a pernicious enemy of highway safety is that it affects us in unpredictable, individualized ways. If 100 drivers were to drink a half pint of whiskey, we could not predict with absolute certainty how many accidents would occur if they all drove over the same route for the same amount of time. There might be no accidents, or there might be many. Some might refuse to drive; others might drive very slowly and carefully. By the same token, if the same 100 drivers had drunk no alcohol whatsoever but had been awake all night long and drove the same route, there might be no accidents, or there might be many. But just as we know with absolute certainty that drunken drivers have more accidents than sober drivers, we know with absolute certainty that sleep-deprived drivers have more accidents than well-rested, wide-awake drivers.

Sleep debt accumulates whenever we are awake. When we do not get the sleep we need over a series of nights, or if sleep is interrupted frequently, sleep debt is not erased completely and carries over from one day to the next. It is best to think of a large sleep debt as a very big load that we carry around. If we are strong, we can carry the load without any help. When we are not strong or when we stumble, the load becomes very difficult to bear and may crush us. The way we feel at any instant is not a reliable index of the sleep debt or load we are carrying. This is because stimulation, excitement, or vigorous exercise can completely suppress any tendency to feel sleepy or drowsy. On the other hand, one very simple life-saving principle should be embraced as gospel truth: *If you become drowsy at any time during the day, you have a sizable sleep debt and you should resolve to be cautious in hazardous situations.* This is particularly true during activities that are repetitive, soporific, or sedentary—driving chief among them.

In 1990, on the heels of their report about the *Exxon Valdez*, the National Transportation and Safety Board recognized that fatigue is the most frequent, direct cause of truck accidents in which the driver is killed. It doesn't take a rocket scientist to realize that long-haul truck drivers are almost by definition severely sleep deprived. However, as the National Commission on Sleep Disorders Research delved into all sorts of issues, I began to wonder how many long-haul truck drivers also suffered from the prevalent sleep disorder obstructive sleep apnea.

In 1991, the second year of the commission's existence, we initiated a study of the overnight sleep of truck drivers. I persuaded the safety manager of a company whose trucks drove all over the United States to allow this intrusion; in retrospect, it is clear he did not know what he was getting into. Accompanying me to the company's transportation hub were Drs. Gèrman Nino-Murcia and Riccardo Stoohs, commission investigators Anna Itoi and L'Ann Bingham, and portable sleep monitoring equipment. Anna Itoi is not exactly tiny, but she looked like a Lilliputian standing beside a burly truck driver.

Led by Anna and L'ann, we would enter the dormitory or cafeteria and ask drivers if they would mind sleeping one night with our equipment. We also had them answer a series of questions about sleep, alertness, and driving. We were able to question 602 drivers, 90 percent males, as well as conduct actual overnight sleep recordings on 200.

The first big surprise was the response to the question "When do you feel you should stop driving?" Eighty-two percent of the drivers replied that they would stop driving when they had a startle resulting from a head drop, or when they saw something in the road that wasn't there (a hypnagogic hallucination). To me, both of these events signal that they had already fallen asleep at the wheel.

The second big surprise was the huge number of drivers who had obstructive sleep apnea. Well over 70 percent were diagnosed with sleep apnea, and 13 percent had a very severe condition. This is about three times the rate found in the general population. Given all the other information we have uncovered about the high rates of accidents among sleep apnea patients, this was alarming news.

When we told the company about our findings, it was as if an iron curtain had fallen in front of us. Everyone in the company suddenly became unavailable to us. The reasons are not clear—skepticism about such dramatic findings, perhaps, or a threat to important economic interests. Of course it did not help that not one driver we encountered, not one manager, not one safety manager or even the three on-site company physicians had ever heard of obstructive sleep apnea or were aware of its significance. In 1991 even fewer people had ever heard of obstructive sleep apnea than today, if that is possible, and no one in the company had any notion that sleep loss accumulates as a debt. We were far enough along in our research to put a paragraph about this study in the final report of the National Commission on Sleep Disorder Research.

The third big revelation for me, although it was not directly involved in our study, was the dispatching system. Fifty dispatchers sat at as many desks in one huge gymnasium, each talking through a headset to an average of 50 trucks all over the United States. The atmosphere in the room was thick with sweat and adrenaline as the dispatchers urged and prodded these 2,500 refrigerated trucks to their destination. The truckers were carrying mostly perishable products that needed to arrive at their destinations "just in time." There was almost a desperation in the voices and behavior of the dispatchers as they wheedled, pleaded, prodded and threatened drivers in order to get the loads to their destinations on time. What I found truly frightening was that there were large bonuses for getting the most loads to the most destinations, being on time the most often, and being late the least often. The dispatcher's function was to egg on the drivers and keep them on the road as long as possible. What this really meant was that drivers were penalized for getting a decent night's sleep or responding to the first signs of drowsiness.

One of the most recent large research project was sponsored by the U.S. Department of Transportation, Canadian Transportation officials, and trucking industry groups, who undertook a $4.5-million several-year study of fatigue and alertness among commercial drivers. The study, which was published in 1997, proved conclusively that poor scheduling of work and rest time and a lack of training for recognizing sleep problems among drivers and managers are major problems in the industry. The study showed that drivers got two hours less sleep per day than they should and that time of day (corresponding to circadian dips of the early afternoon and early morning) were major factors in trucking accidents.

Long hauls are part of the job for truckers, but for ordinary drivers, long trips usually represent some disruption to the normal schedule. Stanford's Christian Guilleminault was one of a group of researchers who, with the help of the French highway patrol, randomly stopped 2,197 automobile drivers one holiday weekend. They found that 80 percent of the drivers were on vacation, and half had decreased their total sleep time before departure that morning. A quarter had lost more than three hours of sleep before their departure.

We're all familiar with this scenario: We wake up earlier than usual to get a jump start on the long drive, or we leave for vacation in a severely sleep-deprived state after extra hours of work and preparation for the trip. Most people have therefore had the experience of fighting to stay awake while driving on vacation. Some actually have nodded off at the wheel, while others take the lesson to heart and find a place to pull off and rest. Yet in my experience, most people claim that they can drive sleepy and handle it. Their attitude is akin to someone being happy to sit on a bomb every day, complacent because it hasn't gone off yet. My response is that it only takes one slip-up to ruin their own lives and the lives of others. When I'm driving and I begin to feel the desire for the delicious relief of falling asleep, I immediately feel intense terror and alarm. It is as if someone has pointed a gun to my head. The indelible memories of stories and photographs of dead children on the highway flash through my mind. I have vowed that I will never be the cause of such an accident. I always pull over and take a nap.

We must never forget, however, that poor scheduling and reduced sleep are not the sole dangers. Many drivers are fatigued because they have a sleep disorder that makes it impossible for them to get an adequate night's sleep. A study of 6,000 patients with sleep apnea, for example, found that 15.6 percent had had at least one car accident, as opposed to only 6.7 percent for drivers in the nonapnea control group who reported ever having an accident. That means people with sleep apnea are more than twice as likely to get in at least one car accident over the course of their lifetime as people without apnea. Even worse, the combination of alcohol use (two or more drinks per day) with severe apnea was associated with a fivefold increase in sleep-related accidents compared to healthy drivers with minimal to moderate alcohol use. I must point out that when patients' apnea is treated, their accident rates fall to the level of the population at large. Yet another reason to diagnose and treat.

It should be obvious by now that the lessons from these studies apply to all of us who are not getting the amount or kind of sleep we need. They apply to anyone who has ever yawned while driving and didn't see it as a warning of danger ahead. It has taken a long time for society to recognize the dangers of drunken driving and to get the word out that driving while drunk is not acceptable. We need a similar public education campaign against driving when sleepy. People in the cemetery or their families don't care if you were drunk or sleepy when you hit them. Over the long term no quantity of coffee and no amount of willpower will keep you awake if your sleep load and your biological clock are working in tandem to put your brain to sleep.

The Anatomy of Fatigue

Some of the consequences of poor sleep can be very annoying or expensive instead of tragic, such as the patient I once had who was so sleepy she loaded her dirty dishes into the clothes dryer instead of the dishwasher. She realized her error only after turning on the machine and hearing the clatter of breaking dishes. Another patient went to great lengths to secure a 50-yard-line ticket to a crucial 49ers playoff game but was so sleepy that he dozed off in his seat in the first quarter and stayed asleep until the game was over. On an everyday level, sleepy people make math errors, drop things, and become emotionally distant from their families, friends, and colleagues.

What's dangerously deceptive is how awake you can feel even

when you're carrying a heavy sleep load. That's because sleep debt is counteracted by arousal—both from the periodic alerting effects of the biological clock and from the alerting effects of excitement or stress. You can stave off the effects of large sleep loads in the short term by staying engaged in stimulating activities—for most of us, it's the pressing demands of the day's tasks. But the weight of sleep deprivation can't be ignored indefinitely. Eventually it catches up with you, usually when you relax a little, or when the body's clock-dependent alerting is at its lowest points during the early morning and the early afternoon. When arousal temporarily subsides, your underlying sleep drive is unleashed like a dammed-up river, and you're in immediate danger of being swamped by sleep, no matter where you are or what you're doing.

A relatively benign example of sleep deprivation is what might be called the Saturday syndrome. Many people work long, hard hours through the week, hoping to catch up on sleep over the weekend. They may collapse into bed Friday night and sleep deeply until late in the morning. Even though they've paid back several hours of sleep debt, they walk around like zombies all day Saturday, barely able to stay awake in front of the televised ball game or at the dinner table. One reason is obvious: You can't pay back a week's accumulated sleep debt in one night. The other, less apparent, reason for weekend fatigue is that the stressful arousal of the weekday workplace is no longer masking sleep debt. Since people tend to drink and eat more on weekends, their sleep-fighting arousal is further suppressed. Many weekend traffic accidents are due to the perilous combination of too much alcohol, unrecognized residual sleep debt, and reduced stress.

To understand how vulnerable we are to the hazards of sleepiness, we need to understand that waking consciousness is an ongoing tug of war. Sleep debt is always driving the brain toward sleep, while stimulation from the biological clock and the environment is promoting wakefulness. As I have explained before, all wakefulness is sleep deprivation. You build up sleep debt over the course of the day, then pay it off as you sleep that night. If you get an hour less than a full night's sleep, you carry an hour of sleep debt into the next day—and your drive toward sleep becomes stronger. Sleep debt accumulates in an additive fashion, so that if you get one hour less sleep than you need for each of eight nights, your brain will then tend toward sleep as strongly as if you'd stayed up all night. Sleep deprivation is the most common brain impairment.

People are often incredulous when I tell them that a typical week's worth of accumulated sleep debt can have a devastating effect on motor and intellectual functions. But lab tests have confirmed this ruthless arithmetic. In his latest research, University of Pennsylvania fatigue expert David Dinges restricted the sleep of volunteers over a two-week period. Dave concluded that when people sleep only four hours a night for two weeks, their performance scores are the same as those of people who were kept up for three straight days and nights.

Dave found that within his test group, individual sensitivity to sleep load initially varied widely, much the way people's susceptibility to alcohol does. But at the end of the two-week period, everyone was seriously impaired by long-term slept debt. Dave and other researchers have demonstrated that chronic sleep loss degrades nearly every aspect of human performance: vigilance (ability to receive information), alertness (ability to act on information), and attention span. In simple terms, a large sleep debt "makes you stupid." People take longer to react to challenging situations, and their reactions are more variable and less effective than when they are well rested.

"It has taken years to create tests that can accurately measure performance," Dave reports, "but as our probes have gotten better, we've found that the effects of sleep deprivation are beyond what we had imagined. Every time we turn a page we find that it's worse than we thought."

The comparison between sleep deprivation and alcohol intoxication is striking in this regard. Researchers in Australia have found that there is more than just a surface similarity between the two. The Australian investigators split 40 volunteers into two groups. One group was kept awake for 28 hours, from 8:00 A.M. until 2:00 P.M. the next day. The other group was given 10 to 15 grams of alcohol every 30 minutes starting at 8:00 A.M., until each volunteer's blood-alcohol level reached 0.1 percent, which is more than legally drunk in most locales. During these periods, both groups were given hand-eye coordination tests. The Australian researchers found that after 17 hours awake (at 1:00 A.M., when biological alerting is declining), the sleep-deprived group had the same test scores as drinking volunteers who had blood alcohol levels of 0.05 percent. After 24 hours awake, the sleep-deprived group had the same coordination deficits as those with the maximum blood alcohol level, 0.1 percent.

When you are extremely sleep deprived, sleep is so beguiling that little else seems to matter. One group of sleep researchers recently studied six female college students deprived of 24 hours of sleep who were given a series of psychomotor finger-tapping tests and asked questions designed to assess their level of motivation to perform the tests. The results suggested that the subjects' motivation to respond, more than their capacity to do so, was the primary factor in the deterioration of their cognitive and motor performance during sleep deprivation.

Time after time, records of various transportation disasters show that people who are sleep deprived react to dangerous situations with indifference. Before a plane crashed on approach to the Guantanamo Naval Base in Cuba—the first major airplane crash to be officially attributed by the National Transportation Safety Board to crew fatigue—the sleep-deprived crew inexplicably pursued a difficult approach instead of an easier one. Before the Chernobyl nuclear reactor melted down—in the wee hours of the morning, when clock-dependent alerting is at its lowest point—the engineers clearly noticed but bizarrely did not respond to critical warnings that should have caused panic. Charles Lindbergh, in his book about the first solo flight across the Atlantic Ocean in 1928, describes this state eloquently. Lindbergh started on the 33-1/2-hour flight after having been up for more than a day and a half already—which meant that by the time he completed the flight, he had been awake for almost 70 hours. Describing the flight, he wrote, "My mind clicks on and off . . . My whole body argues dully that nothing, nothing life can attain, is quite so desirable as sleep." Lindbergh actually did fall asleep on his flight and nearly crashed into the ocean, but woke up in time.

When the brain has been slipping back and forth between sleep and wakefulness, it can go on autopilot, producing what is called automatic behavior. Most people have experienced this at some time. You are driving or walking down the road, and suddenly cannot remember what has happened or what you have seen over the last 10 or 15 minutes, sometimes much longer. You were functioning reasonably well—you were able to avoid bumping into anything—but you are not laying down the usual memory traces. It is almost like sleepwalking, except that it arises out of wakefulness rather than sleep. As sleep debt increases, automatic behavior becomes more common.

Sleepiness Dulls the Competitive Edge

Safety isn't the only area impacted by fatigue. All of the problems that accompany sleepiness—inability to focus, delayed and poor decision making, indifference, lack of motivation—affect the quality of our work. Even if lives are not riding on your decisions at work, livelihoods probably are. Simple miscalculations or overlooked problems can cause figurative train wrecks. Mark Rosekind once gave a workshop on sleep, fatigue, and decision making to a group of private pilots for the MCI Corporation. In the back of the audience were other MCI employees. After the workshop, an executive's assistant asked Rosekind, "This stuff doesn't just apply to pilots, does it?" It turned out that MCI officials were about to travel to London to negotiate a merger with British Telecom. Billions of dollars were riding on these negotiations, yet no one had made plans to ensure that the executives got enough sleep and rest to adjust to the new time zone before they met with British officials. The assistant went back and changed their travel schedules.

Elite athletes are also vulnerable to sleep deprivation and disrupted circadian rhythms. At the Summer Olympics in Atlanta in 1996, investigators studied the effects of jet lag on 12 Korean athletes. After the plane trip from Korea to Atlanta, which spanned 10 time zones, nearly all the Korean athletes experienced fatigue and one-third complained of decreased strength. On average, the athletes required four days of adjustment before they could achieve athletic results similar to their baseline performance in Korea. Notably, half of the athletes were adversely affected by ambient noise in their sleeping quarters, and half also snored regularly or had pauses in their breathing while sleeping.

My colleague Roger Smith has demonstrated that circadian rhythms are an important hidden factor in professional football games as well. The "home-field advantage" is often talked about, but people always have assumed that this advantage lies in the familiarity of the field and the support of the home fans. Smith showed that this is not necessarily true: The advantage goes to the team that is playing at the time of peak circadian alerting. In other words, if the game is played during the midafternoon physiological dip for the local team, but the visitors from the East are already in their period of evening alerting, the visitors will have the advantage. Smith showed that by factoring in circadian rhythms he could, over time, beat the point spread by handicapping teams better than the experts. I couldn't help thinking of his study in December 1997 when the Green Bay Packers kept the San Francisco 49ers out of the Super Bowl by beating them in a playoff game in San Francisco. The 1:00 P.M. game was played just as the Packers' circadian alerting was beginning to rise to its evening peak and the 49ers' clock was falling into the afternoon dip in alertness (1:00 to 4:00 P.M. PST).

Before you rush off to place a bet, consider the broader implications of this research. In addition to demonstrating effects on motor performance, many sports engage skill sets that are essential to business, such as strategy, clear thinking, and quick reactions. Knowing how people are affected by sleep load and circadian rhythms can give you an advantage in any form of competition. Whether you are betting against the other guy, playing against him, negotiating with him, or investing in the marketplace against him, you can use your knowledge of sleep to help you prevail.

Mark Rosekind has now left NASA and started a consulting firm to help companies deal with sleep in the workplace. Mark tells me that the usual sequence of events when clients start learning about sleep is first to deny the problem, then to recognize it and seek a quick fix. He explains that every person needs to tailor his or her own approach to reclaiming healthy sleep, based on a working knowledge of the science of sleep, and the person's individual sleep profile. At some point the idea clicks in clients' heads, and they see how they can use their knowledge to set up meetings for periods when they'll be at their peak, or take catnaps to allow them to outlast others who are working late on a rush project. Negotiators can use knowledge about sleep to best opponents in areas of finances, career, or health. Sleep-deprived people often become indifferent and agree to conditions that would be unacceptable in their more lucid moments. The military already uses circadian factors when choosing when to launch attacks on the enemy—usually between midnight and 4:00 A.M., when the opposition is at its lowest level of alertness. Police could use knowledge of circadian rhythms to apprehend criminals more easily and more safely.

I can think of no better way to conclude and reinforce the material of this chapter than by relating my own near death as a result of obstructive sleep apnea. In November 1996 I had flown on the final leg of a lecture tour to Portland, Oregon, to speak at a conference on traffic safety sponsored by the Washington State Department of Transportation. The actual site of the conference was Skamania Lodge, on the Columbia River about forty miles east of Portland.

The plane landed around noon, and I decided to hail a taxi rather than wait for a limousine. I did not really get a good look at the driver as I climbed into the cab. We crossed the Portland bridge and headed east on a two-lane highway above the Columbia River gorge. I had planned to take a short nap, but some guardian angel kept me awake and saved my life.

About two thirds of the way to the lodge, I suddenly heard the gravel noise of the taxi going off the road. Responding instantly, I yelled and reached over the seat to grab the steering wheel. We veered into the westbound lane, but fortunately there were no oncoming vehicles. I won't quote my angry words to the driver, but when we got to the lodge, I immediately understood. My driver was obese with a relatively small jaw and a thick neck. Using the lobby of the lodge as my clinic, I took a brief medical history:

"Do you snore?" Answer: "Yes. My wife won't sleep in the same room." "Are you tired in the daytime?" Answer: "I don't have any pep at all. I'm driving a cab because the stop–and–go keeps me awake." "Do you have high blood pressure?" Answer: "Yes, I'm taking pills." "Have you complained about being tired to your doctor?" Answer: "Yes, I've even seen other doctors besides my own." "What did they do?" Answer: "Nothing, really."

I had a camera with me, so I took his picture. I made a slide, which I now show almost every time I lecture. My strong point is that sleep disorders are all around us. Make no mistake. Sleep apnea is part of your life in one way or another. No one is safe. If my taxi had crashed into the Columbia River gorge, the accident would have been blamed on brake failure or some other nonsense. That my death was sleep related, let alone that it was caused by obstructive sleep apnea, would never be known. How supremely ironic such a purposeless death would have been.

I warned the driver that he was abnormally sleepy because of a disorder called obstructive sleep apnea, and made him promise he would get off the road anytime he felt the least bit drowsy. The next day I arranged for him to be tested in a Portland sleep center. The results were as expected. Very severe obstructive sleep apnea.

What can we say about this that will make a difference? In many places in America, this person is your school-bus driver, your truck driver, your doctor, your air traffic controller—it might even be you.

PART THREE

When Sleep Works

ONE OF MY great loves in life is jazz music. When I was an undergraduate at the University of Washington, I used to play bass in a jazz
group—partly for tuition money, but also for the sheer joy of playing. Our Seattle jam sessions were well known enough that members
of big bands coming through town would join us. I befriended and
played with Quincy Jones and Ray Charles, among others. I stopped
playing professionally when I went to the University of Chicago—
not because medical school was too demanding but because the
musicians' union dues were too high (about $1,000 in Chicago,
compared to $150 in Seattle). After that I kept playing for pleasure,
but the opportunities were fewer. Although I haven't brought out
the bass much recently, for a number of years I played with amateur
groups at Stanford whenever I got the chance, and even played a role
in fostering an academic program in the Department of Music at
Stanford as chairman of the Committee for Jazz. (For a few years we
had as artist-in-residence one of the all-time greats, Stan Getz. It was
great to get to know and work with him and once, just once, to play
with him—in 1989, in my own living room.)

It has often struck me how much jazz mirrors life. In life there are
certain constants, certain patterns that form the rhythm of our days,
and out of that regularity arise unique events, wonderful chance
occurrences, dazzling interactions and ideas. In jazz the bass and

drums lay down the beat—which becomes the foundation for the melodic improvisation of the trumpet or guitar or sax, thereby creating musical ideas that are rooted in the underlying rhythm and at the same time create something new.

There is another similarity, too. When one player just can't swing with the rest of the group, it makes the whole thing hard for everyone. Everything seems effortless when the whole band is jamming, but one out-of-rhythm musician—even though the audience may not notice—just makes it hard, exhausting work. In the same way, when people are out of rhythm with their sleep cycles, or when a large sleep debt is dragging them down, it makes everything else in life so hard. They may not even feel sleepy, but everything seems more difficult.

When sleep works—and when we allow it to work—our minds and bodies are in tune and working together. By relieving the drag of sleep debt, sleep bolsters us in countless ways, augmenting our feelings of happiness and vitality and enhancing the crucial qualities of mind—pleasure, motivation, memory, and insight—that we need to reach our potential for creativity, productivity, and learning.

In this section of the book I want to give you a quick tour of what is a fast growing field—the scientific study of how sleep (and lack of sleep) affects us biologically and psychologically. In many instances, the things that I am discussing here will not be confirmed by decades of science. Sleep science is young and not well funded—in large part because the need to fight disease is what drives most research in the basic biological sciences. So much of this story is incomplete, a mere preview of things to come. Sleep researchers who are tilling these fields of science face the greatest mysteries about sleep but also have the potential to find its greatest promise. I'm convinced that answers to questions about everyday sleep eventually will improve our lives dramatically and let us really jam.

Chapter 10

What Does Sleep Do?

THE BELIEF that the purpose of sleep is rest the body, particularly the muscles, is still widespread. This is in spite of the fact there is no direct evidence whatsoever supporting this belief. Certain muscles are active continuously without need for rest. For example, the heart doesn't stop beating a few hours every day to rest, nor does the diaphragm take a break from its everlasting job. Even the brain does not rest during sleep in the sense of becoming inactive, and REM sleep is almost the opposite of rest for the brain. Clearly, we sleep to rest the body nor to rest the brain. So, if functional sleep is not a physical repose, then what is it doing for us? Why do we sleep?

It boils down to the question of whether sleep serves a "vital purpose"—is there some critical function that sleep performs, without which we would die? Eating and drinking have a vital purpose: Eating provides caloric energy that keeps life's machinery running, water provides the essential fluid that this machinery needs. But sleep? There are theories, guesses, some very suggestive experiments, but nothing has yet pinned down the precise reason the body must lie still and the mind draw inward for a third of every day. To paraphrase University of Chicago sleep scientist Allan Rechtschaffen: "If the many hours of sleep accomplish nothing, it is the greatest mistake nature ever made." And remember, there are really two kinds of sleep, REM and non-REM. A true understanding of sleep requires an explanation of the purpose for each.

The search for the original cause of sleep has sometimes been called sleep scientists' quest for the Holy Grail. While some of my colleagues wonder if we will ever achieve this knowledge, I believe it is almost inevitable. I can remember when I believed the blueprint for every detail of a human being could not possibly be crammed into the vanishingly tiny nucleus of a single cell. The answer to the mystery of sleep will be found if society is willing to commit the investigative resources required.

The Human Limits of Sleep Deprivation

I once thought that we would discover the fundamental purpose of sleep simply by preventing people from sleeping and observing the result. A huge number of biological functions have been revealed by process of elimination. For example, removing the thyroid in experimental animals immediately demonstrated its important role in metabolism and growth. I have already mentioned the prolonged wakefulness marathon of Peter Tripp, the New York disk jockey. Remember that Tripp's paranoia and hallucinations were probably caused mainly by the stimulants he was given to keep him awake. The initial interpretation was that these abnormal manifestations were caused by the sleep deprivation and that sleep and dreams preserved sanity. The theory was that without sleep, people's minds would break loose from the foundations of reality and be subject to madness.

Six years after observing Tripp, I had the chance to study another person undergoing long-term sleep deprivation. In this case I observed the entire marathon, and it changed my viewpoint about the psychological effects of prolonged sleeplessness. It was January 1965 when I read in a local paper that a San Diego high school student named Randy Gardner was attempting to break the *Guinness Book of World Records* mark for the longest time awake: 260 hours. Randy and two friends had decided that they could do better. I hasten to add that I was skeptical about this record since its holder was not carefully monitored. Randy intended to stay up 11 whole days, or 264 hours, and his friends were going to help him stay awake.

What to most readers must have seemed an interesting but inconsequential news item was to me a rare and golden opportunity that galvanized me into action: a chance to study extreme sleep deprivation in a highly motivated subject. Best of all, it didn't require a grant application. Elated, I immediately called Randy's home, explained to him and his parents who I was, and asked if I could observe him attempt to break the record. Randy had only started day 2 of his wakefulness marathon, with slightly less than 10 more days to go, and I think his parents were glad to have a medical observer to ease their fears that their son's vigil might affect his health. With their consent, I flew south and set up camp at a local motel.

I spent little time in my motel room. Every day, and much of each night, I passed the hours at Randy's house. I found him to be a really great kid and very easy to get along with. At first he found staying awake fairly easy. However, by the third day, it became very difficult, particularly at night. He had to be watched every second to prevent him from inadvertently nodding off. At that point I began spending all night at his house to make absolutely sure he stayed awake. If he began to fall asleep, I would hustle him outside to the small basketball court in his backyard or drive him around the deserted San Diego streets in a convertible with the top down and the radio playing loudly.

A serious problem I did not foresee was that I soon became very sleep deprived myself. On day 5, I turned the wrong way onto a one-way street and almost crashed head-on into a police car. The officers were extremely annoyed. I tried to explain that I was a sleep researcher conducting an experiment, but my story seemed only to increase their annoyance. From the perspective of what I know today about the potential consequences of driving drowsy, I certainly deserved the citation. The epilogue to the story is that I forgot to pay the ticket, and when they finally caught up with me, the fine plus penalties cost me a whopping (in today's dollars) $2,000.

On that day I realized that I needed help if I was to observe Randy safely. I called a fellow sleep researcher in Palo Alto, Dr. George Gulevich, and asked him to join me in San Diego to take a shift keeping Randy awake. We also needed an EEG machine so that we could record Randy's recovery sleep when he ended the marathon. George bought two airplane tickets—one for himself and one for the machine—and flew south with the EEG strapped into the seat beside

him. Randy's friends were still helping a little, but the task of keeping the young man company and keeping him awake fell mostly to
George and me. We traded off shifts, so that one of us was with him
at all times.

I vividly remember that the most arduous time was consistently
between 3:00 A.M. and 7:00 A.M. In the wee hours of the morning,
Randy would become very irritable about the fact that we wouldn't
let him close his eyes. "I'm not going to sleep," he would insist, "I'm
just resting my eyes." We know now that he was certainly having
microsleeps every time he closed his eyes for more than a second or
two, but we didn't know enough about this at the time. When he
appeared dangerously close to unambiguously falling asleep, we had
to shake him over and over and urge him on: "Randy, Randy, you
can't fall asleep." He sometimes got extremely angry, occasionally
even forgetting why he wasn't supposed to sleep. "Why are you
doing this to me?" he would say. During the early-morning hours,
he would get so sleepy that no amount of talking or shaking could
keep him awake. Fortunately, playing basketball always worked. We
almost had to drag him out to the backyard, but once he was there
and got moving, he was much better.

At about midpoint in the vigil, I received a call from LaVerne
Johnson and Ardie Lubin, sleep researchers at the San Diego Naval
Hospital. Ardie had worked on sleep deprivation for the army a
decade earlier at the Walter Reed Medical Center in Washington,
D.C. Ardie and LaVerne offered their facilities to record Randy's
recovery sleep, and they were able to carry out some more sophisticated tests of his psychological and muscular performance.

As Randy's ordeal neared its end, staying awake actually got a little
easier for him because his record-breaking wakefulness marathon
started attracting a tidal wave of worldwide media attention. This was
obviously very stimulating for an 18-year-old high school student.
The phone was ringing constantly. Reporters from newspapers and
magazines were calling from as far away as Europe and Japan, and we
even had inquiries from small-town newspapers in Indiana and Mississippi, as well as other very out-of-the-way places. Reporters and
cameramen began to congregate at his home. Although just an ordinary tired high school student, Randy had the eyes of the whole

world on him. He became much more motivated to keep going—he couldn't allow himself to fail in front of a worldwide audience.

I spent day 10 walking around town with Randy and was generally very impressed at how well he was doing. We went to a penny arcade, where we played innumerable games on a mechanical base-ball machine. He beat me every time. On the last night of the vigil, he easily bested me in several 3:00 A.M. games of basketball. At 5:00 A.M. that morning Randy held a press conference. Even though it was the crack of dawn, all local and national TV cameras that had joined the throng showed up. More than 30 years later, it remains the largest media event I have ever attended. At a lectern bristling with microphones, Randy seemed like the President of the United States. He conducted himself flawlessly, neither slurring nor stumbling over words.

After the press conference, Randy went to sleep. George Gulevich and I were glad we weren't monitoring him ourselves in the motel. With the Naval Hospital folks handling the recording task, we were free to answer some of the many phone calls from around the world. "Will he ever wake up?" "How long will he sleep?"

Randy went to sleep at 6:00 A.M., 264 hours after having awakened 11 days earlier. He awakened spontaneously at about 8:40 P.M. the same day, having slept 14 hours and 40 minutes. After he showered and dressed, there were more interviews and cameras. At about mid-night, he was very wide awake and decided to stay up and go to school in the morning. He knew his fellow students would want to see him—he was certainly the "man of the hour."

After school and dinner the next day, he returned to the hospital and was in bed at about 7:30 P.M. He was awakened, after 10 $^1/_2$ hours of sleep, at 6:00 A.M. the next day in order to get to school on time. On the third laboratory sleep, which was Friday night, he went to bed and fell asleep at about 11:00 P.M. and was awakened at 8:00 A.M. because there was something he wanted to do. He spent three more nights in the Naval Hospital Sleep Laboratory, one each at 1 week, 6 weeks, and 10 weeks after the marathon.

The experience with Randy greatly altered my ideas about the effects of long-term sleep deprivation and mental illness. During Randy's 264 hours of continuous wakefulness he did not become psychotic nor did he exhibit any notable signs of individual psychotic symptoms. Losing sleep did not make him crazy. We could readily attribute any brief lapse to the severe drowsiness itself. Although Randy's record-breaking effort took place more than three decades ago, no one else has stayed awake for a similar duration while being observed by qualified sleep scientists. Today, even if someone volunteered, I believe that a proposed experiment would never get beyond a university human subjects committee, because sleep-depriving someone for such a prolonged duration would be considered unethical.

I sometimes regret that we did not know more about biological rhythms or sleep debt at the time, for we would have done some things a little differently. Judging from the results of his three follow-up nights in the Naval Hospital Sleep Laboratory, it appeared that Randy's sleep requirement was a little less than 7 hours a day. Based on this figure, he lost about 75 hours of sleep, and I doubt that he slept 75 extra hours before he was completely recovered. The follow-up recording at week 1 was almost identical to the recordings at week 6 and week 10. In addition, we were puzzled at the time by his awakening spontaneously after only 14 hours 40 minutes of sleep after 264 hours of wakefulness. In retrospect, I would guess that he woke up not because he had slept long enough, but because it was close to 9:00 P.M. when his biological clock was most strongly alerting his brain.

Ardie and Vern did several working EEG recordings toward the end of the prolonged vigil. Reviewing the data now, I think Randy may have been in the sleepwalking state some of the time. We stayed in touch for at least 10 years, and have since lost contact but I doubt there were any permanent problems. After recently reviewing the movies and audiotapes we recorded and the papers about Randy we published in scientific journals, I can say with absolute certainty that his staying awake for 264 hours did not cause any psychiatric problems whatsoever. I even talked it over with Serge Gulevich and we were in complete agreement that only a sleep scientist would be sufficiently familiar with the manifestations of sleep deprivation that might stimulate true mental illness to be able to tell the difference.

Occasionally someone will interpret my statements about the lack of psychotic symptoms during Randy's ordeal as implying that losing many days of sleep is easy or harmless. On the contrary, Randy and those of us keeping him awake all worked very hard. I am positive that he could not have succeeded without our constant help; staying awake was clearly in dramatic conflict with his mind and body's natural drive to sleep. The necessity of monitoring him closely increased day by day; more and more often we had to shake him awake and to find ever more entertaining activities to pass the long hours. At times, it was very difficult to do what was necessary to keep him awake and endure his anger.

The effects of this long period without sleep were also not innocuous. Randy's analytical abilities, memory, perception, motivation, and motor control were all affected in varying degrees. Even in his most alert periods, he was not entirely unimpaired. At other times his delayed reactions would have rendered him an unsafe driver (even more so than myself!), and sometimes he couldn't even add a few numbers together. He displayed all the disabilities that make the sleep deprived state dangerous.

Besides modifying my assumptions about the psychiatric effects of long-term sleep deprivation, my experience with Randy also changed my basic assumption that I would start seeing signs that pointed to sleep's vital functional role when someone was deprived completely or almost completely of sleep for a week or two. After this experience I no longer thought so, because Randy didn't display any signs that his body or mind was failing, beyond what you would expect during the periods of intense drowsiness. Needless to say, keeping humans totally awake in addition to being comfortable and well fed is very difficult and few people would even volunteer let alone have the intense motivation to stick it out.

Shortly after the Randy Gardener event, a high school senior from our area, whose parents I knew, wanted to break this newest record of 264 hours. As he confronted staying up all night on day three, he threw in the towel. To minimize the difficulty and because there can be much better control of the experiment, recent work has utilized laboratory animals, primarily rodents.

Clues from Other Animals
It appears that all mammals sleep. However, as more and more species are studied, the total amount of sleep and the total time devoted

to non-REM sleep and REM sleep are extremely variable from species to species and are not consistently related to some biological principal. In addition, each species tends to be active at different times of the day. Nearly all mammals (there are some exceptions) show every key sign of sleep: muscle relaxation, changes in brain-wave activity and body temperature, the presence of REM sleep and its unique brain-wave patterns, and most important, the "perceptual disengagement" of the brain as it shuts out sensory stimulation from the outside world. Every creature on Earth, and even every cell in every creature's body, seems to have a cycle of rest and activity. But not every creature can be said to sleep. Somewhere between the evolution of yeast and yak, full-fledged sleep developed. Understanding when sleep evolved may help give us ideas about why we do it.

Cats are excellent sleepers. It seems they can sleep all the time, almost anywhere. They are unusual sleepers in that they nap so much; most animals have a consolidated period of sleep, either during the night or day, and a consolidated period of being awake. But cats nap and are awake during the day and nap and are awake during the night. Actually, some years ago we recorded a number of cats continuously 24 hours a day for several days. Under these circumstances, their total daily sleep time was typically between 13 and 14 hours, but it also tended to be scattered throughout the day. Cats may have evolved this way because they needed to be able to hunt during the day or night. Whatever the reason for their frequent naps, cats' sleep habits made them exceptional subjects for sleep studies. Unfortunately, however, their unusual sleep habits delayed our recognition of clock-dependent alerting, since this process doesn't seem to be very firmly established in cats' brains.

One of the most unusual of mammalian sleepers is the dolphin, that—like other marine mammals—evolved first on land before turning to the sea. In the sea, they evolved a very fishlike form and kept only a few of their terrestrial, mammalian traits, such as bearing live young and breathing air. Another mammalian habit they maintained was sleeping—but not without some extraordinary creative and necessary adaptation. On land, we mammals cede control of breathing to involuntary, autonomic breathing centers in the brain stem. Dolphins have to control their breathing voluntarily—an activity that requires the participation of the waking brain—since they can't afford to breathe involuntarily underwater. The dolphin solves this problem by letting only one-half of the brain go to sleep at a time. First the left side sleeps for two hours or so, and then the right side, and so on until the day's sleep requirement is fulfilled. We can guess that some of the other aquatic mammals share a similar strategy for sleeping, but this has never been proven. To me, the extreme measures that nature has taken to conserve sleep in the dolphin seems to support the idea that there is a vital need for sleep.

Birds also sleep, but their pattern of sleep is different from mammals' and probably evolved independently. For instance, many birds show very short bursts of the kind of activity that is typical of REM sleep—perhaps a sign of REM sleep when it was just evolving. It may be that birds would find it impossible to roost if they had full-fledged REM sleep and the muscle paralysis that accompanies it. The fact that bird species developed their own form of sleep and yet also sleep about eight hours a day may ultimately lead sleep researchers to a better understanding of the basic reason for sleep.

Some of my colleagues have focused on reptiles, which often exhibit a sensory shutting off from their environment during periods of apparent rest—one of the defining qualities of sleep. Light or noise that elicits a response during their active time has to be louder or brighter to get a reaction during their downtime. In general, investigators agree that most reptiles have a pattern of brain activity and behavior that shows some aspects of sleep (although they definitely have no REM sleep). For most lower species, this quiet time cannot really be called sleep in the sense we know it. Insects, worms, and other invertebrates don't show the changes in neurological activity, metabolism, and sensitivity to stimulation that we usually define as the basic signs of sleep. Fish periodically have a quiet time in which they rest their fins lightly on top of a rock or wrap a fin around a piece of seaweed. Many fish species seem to be less reactive to stimulus during this time, which could be a primitive example of sleeplike activity.

I think that one reasonable explanation for quiet time in lower organisms and for what seems to be a state analogous to sleep in reptiles, birds, and mammals is the need to conserve energy. All organisms must meet an energy budget. They cannot expend more energy in growth and activity than they bring in by consuming calories. Each animal best hunts or grazes for these calories under different light conditions. Nocturnal animals usually have very good night vision or great hearing or sense of touch and smell. Other animals, such as bats, operate best during the low light of dawn and dusk. Some animals find the hunting best just after the sun is up, when other animals are out breaking the fast of the night before. In order to meet the animal's energy budget, there is strong pressure to curtail activity when the light and the hunting are not good. When the time of day is wrong for calorie gathering and may even make the organism more vulnerable to becoming someone else's dinner, it's better to lie low and be quiet than risk becoming food. This survival strategy is programmed directly into the genes in the form of a drive to be periodically inactive.

The stakes for survival are especially high for the warm-blooded birds and mammals. As in cold-blooded animals, the strong sleep drive in mammals and birds conserves energy and keeps them from gathering food when it's not most efficient. But warm-blooded animals also require calories to warm themselves, and so they have to consume even more calories to survive. In financial terms, warm-blooded animals are running a capital-intensive business. They must use their larger brains to gather calories more efficiently as well as use their fur coats to hold in warmth. Smaller animals spend proportionally more of their energy keeping warm, because they have relatively more skin (which loses heat) compared to their body mass (which creates heat). Some small animals in cold environments live so close to the edge metabolically that if they run around without food for more than a few hours they starve. In such circumstances it makes very good sense for the brain to create an irresistible urge to sleep.

These facts would seem to favor sleep in animals that need to conserve more energy, and this is exactly the pattern we see. In general, small animals, especially those that live in cold environments, sleep the longest. Larger animals, especially in warmer locales, tend to sleep less. Horses sleep about 3 hours a day, cats about 15, and bats about 20. A few species, such as some marsupials and prosimians, don't fit this pattern (they sleep more than one might expect), but these are typically animals that tend to have a poor diet and need to make extra efforts to conserve calories by sleeping more.

For humans in countries where there is a steady food supply (and, in some places, 24-hour supermarkets), this isn't a factor. If saving calories is sleep's primary purpose, why do the well-fed citizens of postindustrial societies still need sleep? In part because it's only been a second or two of evolutionary time that calorie conservation hasn't been extremely important—and in developing or famine-prone countries, it's still essential. From this perspective, we may someday shed the inherited urge of the sleep drive or eliminate it through genetic engineering. In any case, regardless of whether calorie conservation was the original purpose of sleep, the brain has created additional uses for it.

I recently attended a meeting where my friend Jerry Siegel, one of our very best basic sleep researchers, gave a truly fascinating lecture bringing us all up-to-date on progress and describing sleep in widely diverse species. The differences were mind-boggling to say the least, and to understand these variations will be a great challenge, but is likely to yield a greatly important fundamental understanding.

The Budding Brain

Nested within quiet slow-wave sleep is a completely different kind of sleep—REM sleep, the generator of dreams. Whatever its purpose, the intense activity of the dreaming brain is so important to us that the brain actively paralyzes the body's muscles to accommodate it. To find REM sleep's purpose, one of the first places we have looked is in the budding brain of infants.

Recall that in 1960 Howie Roffwarg and I did standard polygraphic wave recordings of infant sleep and were astonished to find that infants spend about 50 percent of their sleep time in REM sleep, vs. about 25 percent for young adults. But the percentage does not tell the whole story, since newborn infants sleep about sixteen hours a day. This means they can spend a full eight hours in REM sleep. Howie and I hypothesized that fetuses and infants have such a large proportion of REM sleep because REM activity is crucial to the developing brain. We already know that the young brain is shaped by the nerve signals generated by sights, sounds, smells, and other sensations. Even in the womb, fetuses will be exposed to sounds, pressure on the skin, and smells and flavors in the amniotic fluid. As these nerve pulses travel through the brain, they are routed through various pathways. The nerve pathways that most efficiently connect cells and are used most often become stronger, much as well-traveled high-ways are expanded into interstates. On the other hand, like back roads that fall into disrepair, the nerve networks that are not used often, or don't work well with other cells, are weakened or elimi-nated. Nerve cells that don't fit in are destroyed. After about four months of gestation, the human fetus has grown 200 billion nerve cells in the brain, twice as many as it needs. The excess is eliminated during the first year of life. The brain cells that are killed off are the ones that don't fit in during the early brain activity.

When nerve systems don't get the proper stimulation during cer-tain critical early development periods they never function properly, even if they get plenty of stimulation later. In those rare cases where infants have cataracts, for example, part of the visual field that is blocked by the cataracts will atrophy and never develop if the cata-racts are not treated immediately.

Remember that during REM sleep, an area at the base of the brain sends out pulses of nerve activity that filter up through the rest of the brain and stimulate higher centers as well as the cortex, the brain's thin outer layer where most cognition takes place. It may be that REM sleep provides the developing brain with a regular workout and produces much more nerve stimulation than the fetus or infant would get simply from sensory stimulation. This self-stimulation by the brain may lay the foundation for its own organization by creating proto-sensations that train the brain and prepare it for the real-world sensations to follow.

That is our theory, at least. Howie and I first published this hy-pothesis in the prestigious journal *Science* in 1966, and so far it has been neither completely proven nor completely disproven, mostly because it is extremely difficult to test. However, the last decade of neurological research provides evidence that the fetal brain uses arti-ficial stimulation to help its visual system develop. Since the womb is dark, the eyes can't send messages back to the visual areas of the brain and give them the workout they need to develop. And yet immedi-ately after birth, the eyes and the visual areas of the brain work fine. This is possible because the eyes of fetuses create their own nerve signals, just as they would if activated by light. These signals then pass from the retina to the visual areas of the brain and give them the stimulation they need to form images later. This allows the visual system to organize itself so it can make meaningful images from the first patterns of light that hit the eyes after birth.

In recent years Roffwarg investigated this phenomenon by covering a kitten's eye for just one week. This was not long enough to permanently impair vision in that eye, but the nerve cells did start to atrophy and become less reactive to light. Roffwarg found that if—in addition to covering the eye—he also interrupted REM sleep, development of the visual system was more severely affected. Without the stimulation of either light or REM sleep signals, the visual nerve cells atrophied even faster. This suggests that REM sleep continues to be an important part of visual development after birth, exciting brain cells in a way that complements the stimulation from light.

Since REM sleep excites nerve cells elsewhere in the brain, not just in the visual system, it also might help other areas of the brain develop. It's possible that in the womb, REM stimulation of the brain pairs with the stimulation provided by the sound and motion of the mother. Some of the biochemical signals that the mother produces when she is relaxed, hungry, excited, or stressed pass over the placenta and become another source of stimulation for the fetus's growing neural and hormonal systems.

The idea that REM sleep is important for brain development fits nicely with the evolutionary pattern of brain development we see in other animals. Extended periods of REM sleep are found only in mammals, the animals with the greatest mass of brain tissue—specifically the greatest proportion of neocortex. The neocortex is the most advanced part of the brain, where most thinking takes place. Reptiles and fish have a neocortex, but it is very small. Birds, which evolved after reptiles and have a slightly larger neocortex, show evidence of ephemeral REM-like activity: short bursts that last only a second or so. It seems possible that during the course of evolution, the most efficient way for mammals to develop a large neocortex was first to acquire self-created nerve activity.

The platypus—the strange, duck-billed, egg-laying mammal native to Australia—is an interesting example of REM sleep on the evolutionary scale, because it is one of the most ancient mammalian species alive today. An Australian scientist in Los Angeles recently discovered that the platypus's forebrain is inactive during REM sleep. The forebrain is also inactive in human infants during REM sleep until the brain develops a little more. In human adults, the forebrain is very active during REM sleep. This finding suggests that the location of REM activity in human infants may retrace evolutionary development as they grow.

According to the Roffwarg-Dement theory, the primary purpose of REM sleep is to help the brain develop, which I admit poses a problem. It should mean that once the vast majority of physical brain development is completed at about age five, the brain no longer needs REM sleep. So why do we maintain REM sleep and dreaming until the day we die? Howie and I speculate that REM sleep may be a holdover of the brain development stage. Even though REM sleep is no longer important for adults, it is so important to infant brain development that adults continue to have it anyway.

Another possibility is that REM sleep still continues to help our brains develop. Studies in animals and humans suggest that sleep deprivation may impair the formation of some long-term memories. As new memories form, the related brain cells change the way they interconnect, in the same way that the brain cells of the developing brain strengthen or eliminate their connections. Perhaps during REM sleep, as our brains sort through the experiences of the day, the showers of nerve activity help nerve connections change and create the new memories.

I also wonder if the function of REM sleep isn't confirmed by the recent discovery that the adult brain is able to grow new brain cells—a finding in direct opposition to the long-standing dogma that, after infancy, the brain does not generate new cells. Perhaps the brain never truly stops developing, and we need REM sleep to integrate new brain cells and to shape the connections made by existing ones. I would guess that further research will give us the answers.

Going back to REM sleep deprivation and mental illness, as soon as I realized that sleep consisted of two entirely different states, I hypothesized that each should have a different purpose or purposes for existing. The normal sequence in which non-REM sleep always precedes REM sleep and lasts for about an hour made it possible to deprive volunteers selectively of REM sleep by waking them up at the onset of each successive REM period. I then spent about 10 years trying to discover the unique purpose of REM sleep by the method of selective REM sleep deprivation. As I mentioned in Chapter 2, my early assumptions were dictated by the psychoanalytic thinking of the time. The hypothesis that dreaming and/or REM sleep might be necessary for mental health was not confirmed. On the contrary, our REM sleep-deprived human volunteers and experimental animals seemed to be energized by this procedure. My conclusion at the time was that selective REM deprivation enhanced brain processes underlying motivation and drive-oriented behavior. This was a very counterintuitive result because it suggests that the more REM sleep one has, the less motivated one would be.

During the years that selective REM sleep deprivation was one of my high research priorities, we had not yet developed a clear concept of daytime sleepiness and we had developed no method to quantify it either with subjective scales or with the Multiple Sleep Latency Test. A couple of studies were reported in the 70s suggesting that both kinds of sleep had pretty much the same effect on daytime sleep tendency. Even so, as we did more and more work with the Multiple Sleep Latency Test and the role of nighttime sleep on daytime alertness, I could not fully accept that two widely desperate states could have an identical function in anything. I wondered if the effect of sleep loss was somewhat buffered by REM sleep loss. Just recently, my friends Tom Roth, Tim Roehrs and their associates, carried out experiments that support this idea. In their excellent study, paired subjects were "yoked" during sleep, so that every time an experimental subject was awakened to prevent the occurrence of REM sleep, the yoked control was also awakened. Thus, the two groups had identical sleep disturbances and were different only in the amount of REM sleep. The total time of both groups was reduced by about two and a half hours. However, the yoked controls had an almost normal amount of REM sleep.

The results were striking. The daytime sleep tendency did not change in the REM-sleep deprived group in spite of two nights of partial sleep loss, whereas the yoked control group (which lost much more non-REM sleep) became significantly sleepier in the daytime. The investigators are naturally very cautious about this result partly because only two nights of REM deprivation were carried out. For my part, given the vast experience with selective REM deprivation, I feel certain that a new level of complexity for the role of sleep with regard to daytime alertness is about to be added. However, for the time being our concerns about sleep deprivation and daytime alertness must remain the same. It may be that REM sleep is treated as wakefulness by the sleep homeostat. At the very least, I'm absolutely confirmed in my belief that there are two different states of sleep, and that it will eventually be shown that they play different roles in our lives.

Dispensing with Sleep

Every once in a while, there is a newspaper story about someone who is said never to sleep. Is this possible? As I have stated, not all people have the same need for sleep, and a very few people seem to need either a huge amount of sleep each day or very little. In 1977 London psychologist Ray Medis searched for individuals who claimed to sleep less than an hour each day. After advertising widely for very short sleepers, he located a young woman who appeared to sleep approximately 70 minutes a night and agreed to undergo a sleep recording. Medis also found two other adult individuals who averaged perhaps 30 minutes of sleep per day and appeared to be in excellent health, with no complaints about fatigue or concern about not sleeping.

In 1978 I visited Professor Medis and I met two of these three people. I met them in the middle of the night, and they were perfectly alert and energetic. Both of them were very convincing and stated that they had jobs both in the daytime as well as the night. Nonetheless, I tried very hard to persuade them to come to Stanford for round-the-clock observations so we could prove beyond a shadow of a doubt that their remarkable claims were true. If there really is some vital need for sleep, then extremely short sleepers must be fulfilling that need in a very short time. Perhaps sleep in the rest of us has just been expanded by evolutionary forces to fit the eight dark hours of the day.

This effort to study short sleepers should be repeated with adequate resources and a set of experiments that everyone agrees would settle the issue of whether short sleepers really sleep extremely little over the long term. According to Medis, it was a major effort to advertise for volunteers, screening huge numbers to eliminate frauds, cranks, crazies, and probably individuals with sleep-state misperception, and to persuade the truly short sleepers to submit to observation. Today, the Internet would greatly simplify locating people who claim to be very short sleepers. Screening, however, would still be difficult, and observations would have to be carried out long enough to be completely sure that the supposed short sleepers actually slept very little every night and enjoyed normal mental and physical health.

In the attempt to uncover what critical functions sleep and dreams may perform, researchers have deprived rats of all sleep, and sometimes just REM sleep, for many days at a time. Allan Rechtschaffen and his colleagues at the University of Chicago found that as total sleep deprivation progresses, rats appear unkempt and develop sores on their bodies that won't heal. Soon they lose their ability to regulate their body temperature, and it begins to drop. They lose weight, even though they are eating more than usual. The inevitable result is death, usually in about 16 days. When Rechtschaffen allowed the rats to get some non-REM sleep but no REM sleep, the rats still died, but it took around 40 days. We have no idea what would happen to human beings under the same conditions, but unconfirmed reports, torture victims not allowed to sleep for many days usually die. While the Rechtschaffen experiments might seem to clinch the case that both non-REM and REM sleep serve some vital need, the results aren't that clear to me. Yes, the lack of sleep and the accumulation of sleep debt could be killing the rats, but it is also very hard to remove stress completely from this sort of experiment. We know that extreme, long-term stress can cause tissue destruction and death.

Just suppose that the primary purpose of sleep is energy conservation and the sole purpose of REM is to help the brain develop in infancy. Let's suppose that in adults sleep serves no truly vital purpose. Conceivably one day scientists could eliminate sleep. After all, the sleep drive may be less like the drive to eat than it is like the sex drive: Going without sex is unpleasant, but unlike going without food, it won't kill you. I believe that there must be a specific structure or center in the brain that creates the sleep drive, much as the brain's suprachiasmatic nucleus alerts us and opposes the sleep drive. Then the question is whether it is possible to deactivate this sleep center and be awake all the time.

New drugs like modafinil—which is used in the treatment of narcolepsy—eventually may help end the search for sleep's vital role, if in fact it has any vital role. Because wakefulness caused by modafinil, and perhaps even more effective drugs of the future, doesn't cause an accumulation of sleep debt, we might be able to keep rats or humans awake for long periods without inducing extreme stress. Until long-term studies of the potential side effects of chemically induced sleep-lessness are conducted, however, we must assume that humans won't be able to dispense with sleep anytime in the near future. The fact is that the body has adapted sleep to serve too many other functions. During sleep, hormones like growth hormone, prolactin, cortisol, and many others we aren't aware of are released into the blood-stream. Sleep affects the immune function, and vice versa. As I will show in the rest of this book, sleep is woven into the fiber of our well-being and affects us in many ways.

Sleep touches on nearly every aspect of our physiology and psy-chology, of our interaction with the world and with others. It may be that sleep's original purpose is no longer its most important one. Hundreds of biological processes go on during sleep, making it im-possible to separate sleep from the process of living. Whether we theoretically need sleep or not, for the foreseeable future we will need to work within the boundaries built by our need to sleep. For our health and happiness, we need to learn as much as we can about what kind of sleep we need for physical and psychological health.

I have to admit that I sometimes find the idea of not needing to sleep pretty appealing, since there are so many experiments to run, so many grants to write, so many patients to take care of, so many students to teach, and so little time—particularly as I grow older and my days become more and more precious. But I think I would miss sleep. I like the cycles it imposes. I like the forced rest, the require-ment that we have some downtime every day. Besides, it might be okay if I didn't have to sleep, but if everyone didn't have to sleep, my guess is that society would only find more work for us to do. I enjoy the delicious feeling of giving myself over to sleep in the night and, most of all, enjoy getting up in the morning and feeling the pulse of the new day. I cannot imagine being without the daily opportunity to begin anew, to start over, to have left the old day behind. I am sure this feeling is more likely when you are a lark, but even owls must have some feeling of wrapping up one day's task and having the delicious buffer or demarcation before starting the next. Even though scientific honesty compels me to consider the possibility that sleep is not vitally necessary, and that individual findings so far may have alternative interpretations, I think in the aggregate, the widely diverse findings favor vital functions that are yet to be discovered or hints that are yet to be absolutely proven. Just last fall, I attended an NIH conference entitled "What is sleep, what does it do for us" and listened to a dazzling array of creative new approaches from trying to define sleep and wakefulness in the fruit fly with considerable success, to the fascinating differences among species, to the latest data on early failure of the immune system when animals are deprived of sleep. Certainly from the point of view of sleep research and from one perspective of all of science, the basic biological function of sleep is one of the greatest of scientific questions ranking alongside the nature of matter, the nature of consciouness, how genes operate, and so forth.

So I think the question of whether we can do without sleep is not as interesting as it first seems. After all, if we could take pills instead of eating, how many people would give up food completely? Sleep is a joyous thing in itself, a restorative for the soul and spirit. Apparently, my appreciation for the pleasures of sleep are nearly universal; in a recent survey of my several hundred undergraduate students at Stanford, an astounding (to me) 97.2 percent said that they "love to sleep."

Chapter 11

Sleep, Longevity, and the Immune System

JUST BEFORE I STARTED writing this chapter, I happened to visit the man who started me off in sleep research. Nathaniel Kleitman was born in 1895, and at 102 years old he was still a sharp and thoughtful conversationalist. He didn't move as quickly as in previous years and his hearing was a little impaired, but he got around pretty well. Dr. Kleitman doesn't complain about his sleep, so I guess it is okay. I have always been happy to follow in the footsteps of such a dedicated, bright, and congenial person; I can only hope that I will follow his lead in terms of healthy longevity. Like most people, I try to watch my health. And like most people, I don't do as much as I probably should to get enough exercise and watch my diet. But I do keep a close eye on one thing that most people don't: sleep.

From the perspective of longevity, sleep may turn out to be more important than most people think. There is plenty of compelling evidence supporting the argument that sleep is the most important predictor of how long you will live, perhaps more important than whether you smoke, exercise, or have high blood pressure or cholesterol levels. In the 1950s the American Cancer Society did a massive study of such factors. Volunteers surveyed over 1 million Americans representing every county and parish in the United States about their exercise, nutrition, smoking, sleep, and other health related habits. Six years later, the volunteers repeated the survey clearly identifying all of the respondents who had died since the original survey. Out of all the factors in this gigantic study, stated habitual sleep time had the best correlation with mortality. However, the correlation was not linear. The highest mortality rates at all age levels occurred for those who said they slept four hours or less, and for those who said they slept nine to ten hours or more. The lowest mortality rates were seen for those who said their habitual nightly sleep time was around eight hours. Other investigators carried out a very similar study with a smaller sample and a nine-year follow-up, and the results were essentially the same.

Just as the American Cancer Society study shows a significant association between sleep and longevity, a more recent Finnish study suggested there is a link between good sleep and good health. Finnish researchers sampled 1,600 adults in Tampere, Finland, ages 36 to 50, and determined their health status and the length and quality of their sleep. The results were unequivocal: Compared to good sleepers, male poor sleepers were 6.5 times more likely to have health problems, and female poor sleepers were 3.5 times more likely to have health problems.

At first glance, one possible explanation for this finding is that the ranks of the short sleepers or the long sleepers are filled with people who are chronically or terminally ill. Serious health problems such as cancer that cause a great deal of pain or discomfort go hand in hand with poor sleep, for obvious reasons. But over the years scientists have gone back to the original data and worked these factors into their calculations. The original results still stand: Although sleep needs vary, people who sleep about 8 hours, on average, tend to live longer. For the long sleepers, we speculate that they are more prone to die because they have undiagnosed sleep apnea or some other disorder. In a sense, the people who have sleep disorders and spend many hours in bed are not really "long-sleepers." Their sleep is disrupted repeatedly by short, unremembered awakenings that severely cut down on real sleep time. Apnea and other disorders excessive daytime sleepiness that can be life-threatening health problems.

None of the aforementioned studies prove a casual relationship between amount of sleep and life span, but the results are extremely suggestive. Could shortened or lengthened sleep actually shorten life? One possibility is that the answer lies in the immune system.

There seems to be an intriguing and mysterious connection between sleep and the maintenance of our bodies through immune function and cell repair.

Sleep and the Common Cold

From everyday experience, people have the preconception that lack of sleep increases our susceptibility to illness. A student stays up all night cramming for exams and then comes down with a cold. A parent gets up every few hours to attend to a newborn and then gets a sore throat. An executive stays up two consecutive nights negotiating and then falls ill. But is there truly a connection? Lots of students who cram for exams don't get colds, and lots of parents stay up with their newborn baby and don't get a sore throat. When people fall ill, they have a marked tendency to look for a cause and to blame any event that preceded the illness, if it seems remotely possible.

Searching for answers, some immunologists have been trying to learn not how to cure the common cold but how to give it to people. An early example of this was set in a very unlaboratory-like spot in the bucolic countryside of southern England. There seemingly happy vacationers each received an all-expenses-paid week in pleasant country cottages, free to read, paint, or roam the nearby glades and woods. But in return for the free holiday these volunteers "paid through the nose." Upon arriving at the Medical Research Council's Common Cold Unit, the visitors snorted a noseful of aerosol containing common cold virus. Researchers then spent the week observing the subjects and monitoring their response to the virus. Many subjects found it a pleasant week. The setting was beautiful, everything was free, and there was a good chance they wouldn't get sick at all. The virus didn't even infect one out of 10 people exposed to it. Among those who became infected, only 30 percent got a bad cold, 30 percent got a mild cold, and 30 percent didn't get sick at all. What immunologists and virologists have done at the Common Cold Unit and in other, less resortlike laboratories around the world is monitor people's diet, exercise, stress levels, smoking habits, and myriad other factors to find out what determines whether someone gets sick or not.

The results of some of these experiments have surprised some immunologists: Quality of sleep before infection is a statistically significant factor in determining whether someone gets a cold. As Sheldon Cohen of Carnegie Mellon University and William Doyle of the University of Pennsylvania found, sleep seems to affect how sick people get and how much mucus they produce. The pair found that sleep is one of many minor, but statistically significant, factors that affect someone's susceptibility to cold virus. The result stands even when factors such as stress are taken into account. These are the kinds of tests that I've advocated doing for many years, and sleep scientists themselves need to do a lot more of such studies to make this result really solid.

The Immune System's Defense Network

To understand how sleep and the immune system might affect each other, it's helpful to know a little about how our bodies fight disease. Imagine an average five-year-old covered with grime after a long day playing. Every moment of the day, her tissue is under attack by thousands of types of viruses, bacteria, protozoa, and fungi. The scaly armor of her skin cells traps bacteria and then sheds itself. Blinking washes the eyeballs with tear-water, constantly sweeping organisms into tear ducts to be destroyed. Mucus in the nose traps and annihilates airborne nasties, and if she already has a cold, the mucus runs free to wash out the virus. Acid in the stomach and immune cells in the intestines attack the millions of dangerous microbes that munch on the food she has eaten. Without immune defenses, she would be as defenseless as the lump of food she has just ingested and would succumb quickly to pathogens.

Our bodies keep these organisms in check through the action of special cells that recognize whether other cells are part of the body or foreign. The immune system also recognizes and destroys mutant cells, those that are or can become cancerous. Immunological attack is probably behind occasional miracle recoveries from cancer, when well-developed tumors shrink and disappear without treatment, or after all treatments have failed. Scientists now are trying to harness the immune system as a way of fighting cancers.

When the body detects invaders, immune cells release a family of substances called interleukins. These chemical messengers are a call heard throughout the body, mobilizing many kinds of immune cells to multiply and arm. Special proteins called immunoglobins are sent forth like foot soldiers to engage foreign matter. If a cell is found to be foreign, cancerous, or infected with a virus, the body calls in the tanks—immune cells like T-cells, macrophages, and the vicious-sounding natural killer cells. Natural killer cells attack cancers and viruses in particular. They act by sidling up next to the mutant or infected cells and releasing enzymes that dissolve holes in the enemy's cell membrane, blowing up the target cell. In acquired immune deficiency syndrome (AIDS), the immune system itself is under attack by the human immunodeficiency virus (HIV). The immune system is not in abeyance but rather is very active in the early stages of the disease, mobilizing in high quantities a particular kind of immune cell, the helper T-cell. Despite the immune system's valiant struggle, however, HIV eventually destroys T-cells and thereby opens the door for other organisms to invade the body. The immediate cause of death for AIDS patients is typically an illness like pneumonia, which would not be fatal in uninfected individuals.

The Sleeping Cure

Once we fall prey to an infectious disease, all the elements of the immune defense network go into high gear. Interleukins and other immune molecules spur a massive mobilization among the immune cells. One result is fever. Scientists have found that if they inject the body with interleukin-1, it acts on the brain's thermostat to raise body temperature a few degrees. Some scientists theorize that fever protects the body because foreign organisms often live best at our normal body temperature. When we are sick, in addition to getting fever, headache, and aching muscles, we get very sleepy. All we want to do is find a place to lie down. People often say they feel "wiped out," "knocked out," or "knocked flat on their back" by sickness. Even a cold that is not bad enough to cause a fever will make us feel groggy and tired. This also seems to be largely the effect of interleukins, which act directly on some part of the brain (probably the hypothalamus) to increase our brain's pressure to sleep. If test animals are given interleukin-1, they will pass more quickly into slow-wave sleep. If interleukin-1 then is blocked chemically, the animals will return to wakefulness.

Increased sleepiness doesn't always mean more sleep, however. People and lab animals tend to sleep more at the start of an infection and then less as the illness continues. During the peak stages of sickness, people tend to sleep fitfully. We stay awake for a few hours, then sleep for a few more, then wake again for several hours. This resembles the pattern we see when we disable the biological clock in animals. Therefore, it seems that interleukins and other immune messengers also may act directly on the body clock, perhaps even turning it off or blocking its alerting impact. Sleep disruption and sickness–induced desire to sleep more than usual can be a one-two punch that makes being sick all the more fatiguing and debilitating. In addition to the fact that sickness can feel like sleep deprivation, sleep deprivation sometimes can feel exactly like getting sick.

I remember once some years ago I was giving instructions to five or six research assistants who were seated in a semicircle in front of me. At about 2:00 P.M., I began to feel tired and achy and suddenly could hardly keep my eyes open. I thought, "I can't be getting the flu now, this is too important!" Nevertheless, I was beyond any ability to manage further, so I went home and went to bed. I slept about 14 hours. When I woke up, I felt fine, as if nothing had ever happened. Perhaps I had some low-level infection that simply went away in 14 hours. However, I feel it is more likely that long hours of sleep research had built up a sleep debt so large that my system shut down. In this case, I felt physically drained, foggy-headed, with zero motivation—all common symptoms of the flu. The fact that sleep debt can make you feel unwell is backed up by other observations. Sleep deprivation can cause stomach upset, increased sensitivity to pain, and decreased ability to ignore bothersome stimuli—some of the main symptoms of common illnesses. It may be that many cases of the so-called 24-hour flu are in fact sleep deprivation, and this "viral infection" is in fact cured by going to bed and getting some sleep.

While being sick clearly increases our desire for sleep, a few physiologists also have wondered if sleep can help the body fight microbes once we are infected. A few years ago Carol Everson, a physiologist then at the National Institutes of Health in Bethesda, Maryland, took a new look at why rats totally deprived of sleep died after about 40 days of sleep deprivation. As I explained in the last chapter, it is difficult to make a strong case that the rats had died from metabolic or neurological problems or stress. Everson wondered what might have caused the wasting away that preceded death and thought it resembled terminal cancer patients she had seen. In the last stages of the patients' illness, at the end of their physical reserves, they succumbed to massive bacterial infections. As with AIDS patients who die of pneumonia, in the end it was the bacteria that killed the patients when their immune systems began to fail. Everson did autopsies on rats sleep deprived by the Rechtshaffen method and found greatly enlarged lymph nodes and a massive amount of bacteria living in the blood. In order for these bacteria to have multiplied so rapidly in the rats' bodies, she concluded, the immune system must have broken down as a result of the extreme sleep deprivation.

Everson has been studying rodents at shorter and shorter durations of total sleep deprivation. Recently at a symposium she reported finding live E. coli bacteria in abdominal lymph nodes after as few as four or five days of sleep deprivation, when the rats still appeared to be perfectly healthy. It is as if the first line of defense is in some way enfeebled and that the all-out, hugely complex immune response with the formation of antibodies, release of interleukins, and the proliferation of killer and helper t-cells is called into play but eventually begins to weaken. In other words, bacteria multiply in the bloodstream because the body's front-line defenses have been weakened, forcing other defenders to come into the fight. Because that fight is ultimately successful we often don't notice the negative health effects of reduced sleep. Everson feels that sleep deprivation may be analogous to food deprivation. "If you deprive someone of food for a short time they get hungry, but you don't really see any nutritional problems. Only when someone has a restricted diet for a long time do you see nutrition problems becoming obvious."

There is some evidence indicating that sleep may help sustain the activity of certain immune cells and chemicals. Whenever we fall asleep the level of immune system molecules such as interleukin-1 and tumor necrosis factor (TNF) rise in the blood, then drop in the morning as we wake up. TNF is a potent killer of cancer. Both TNF and interleukin-1 behave like sleep medication when injected. Even when we are completely healthy, circulating TNF naturally increases tenfold while we sleep and then drops again when we awake.

Natural killer cells may be particularly affected by lack of sleep. Staying up all night doesn't appear to affect their levels during the sleepless night itself, but the next day the number of natural killer cells available to fight off invaders can be severely reduced. Investigators in San Diego and elsewhere have found that people who simply stayed up until just 3:00 A.M. before falling asleep had a 30 percent reduction in the number of natural killer cells the next day and depressed activity in the natural killer cells still present. In addition, the production of interleukin-2 was diminished. This suppression of immune function could result in a greater susceptibility to viruses such as those that cause colds. Since these immune cells also protect the body against tumors, it is possible that chronic sleep deprivation increases cancer risk.

These are all tantalizing findings, suggesting a tremendously complex, undiscovered interaction among the immune system, the brain, and sleep that is just beginning to unfold before our eyes.

Sleep and Cell Repair

We tend to think of healing as something that happens only when we are injured, when a cut or abrasion rends tissue and destroys cells. The truth is that cells in the body constantly are replenishing themselves, repairing not only cuts and bruises but also the wear and tear of daily living. This has become more obvious to me as I get older: Small sprains or joint soreness that would have lasted barely half a day when I was younger now can linger for a week. Much of this repair is the job of growth hormone, which stimulates protein synthesis, helps break down the fats that supply energy for tissue repair, and stimulates cell division to replace old or malfunctioning cells. The concentration of growth hormone released during the night's first period of stage 4 sleep suggests that deep sleep is important for this repair process and that the disappearance of deep sleep may contribute to the physical decline we experience in old age.

Growth hormone is released into the bloodstream through the action of the logically named growth hormone–releasing hormone (or GHRH). It turns out that GHRH is a sleep inducer. When levels of GHRH are artificially increased in the body, sleepiness increases. In animals, administering drugs that specifically block the release of growth hormone tends to keep them awake longer, even after they have been sleep deprived and are very sleepy. In other words, the process of releasing growth hormone into the bloodstream, is not just a response to sleep but seems also to foster sleep, via the action of GHRH.

Growth hormone, growth factors and immune regulators seem to work with each other to foster sleep, the best state for doing their jobs. As we fall asleep, our bodies turn to the task of energy and tissue conservation. Body temperature decreases, conserving energy, sugars are stored away, growth hormone fosters the repair of tissue, and the immune system is bolstered. As we wake up and work through the day, our bodies are outfitted for action, and the opposite biochemical profile is put in place. Stress hormones rise, mobilizing stored sugars to make energy available and raising our adrenaline levels and general excitability. Stress hormones also are known to work against interleukin-1 and other immune factors, further encouraging wakefulness. Growth hormone levels drop, possibly because cells switch from reproduction to other functions, such as processing food or muscular action. Added to this daily cycle are the psychological stresses in our lives, which tend to interfere with sleep and also aid the suppression of our immune system.

In this complex and roiling symphony of interaction, it is impossible to separate cause and effect. Does sleep prompt tissue growth, or does the process of tissue growth, through the action of growth hormone releasing hormone, prompt sleep? Does the immune system govern sleep, or does sleep govern the immune system? The more we study sleep, the more it emerges as an integral and inseparable part of the body's vital cycles—of energy storage and use, of defense against enemies within and without. Hormones, immune chemistry, the metabolic machinery, and sleep are all tied together in a complex web of biochemical interaction. Our bodies oscillate between the needs of waking life—to work, to use energy, to expose our body to wear and tear—and the necessities of renewal, when energy is stored, tissue repaired, and the immune system prepared to fight another day.

I don't want to offend those individuals who have done outstanding work on sleep and immunology. Nonetheless, I feel that there still is not an absolutely unambiguous answer to the question "If we do not sleep, will we inevitably get sick?" If the answer were an absolutely unambiguous yes, then the homeostatic drive to sleep could be viewed as a protection against extreme sleep debt that would allow the immune system to fail and deadly illness to attack. But very long wakefulness marathons such as Randy Gardener's, where illness did not occur, contradict this. If this question were a really high priority for the health research establishment, funds would be made available to try a vast array of challenges to the immune system in sleep-deprived organisms and normally sleeping organisms and we would get the answer. The public should demand an answer. My colleague Jim Kreuger has been astoundingly productive in this area for more than 30 years. Adequate funding would make it possible to prove or disprove Jim Kreuger's and Carol Everson's hypotheses beyond a doubt. Long-term studies of sleep loss could document the putative breakdown of the immune system.

For the time being, I believe I will remain healthier by monitoring my sleep needs than I would if I didn't. Not only am I betting that sleep helps preserve my body, but I am treating sleep as a reliable barometer of my body's tenor, an indicator of whether I can expect fair or heavy weather ahead. In a recent general wellness test in which people assessed their own feelings of health and well-being, researchers found that sleep quality was one of the key components in determining how well or ill people felt in general.

Sleep is tightly woven into healthy neurological and hormonal function, like the warp and woof of cloth, and I strongly believe that taking a holistic approach to good health means that I must work on sleeping well and enough. Of course, as with many other aspects of life, sleep quality is the product of genes and environment, nature and nurture. So I can only hope that I acquired the sleep skills of Nathaniel Kleitman and inherited the genes of my mother, who lived past the age of 104 and, I am quite certain, slept well until her final years.

Chapter 12

Mood and Vitality

A BIOCHEMISTRY PROFESSOR I know at the University of California, San Francisco, School of Medicine spends every August in the mountains. The late-summer sun sets at 8:00 P.M. and the small, primitive cabin with no electrical power soon thereafter becomes wrapped in darkness. The few kerosene lanterns he lights are too dim to shift his internal clock, and he feels sleepy soon after dusk. By 9:00 P.M. he has trouble staying awake. At the beginning of his vacation he sleeps a good 10 or 11 hours per night, getting up at 7:00 or 8:00 A.M. and even manages to nap. After a few days he starts waking at 6:00 A.M. and feeling great, having slept about nine hours. His pattern at home is to retire around midnight, giving himself seven hours in bed, maybe six and a half as actual sleep time. But every year during his mountain sojourn he can feel vitality seep back into him. By the time the vacation is over, he has paid back a huge amount of his sleep debt and established a rhythm that works best for his body. He returns feeling reborn, energized, reminded of the reasons he loves medicine. Undoubtedly his emotional reconstitution is partly due to escaping the stresses of work. But even more significant is the fact that he follows the schedule his body sets. Without artificial lighting to encourage sleep loss, he allows his body to work off the sleep debt that he had accumulated back in the city. He returns to that simple harmony between the rhythms of the planet and the rhythms of his body.

Healthy sleep prepares the brain for the next day and renews our mental balance. At one time or another nearly everyone has experienced something like the following: After a good night's sleep you rise feeling fresh and renewed. Your senses soak up simple pleasures, such as the clean smell of the air, the singing of the birds, the texture of the morning paper. You are rested and relaxed but not bored or sleepy. You are interested and pleasantly aware of your surroundings but not overwhelmed. You are engaged with the world. Confident that you are ready to tackle the day ahead, frustrations seem minor, challenges exciting rather than foreboding. You can focus your mind like a laser on any problem, tackling it with exhilaration and confidence, and you can concentrate at the highest level while your body is at rest. If you remember these feelings, you may also realize it's been a very long time since you last had them.

In addition, it is easy to understand how easy it was to believe in the old notion of a hypnotoxin (a sleep-producing poison that built up in the body during daytime). People often felt so tired (poisoned) at night and so good (hypnotoxin detoxified by sleep) in the morning that this notion was supremely reasonable. Sleep debt itself could be thought of somewhat in this manner: building up during wake, being reduced during sleep.

Shakespeare—who, to judge from his writing, probably suffered some insomnia—created the most poetic description of sleep's benefits in Macbeth's paean to lost sleep:

Methought I heard a voice cry "Sleep no more!
Macbeth does murder sleep," the innocent sleep,
Sleep that knits up the ravell'd sleeve of care,
The death of each day's life, sore labor's bath,
Balm of hurt minds, great nature's second course
Chief nourisher in life's feast.

Only when it was too late, after he had murdered his king and realized he would never again be blessed with untroubled, innocent sleep, did Macbeth become a connoisseur of all that sleep represents and all he had lost. Shakespeare understood that the feast of life might be its waking hours, but its nutritional value, the nourishment that sustains and heals the mind, somehow lies in our sleep.

Sleep is both medicine and sustenance. It's a balm we would like to be able to bottle and pull out on demand, the kind of feeling we wish we could make last throughout the day, every day. What sleep sets us up for is arousal, a heightening of the senses and motivation, a feeling so good that people seek it out, whether from a good night's sleep, a cup of coffee, or a hit of cocaine. The resulting sense of vitality is what we are built to strive for. It's what being awake is all about. Many of us are dead tired by the evening, having looked forward all day to the respite of going to bed. But how many times do we end up postponing bedtime long after a prudent hour, glued to the TV or engrossed in a book? We all have retained a bit of the desire to stay up late, to have time to ourselves after the kids are in bed and the chores are done. We so crave stimulation that it can be difficult to put away our entertainments tonight for the sake of securing tomorrow's well-being.

This sense of stimulation that we all seek is a product of the way the brain is created. The human organism is wired to be energetic when faced with challenges. We need to be fired up to best accomplish life's basics, the four Fs: foraging, feeding, fighting, and fooling around. Vitality, this feeling of mental and physical energy, is also a key ingredient of motivation, the internal psychological push that drives us toward a goal. Without it we may feel dull, listless, apathetic—in a word, depressed.

Many people clearly recognize how badly they are affected when they don't get enough sleep. The National Sleep Foundation's 1998 Omnibus Poll reports that about a third of all adults feel that daytime sleepiness interferes with their social lives, their relationships with friends and family, and their recreational activities. These same people feel that their enjoyment of these activities is reduced by at least half when they feel sleepy during the daytime. Because people generally don't recognize the severity of their own sleepiness, I would bet that inadequate sleep diminishes the quality of many activities to an even greater degree than reported.

In study after study, sleep researchers have found that good sleep sets up the brain for positive feelings. When we don't have enough sleep, we have a sour view of circumstances: We are more easily frustrated, less happy, short tempered, less vital. In addition, sleep deprivation increases complaints about other bodily problems— headache, stomachache, sore joints or muscles. The fact that extreme sleep deprivation makes people grumpier has long been apparent. Anyone who has had to stay up one or two nights in a row knows this. Keeping someone awake during a long period of total sleep deprivation requires an enormous amount of nagging: "Keep your eyes open, keep your eyes open, keep your eyes open, open your eyes, open your eyes, come on now." Many many times my nagging has elicited an explosion of anger from a volunteer subject. What is less clear is how mood is affected by partial sleep deprivation over many nights. How are we affected when we get some sleep for several nights, but never a full night? This question is more relevant to the general population, since staying up for more than 24 hours is relatively rare, while shorting oneself on sleep for many nights is more common.

As part of his comprehensive program studying partial sleep deprivation, David Dinges and his colleagues at the University of Pennsylvania limited subjects' sleep to four and a half hours per night for one week, giving the subjects a number of performance tests and assessments of mood, feelings, and emotion during the day. The sleep-deprived volunteers were rated on scales of stress and calmness, happiness and unhappiness, healthiness and sickness, physical exhaustion and energy, mental exhaustion and sharpness. They were also asked to list any significant problems or complaints they might have, an open-ended question that was intended to catch physical, cognitive, or emotional problems. This was important, because we often complain about stomach problems, fuzzy thinking, or other physical or cognitive problems, when our real complaint is just feeling down.

Dave's experiments showed conclusively that people who get less than a full night's sleep feel significantly less happy, more stressed, more physically frail, and more mentally and physically exhausted as a result. Overall scores for general mood and vigor declined steadily over the test days. When the volunteers were allowed to get more sleep again, their mood scores quickly bounced back to near what they had been before.

A significant, and for me, gratifying result of this experiment was the close parallels between mood and the daily increase of lapses in performance. Dave pointed out that the lousiness of the volunteers' mood rose right along with their accumulating sleep debt. This fact implies that even a little sleep debt will make us feel a little down, a little stressed, a little less happy than we would be if we got more sleep. It's much harder to test for these subtle mood differences, but the strong implication is that they are there.

I recently visited Dave at U. Penn where he is in the midst of an exciting new study that restricts subjects' sleep to four hours a day for two entire weeks. The effects during the first week look essentially the same as those just reported. However, according to Dave, there is a strong suggestion that the impairment accelerates in the second week!

After talking to Dave, I found myself terrifically excited. Many of us in sleep research have long been convinced that human beings can never adapt to short sleep. It looks like Dave's research is going to prove it beyond the shadow of a doubt. I remember a visit more than 10 years ago when he earnestly sought my counsel about the future possibilities of a scientific career studying sleep deprivation. I couldn't have been more enthusiastic, but regardless of whether my encouragement made a difference in his career direction, everyone will benefit from Dave's scientific contributions.

Two other researchers, June Pilcher and Allen Huffcutt, reexamined 56 sleep studies with a statistical tool called a meta-analysis. By combining the results from many separate studies, a meta-analysis can demonstrate a clear pattern that is more revealing than the information offered by any individual study. The meta-analysis revealed that mood is affected more by sleep deprivation than are either cognitive skills or physical performance.

Earlier I discussed research which demonstrates that most of us are walking around with a significant amount of sleep debt without knowing it. What Dave Dinges's experiment implies is that most of us also are walking around feeling lousy without understanding that this isn't how we have to feel. Just as people think that it is normal to feel sleepy while driving, while sitting in a hot room, or after a meal, we probably think it is normal to feel as cross as we do, to be easily irritated at small annoyances, to feel as if we are just going through the motions all day long. This research suggests that lowering sleep debt can make us feel better, happier, more vigorous and vital.

Another very recent experiment that might support this idea was carried out by Eve Van Cauter and her colleagues at the University of Chicago and Harvard University. Van Cauter tested mood and cognitive function in a group of volunteers who were allowed 8 hours of sleep for three nights, then were restricted to 4 hours of sleep for six nights, and finally allowed 12 hours of sleep for seven nights. As with Dave's experiment, over the six nights of partial sleep deprivation, the mood scores dropped significantly, and there was a marked increase in sleepiness, as measured by the Stanford Sleepiness Scale (a self-rating questionnaire). Then came the recovery sleep. The volunteers had accumulated more than 24 hours of additional sleep debt during their period of sleep deprivation, but with 12 hours of sleep over a seven-night period, they had the opportunity to make up 28 hours of sleep debt, slightly more than they had accumulated during their nights of shortened sleep. Thus they had the opportunity to work off some of the sleep debt that they had taken into the experiment. It is therefore not suprising that, after the full period of recovery sleep, the volunteers had slightly lower scores on the Stanford Sleepiness Scale (indicating less sleepiness) and slightly higher scores on overall mood tests than they had during the baseline testing at the beginning of the experiment. In addition, the mood scores on the day following the extended sleep showed a more pronounced evenness interrupted by fewer ups and downs than at the beginning of the experiment. In simple terms, people who got more sleep were happier and more even-tempered. This is a major result in sleep research.

A few years ago I took my seat on a plane and found myself next to a regal-looking black woman who seemed familiar, although she obviously didn't recognize me. This feeling of familiarity continued to nag at me, however, and after an hour of thinking "I know I've seen her somewhere," it came to me. I had seen her on television in an arresting interview on CNN. She was Madeline Cartwright, the passionately committed principal of an elementary school in a Philadelphia ghetto who, by the sheer force of her personality and character, had made the school a shining oasis of education in which well-behaved and happy students were learning at a very high level. After I introduced myself and told her of my mission to persuade students to get more sleep, she told me a very interesting story.

One morning she was standing in the schoolyard greeting arriving students. As they passed inside, the students would say, "Good morning, Mrs. Cartwright," and then several asked slyly, "Did you see Arsenio last night?" She had no idea who Arsenio might be. She finally discovered that "Arsenio" was Arsenio Hall, the host of a popular late-night talk show, and that the previous night he had been poking fun at elementary school principals. She also found out that the show started at 11:00 P.M. and finished at midnight. She was shocked to realize that many of her elementary school children must be staying up to watch the show. This remarkable woman had developed good relationships with the parents in the neighborhood, and she immediately requested that as many of them as possible attend a special meeting. She explained that the children weren't getting enough sleep and insisted that they had to be in bed by 9:00 P.M. The parents responded. No more Arsenio for 6- to 12-year-olds! According to Mrs. Cartwright, the result was an absolutely unquestionable improvement in the children's mood and a striking decrease in quarrels and irritability.

I think this and many other examples I have heard demonstrate that the general problem of sleep deprivation and mood among normal individuals needs much more attention. The conventional questions about sleep and mood focus on clinical depression. The effect of sleep deprivation on mood in the average healthy person is potentially a huge, invisible problem. Sleep-deprivation studies have shown consistently that sleep-deprived subjects are more irritable, more volatile, and more depressed than control subjects. Accordingly, we can hypothesize that some of the violence and depression in today's society is related to pervasive chronic sleep deprivation. Unfortunately, here again we are not able to mobilize the resources to address this problem, even though it should not be difficult to do so.

The Biological Clock and Mood: The True Font of Vitality

Sleep releases the natural vitality that we have in us, but it doesn't directly create that good feeling. This is a subtle but very important point: Sleep debt is what makes us feel lousy. The main benefit of sleep, what sleep actually does to make us feel better, is to erase sleep debt. The notion that sleep itself actively restores and energizes is so ingrained that most people find it difficult to understand that anything that gets rid of sleep debt or covers it up can lift one's mood. This is true whether sleep debt is paid off through sleep, or covered up via a cup of coffee or amphetamines. It is also hard for people to see that one other factor besides sleep affects our mood on a daily basis: the alerting effect of the biological clock. In other words, the daily pull of sleep debt and push of clock-dependent alerting is a major factor not only in whether we are asleep or awake but also in how we feel emotionally.

Often even I find myself taking the semantical shortcut of saying "Sleep does this or that," without mentioning the role that the biological clock plays in the equation. But the effects of the biological clock are very easy to see when you know what you are looking for. Some years ago I had the chance to observe a completely unambiguous and beautiful episode of clock-dependent alerting at work on mood. It occurred while I was visiting my daughter, Cathy, who was then a student at Harvard. We were sitting in her room after a late lunch and I was attempting to satisfy my parental curiosity about how things were going, what classes were most interesting, how her social life was, and so on. Her monosyllabic, almost sullen answers conveyed no worthwhile information besides the impression that she was not happy. Indeed, she was almost alarmingly apathetic and seemed to be totally uninterested in my visit. I was even beginning to ask myself why I had bothered to make the trip. Anything would be better than the nonconversation we were having, so I suggested we take a walk. It was about 4:00 P.M. on a sunny late-spring afternoon.

After we had strolled silently along the banks of the Charles River for about half an hour, Cathy began to speak a little. Over the course of perhaps 20 to 30 minutes she metamorphosed into a talkative, informative, smiling, even vivacious person. This continued through dinner until I departed at about 8:00 P.M. We had a great time, and I learned all I wanted to know about how things were going and more. Had I left at 4:00 P.M., it would have been a lousy visit. But Cathy was at the age when even a heavily sleep-deprived college student will have a late afternoon/evening period of strong clock-dependent alerting. In her case it was able to abolish her fatigue completely. This marvelous transformation occurred in the complete absence of any outside stimulation; it was entirely internal and spontaneous.

Chuck Czeisler has explored this interaction through a series of experiments that have demonstrated the power of the effect of clock-dependent alerting. First, when he tested people's mood at the same time each the day, it correlated strongly with their recent amount of sleep. But when the amount of sleep was held constant, mood varied throughout the day, as clock-dependent alerting rose and fell. For either owls or larks, clock-dependent alerting can overcome the mood-dampening effects of sleep deprivation.

Although someone who feels great during certain parts of the day can feel horrible hours later when clock-dependent alerting is not as active, those good parts of the day unfortunately can make it harder to see the negative effects of lack of sleep. Owls barely dragging themselves out of bed in the morning or larks who are tired and sleepy right after dinner can rationalize that they are just "not morning people," or "not evening people." If such individuals would lower their sleep debt, they would find that the "bad" parts of the day would become much better. They might even be wide awake and full of energy throughout the entire day rather than just a part of it.

The Excited Brain

The neuroscience of emotion is still in a fairly early stage of development. For thousands of years, people have been thinking about what sorts of things make us feel happy or unhappy, elated or depressed. While it is not known exactly how sleep and sleep debt help the brain create good feelings and bad, we are learning how the brain puts itself in an "up" mood and how addictive drugs create a "high" by stimulating the brain's pleasure centers. We also have a simple model of how the brain becomes activated and fully conscious during waking and dreaming activity. What we have found is that the biochemistry of wakefulness and sleep is intimately tied in with the state of the emotional part of the brain. The waking brain naturally excites and primes itself for vital interaction with the external world, while the sleep-deprived brain suppresses that natural buoyancy by damping the brain's neurochemical activity.

A brain circuit called the reticular activating system plays a major role in arousal. It is highly likely that the biological clock operates on this system to wake up the brain and keep it awake. The reticular activating system is a small collection of nerves that originates deep in the brain stem, the most ancient and primitive part of the brain. A relatively few cells in the brain stem reach out and touch nearly every cell in the brain. These cells carry neurotransmitters, that relay activating signals from the reticular activating system. These neurotransmitters are norepinephrine, dopamine, and acetylcholine. Norepinephrine is one of the key neurotransmitters for arousal, acting as the brain's form of adrenaline. Dopamine is known to be involved in body movement and pleasure. Acetylcholine also acts as a prime arousal chemical and is known to be important in carrying signals concerning muscle movements. Another neurotransmitter, serotonin, also has a strong effect on mood.

These excitatory neurochemicals prepare the brain's 100 billion nerve cells to react more quickly. It is also no surprise that they interface closely with the limbic system, which is sometimes called the emotional brain. This is because we must be wired not only to react quickly to challenge in a purely mechanical way but also to be motivated emotionally to face challenges. The reticular activating system sets the emotional brain on edge, as when runners ready to start a race get down on their hands and the balls of their feet. The activating system doesn't so much create feelings as set an emotional tone for any stimulus that filters into our brain.

The activity of the limbic system is like the background music in a movie. The screen shows someone creeping down a hallway at night toward a closed door. If the background music is tense, perhaps in a minor key, with a few discordant notes thrown in, we interpret the scene as suspenseful and feel anxious about what might lie behind the door. If the music is bouncy and jovial, like something out of an old Charlie Chaplin movie, we interpret the same scene quite differently. We are prepared for humor and might imagine the doorknob coming off when the person tries to open the door. If a monster does pop from behind the door, we might think "What a silly monster suit."

Now consider the movie that constantly plays in your head—the images of the world around you that sensory stimulation tells you is "reality." The nerve cells sprouting out of the base of the brain are creating the mood music inside you by acting directly on all the other brain cells, making them more or less reactive to the scenes that are coming in from the outside world. When we get a good night of sleep, and the reticular activating system is priming the emotional brain properly, our norepinephrine and dopamine infusions create a positive, energetic "background music." The result is a feeling of mental and physical energy we call vitality and an internal psychological push called motivation. Without them we get depressed. (I should note that clinical depression is very different from feeling low or down. In clinical depression, the brain's natural biochemistry is seriously altered.)

One major hypothesis about how sleep affects mood is that sleep somehow replenishes these excitatory neurotransmitters in the brain. Over the course of the day, neurotransmitters are released from nerve cells. Some are recycled back into the cell and others are lost. By keeping brain activity high, sleep deprivation may prevent the brain from replacing lost neurotransmitters. When nerve activity is decreased, alerting is impaired. Your thoughts don't flow as smoothly as they should. You feel down.

To counterbalance the brain's accelerators, other nerve cells and neurotransmitters act as the brain's brakes. The most widely distributed nerve cell receptor in the brain is GABA, the receptor that alcohol and benzodiazepine sleeping pills act on. An activated GABA receptor makes a nerve cell much less reactive to stimuli, slowing the rate of information processing, and uncocking the hammer in the emotional brain.

Another of the brain's primary braking mechanisms is adenosine. Adenosine is one of the molecules that results when the brain breaks down its primary energy source, adenosine triphosphate, or ATP. When the brain is very active and using a lot of energy, more adenosine is present in the brain. This surplus of adenosine acts as a natural governor, reining in brain activity so that it doesn't run too fast. Increasing adenosine concentration in the brain may be part of the reason we feel mental fatigue when we face emotional or mentally challenging situations. The increased brain activity may create a lot of free adenosine, which then depresses brain activity.

One school of thought holds that the sleep drive actively supresses brain activity through this braking mechanism, thereby linking sleepiness and mood. The more time we are awake, the more the inhibitory circuits of the brain damp down the stimulation of the reticular activating system, as if the nerve excitatory and dampening systems are fighting for control of the brain. As various areas of the brain are slowed down by this braking action, the effects show up in how we act, think, and feel. The dampening of nerve activity of motor areas makes us less coordinated; the dampening of nerve activity in the cerebral cortex makes us slow in thought; and quenching nerve activity in the emotional brain makes us feel less vital, less motivated. To counteract this we can walk around, concentrate harder, and give ourselves a pep talk, but eventually the brain's sleep drive triumphs. At some point no mental trick will stimulate brain activity in the areas we need to stay awake—it's like trying to light wet sawdust with a match. We have to fall asleep.

After we sleep, the brakes are off again. Dopamine and norepinephrine release in the brain increases. We feel alive again. Of course, some people skip sleep and turn to a chemical.

Vitality in a Bottle
The energized feeling you get when the sleep-satiated brain is turned on by clock-dependent alerting in the morning can be so good that you want to bottle it, and every generation throughout civilized history has tried to do just that. Each era seems to have had a preference for a stimulant that resists the sleep drive and boosts mood. Over the centuries commercial empires have been built through trade in caffeinated goods such as coffee, tea, chocolate, and soda. Much of Latin America, India, Indonesia, and East Africa were colonized to grow coffee or tea. In this century, cocaine and amphetamines, or "speed," have each had their legal heyday before the dark side emerged. The human craving for a "boost" will never go out of fashion. It's important to understand the history of drugs that affect sleepiness and mood, because new pharmaceutical agents may force us to radically change how we view stimulants.

Artificial stimulants work by modifying how the nerve cells in the brain send messages to each other. Nerve cells communicate when neurotransmitters are passed from one cell to another across a gap called a synapse. (See Figure 12.1.) After the neurotransmitters norepinephrine and dopamine are released into the synapse, the cells usually recycle them rapidly, snatching them back into their source cell. Cocaine blocks this process, causing dopamine and norepinephrine to stay in the synapse long after they should have left the scene and keep stimulating other nerve cells during this time. Amphetamine stimulates the same neurotransmitters, but through a different route, actually creating brain signals where cocaine simply makes normal brain signals more potent and longer lasting. Similar in structure to the neurotransmitters norepinephrine and dopamine, amphetamine works by penetrating nerve cells and ejecting dopamine and norepinephrine out into the synapse where they excite adjacent cells. Since the norepinephrine and dopamine systems reach deeply into the emotional part of the brain and provide "background music" for our experiences, the result of both chemicals is a general feeling of high energy and euphoria. Dopamine, in particular, is the main neurotransmitter involved in the brain's pleasure centers. When dopamine is released in these parts of the brain, we feel wonderful and want to re-create the events that led to this reward. Sex, love, a thrilling ride, or a great purchase can all stimulate that dopamine-generated burst of pleasure. More and more, it seems that all addictive drugs are addictive precisely because they cause dopamine release, either directly or indirectly.

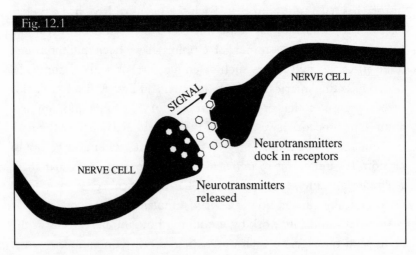

Fig. 12.1

NERVE CELL

SIGNAL

Neurotransmitters dock in receptors

NERVE CELL

Neurotransmitters released

Cocaine is derived from the leaves of the South American coca plant which the Inca chewed to allow them to work longer at high altitude. The Inca regarded the coca plant as a gift from the gods, one that banished hunger, supplied vigor, and made the unhappy forget their troubles. The leaves and their effects were introduced to Europeans after the Spanish conquest of the Inca in the sixteenth century. Not until the Corsican chemist Angelo Mariani added a coca extract to wine in 1863 and named it Vin Mariani, however, did coca become popular in Europe. The tonic wine became the toast of Europe and, later, America. It was recommended in advertisements as a treatment for all sorts of ailments, including "general debility, exhaustion, profound depression, overwork, throat and lung diseases, consumption and malaria." Mariani became rich and famous.

A few decades later George Pemberton, an American chemist from Georgia, developed a beverage containing coca extract, undoubtedly in imitation of Mariani. At first he toyed with adding wine to the drink, but it was 1884, and the temperance movement was growing in the United States. Pemberton saw a market for a nonalcoholic, sweetened health tonic. Finally settling on an extract of the kola nut to supply flavor, he added carbonation and named the drink Coca-Cola. Like Vin Mariani, the coca-laced Coca-Cola was hailed as a healthy, refreshing elixir. (Now, of course, Coca-Cola uses caffeine, a less potent stimulant, instead of cocaine.)

Sigmund Freud was among the first in the medical community to become a promoter of purified cocaine, the active ingredient in the coca plant. Ethnopharmacologists have found that people who chew coca leaves or sip drinks with coca extracts don't become addicts or show other behavioral problems, but this is not the case with cocaine. At first, cocaine seemed harmless. Freud tested the drug on himself and his patients, convinced that it was a wonderful short-term energizer with fewer side effects than alcohol. In "Über Coca," a widely read paper Freud published in 1884, he wrote that cocaine "wards off hunger, sleep, and fatigue and steels one to intellectual effort." Cocaine was soon widely dispensed, almost as a panacea. Users develop a tolerance for the drug, whereby larger and larger doses are needed to get the same effect, a route that ultimately leads to outright psychosis. After cases of psychosis became widespread,

Freud was roundly criticized and cocaine was denounced as a scourge equal to alcohol and morphine.

Amphetamine was also first thought to be a harmless fatigue fighter. But where cocaine was a natural substance in search of a medical application, amphetamine was a synthetic drug developed to treat a specific ailment, asthma. In the 1920s pharmacologists at the American drug company Eli Lilly discovered that one of the ingredients in the Chinese herb *Ephedra vulgaris* helped asthmatics breathe easier, much like the traditional treatment, adrenaline. They named the drug ephedrine, and its synthetic version pseudoephedrine is still used in over-the-counter cold medications like Sudafed. It was hard to get enough ephedra plants, so in the 1930s chemists went in search of a synthetic substitute and arrived at a drug they named amphetamine. Under the trade name Benzedrine, amphetamines were sold as a nasal decongestant in inhalable form without prescription.

People quickly learned that you could break apart the inhaler and ingest the Benzedrine inside. When I was working the overnight shift in a Walla Walla pea cannery in the late 1940s, someone showed me this trick. Once you broke apart the inhaler, you could remove the little piece of paper that contained the drug. Drop it in a cup of coffee or water, dissolve the amphetamine, and drink. At the time, amphetamines were used by militaries worldwide to keep soldiers and pilots awake. During World War II Japan encouraged the civilian population to use amphetamines in order to boost production. Amphetamines were so easy to get and widely embraced around the world that by the late 1940s, an epidemic of addiction was blooming. By the early 1950s the epidemic was impossible to ignore. The most shocking example was in Japan, where 25 percent of the population between ages 16 and 25 were addicted to the drug. Soon authorities were cracking down.

When I was in medical school in the early 1950s, medical students could still simply go to the pharmacy, show their student card, and get 50 to 100 pills. Occasionally I used amphetamines to increase available study time before big exams, although I'm not certain I actually performed better. Of course, enforcement of drug laws hasn't ended amphetamine and methamphetamine addiction. There was a jump in cases during the 1960s and today it is estimated that approximately 1 percent of the population illegally uses amphetamines.

Of course, caffeine is the brain stimulant of choice in the civilized world. Its psychological effects are less intense than cocaine or amphetamine. Caffeine has become a pervasive stimulant in modern society. Every day billions of people around the world use coffee, tea, and other caffeinated beverages. I, for one, am very happy we have these drinks—one or two steaming cups of coffee are an important part of my morning. But even if you refrain from coffee and tea, it is very difficult to avoid caffeine. Sometimes, when I am speaking before an audience, I ask if there are people who abstain from caffeine. Usually about 5 to 10 percent of the audience raise their hands. "No caffeinated coffee or tea?" I press. "No caffeinated sodas?" Some of the hands drop. "No chocolate?" I ask, and nearly all of those with hands still raised drop their hands. Manufacturers even add it to some aspirin and cold medications.

Caffeine stimulates the brain and body because its chemical structure is similar to adenosine, one of the molecules that act as a neural brake, though its effect is dramatically different. Because the caffeine molecule is shaped like adenosine, it actually blocks adenosine's access to its receptor, so that this brain brake is not allowed to engage. As with other stimulants, the energy we get from caffeine is not without cost. Its side effects are well known: It can make us jittery if we overuse it, or unable to sleep if we consume it late in the day. It has long been known that we tend to become habituated to caffeine, needing more and more to get the same effect, until we become mildly addicted and face headaches, irritability, and discomfort if we stop using it. Most of my colleagues agree that if caffeine were a new drug, it would never get approval for human use from the Food and Drug Administration because its side effects outweigh its benefits as a stimulant.

Nicotine, usually taken by consuming or smoking tobacco, is another common stimulant. Nicotine mimics another key activating neurotransmitter, acetylcholine, thereby stimulating brain activity. Scientists have known about this activity of nicotine for a long time, but recently they have discovered that nicotine acts a lot like cocaine in the reward centers of the brain, by stimulating dopamine release. It is nicotine's effect on dopamine that ultimately may be the biggest reason that cigarettes are addictive. Like caffeine, nicotine has a lot of side effects, and over time people need to take more and more to get the same stimulating effect. Tobacco, of course, also causes a number of health problems; one can hardly imagine cigarettes getting through the current regulatory approval process if they were invented today.

Cocaine, amphetamines, nicotine, and caffeine are only some of the many artificial stimulants that people have taken throughout history. The desire for stimulation is so strong that every year 1 in 25 people in the United States is willing to face harsh legal penalties to abuse stimulant drugs. There are still truck stops in the Midwest where drivers can plop down $18 for "trucker's coffee," a cup of regular coffee into which is stirred a spoonful of methamphetamine-laced sugar. These illegal stimulants are dangerous in part because they deplete neurotransmitters in the brain, so that after the drugs wear off, the brain crashes.

So far, all of the drugs I've mentioned merely postpone the inevitable demands of the sleep drive. You may be able to stay up later, but eventually you will have to sleep extra to pay off the debt you build up during that time. But what if sleep researchers came up with a new drug that would allow us to go without sleeping and not accumulate debt? What if you could take a pill at 10:00 P.M., stay up all night, and still feel completely normal the next day?

Wonder Drugs That Affect Sleep Need?

One Stanford Sleep Research Center team led by Dale Edgar is currently investigating the properties of a different kind of molecule that may stimulate the body's natural arousal processes or block its natural sleep processes, or both. It was developed in France in 1976. This drug is modafinil, which I introduced earlier in the book as a treatment for narcolepsy. What is really interesting is how non-narcoleptics feel when they take it. Modafinil just seems to wake people up. Not jack them up like amphetamine. Not get them wired. Just wake them up. A few years ago French sleep scientist Michel Jouvet gave me a sample of modafinil. When I tried it I didn't feel as if I had taken a stimulant. I just felt awake. Neither our group here at Stanford nor any of the other groups involved in the

FDA testing process has yet to find a major negative side effect or a potential for addiction.

What really makes modafinil of great interest to us is that it seems to both suspend the need for sleep in the short term, as well as delay or diminish the need to pay back sleep debt. If you forego sleep for a long period, with or without the aid of drugs, you'll need a long recovery sleep to repay the large sleep debt. But when Dale keeps test animals awake with modafinil for more than a day, he reports that they don't "crash" and need to sleep longer to make up sleep debt accumulated while the drug was working. This means that modafinil and similar drugs are not stimulants at all but a new class of drugs that we have called "somnolytics" rather than stimulants.

Dale has suggested that modafinil acts at the nexus between the brain's sleep homeostat and its clock-dependent alerting system. The drug may work by modifying the inhibitory action of the GABA receptor to block the particular receptors that mediate between the excitatory action of the biological clock and the dampening action of the sleep homeostat. If modafinil does target a small subgroup of receptors like this, it would explain why the drug staves off sleepiness and affects how sleep debt is accumulated and paid off. But this is still just theory. Dale believes, as do I, that modafinil or similar compounds eventually may offer us a tool to find how the brain keeps track of sleep debt, one of the most important and interesting questions in sleep science.

Modafinil is now being used clinically in France to treat narcolepsy and idiopathic hypersomnolence (excessive daytime sleepiness without known cause). In the United States, the FDA has approved the compound as a treatment for narcolepsy. Once the FDA approves a drug, a doctor can prescribe it to treat any ailment, not just the condition for which the drug is approved. The medical community views this freedom of "off-label" prescribing as a sacred cornerstone of doctors' autonomy.

In this climate, modafinil may be prescribed for other reasons, not just narcolepsy or hypersomnolence. Assuming that modafinil and similar compounds prevent sleep without engendering the euphoria that underlies the abuse of other stimulants, these drugs could certainly be useful for individuals dealing with all kinds of emergencies:

soldiers in combat, surgeons during very long operations, and leaders during national and international crisis, even the President of the United States. The U.S. Air Force already has studied the use of modafinil, and Canadian troops used it successfully in operations during the Persian Gulf War.

I wonder though what will the development of even more powerful somnolytics in the future will mean for society. If such a drug truly would be able to turn off the homeostat, even if only for a day or two, without side effects and without risk of addiction, would that be bad? What would happen if such a future drug becomes widely prescribed, or even available over-the-counter, so you can take it as casually as you now drink coffee. Would everyone take it to work more? If you decided to sleep anyway, would your career suffer because you allowed yourself the luxury of sleep, while Mr. Jones in the office next door took the wonder drug every night and accomplished twice as much? In the book *Brave New World* by Aldous Huxley, people take a drug called Soma to stay happy and unquestioning of the government. What if the first country that distributed "Somnolyrica" freely to its citizens became the wealthiest and most productive in the world?

I am a believer in the power of science and medicine to improve our lives. Medical technology has created truly miraculous cures for some of our most frightening physical and mental illnesses. It has spared us the anguish of previous generations of parents who watched their children become crippled by polio or killed by tuberculosis. Yet our accelerating power to manipulate our body chemistry and genes makes me uneasy. Drugs that enhance fertility, memory, mood, and even virility are fast becoming fixtures of our cultural medicine cabinet. How best to use these biotechnologies may become the preeminent moral and medical question of our age. Bioethicists can help us frame the issues, but only open and honest public debate can lead to wise decisions. Most technological leaps come with a price to society, whether the leaps are electric light or internal combustion engines. But as individuals and as a society we must weigh freedom of choice carefully against the dangers of ceaselessly expanding the limits nature imposes. Any reasonable person would advise caution. One day our children may wax nostalgic for a time when people daily were forced to put down their labors to mend mind and body.

For now, the body's own natural chemistry is the most reliable, sustainable way to set the brain up to enjoy life. Without excessive sleep debt to hold it back, the healthy brain is practically a vitality machine, creating the chemical environment necessary for vigorously engaging and conquering life's challenges. Artificial stimulants may be beneficial in the short term to level out the swings of the biological clock or to deal with emergencies. But until proven otherwise (which may never happen), healthy sleep is the best long-term strategy for spurring brain activity and lifting our spirits.

Chapter 13

The Real Life of Dreams

I USED to be a very heavy smoker. What started as an occasional indulgence in my army days had, by the early 1960s, become chain smoking. I was smoking two packs a day, maybe more, and it seemed like I always had a cigarette in my hand. Like many heavy smokers, I had developed a chronic cough, known as a smoker's hack. One day in 1964 I was coughing into a handkerchief and noticed with a chill that the little flecks of sputum on the white cloth were reddish pink. Those were the good old days before managed care, when doctors freely exchanged services without paperwork or delay, so I sought out a radiologist friend and asked him to order a chest X ray. The next day I went back to his office, full of dread. I will never forget the grim expression on his face as he motioned me to the light box behind his desk. Without a word, he turned and clipped my chest film onto it. Immediately I saw that my lungs harbored a dozen white spots—cancer. The wave of anguish and despair that I felt was overpowering. I could barely breathe. My life was over. I wouldn't see my children grow up. All because I hadn't stopped smoking, even though I knew all about smoking and cancer. "You utter fool," I thought. "You've destroyed your own life!"

And then I woke up.

The bloody sputum, the X rays, and the cancer had been a dream—an incredibly vivid and real dream. What a relief. I was reborn. I had been given the chance to experience having inoperable cancer of the lung without having it. I stopped smoking right then and have never lit another cigarette.

This is exactly the kind of powerful, realistic dream that has fascinated people since at least the beginning of recorded history. This experience is the archetype of the dream as a personal warning, as the embodiment of repressed anxiety, as prophecy. Such dreams have an intense power over human beings. We can be living a normal life, seeming to move from one relatively untroubled day to the next, and then have a dreaming experience that literally changes our lives.

Think about it. I believe this dream saved my life, that I am alive and breathing today, 35 years later, because of something that never really happened. I have speculated that dreams may be a distant early warning. Maybe there were actually a few cancer cells or cells beginning to undergo the malignant change under the daily battering of cigarette smoke, and my brain somehow picked up on that.

I've told the cancer story often, and countless times people have come up to me to recount their own life-changing dreams. Often it's a variation on something like this: "I couldn't decide whether to marry Mike or Jim, but then I had a dream that I married Jim and it was terrible, so I married Mike and we've been happily together for 20 years." More recently a student in my class said that she had been accepted for admission to the University of California at Berkeley and at Stanford. She couldn't decide which one to attend. Then she had a dream that she had accepted admission to Berkeley and was having an awful time. In her dream, she said, "Oh, I wish I had chosen Stanford." So, in real life, she did, and she testified in class that she could not imagine being happier.

To some it may seem amazing that people will take drastic action as a result of something that didn't even happen. But the emotional impact of dreams can be so powerful that they might as well really have occurred. Suppose that I dreamed that I lost track of my daughter at the beach, and that my anguish and despair had been multiplied a hundredfold as my daughter's lifeless body was discovered. What if I actually experience holding her in my arms in utter despair, cursing that I ever took my eyes off her, and then I woke up? You may be absolutely certain that I would have been even more careful in the future to avoid this happening in reality. As with my dream of cancer, I would experience it as some kind of miraculous second chance to avoid the circumstances that led to disaster.

The logical part of the awake brain knows that the dream was not real, but the emotional part of the brain cannot set it aside. As far as our brains are concerned, what we dream really happens to us. After I awoke from my smoking dream I knew it was a dream, but you better believe I got a chest X ray in the real world with some trepidation, although I had not really coughed bloody sputum. The emotions I had experienced in the dream were real, even if the events were not. The physical feelings seemed as real as could be. Having experienced that awful moment when I learned I had cancer—not just imagined it as if in some daydream, but really lived it—I had been given a second chance, and there was no way I could keep smoking. This possibility of really experiencing two alternatives or experiencing what may be the consequences of a very important choice not as a fantasy or illumination but as a real experience may someday be of enormous importance. I think it is quite possible that someday we will be able to enter the dream world more or less at will.

Many people consider dreams the most important part of sleep. The idea that dreams are, as Freud said, "letters to ourselves," supplying crucial information about hidden emotions, continues to have strong popular support. It was dreams that first attracted me to the science of sleep, and I launched my research career studying the connection between dreams and REM. Decades later I continue to be fascinated by the power and mystery of dreams.

Not all my fellow sleep researchers feel this way. Some regard dreams as merely an epiphenomenon of the sleep process. Dreams, according to sleep researcher, psychologist, and colleague Bernie Webb, are "just the foam on the beer" of sleep. Two prominent neuroscientist sleep researchers ignited controversy by marshaling evidence to support their hypothesis that dreams are nothing more than random nerve activity in the brain with no real purpose or meaning.

But I continue to be drawn to dreams, because I think they can signify much more. Dreaming is like another world, an alternate reality with its own rules and lessons. I believe the answer to the question "Why do we dream what we dream?" holds profound implications not just about ourselves but also about the nature of consciousness and the deepest workings of the human brain.

The Physiology of Dreams

Some studies suggest that dreaming sometimes can take place during non-REM sleep, but I believe this depends on how you define "dreaming" and how you ask people about dreams. If you wake someone and ask, "What was going through your mind just now?" the person more often will have a narrative to relate than if you ask "What were you dreaming?" Still, recall of vivid dream imagery is reported only about 10 percent of the time when people are awakened in non-REM sleep, whereas people report vivid dreaming more than 80 percent of the time when awakened during REM sleep.

In my early days with Nathaniel Kleitman, I often served as a research subject, partly because there was no money to induce lots of others to volunteer but mainly because it was an amazing experience to be repeatedly awakened and vividly remember a lengthy dream every time. Furthermore, in at least 100 awakenings from non-REM sleep, I never recalled dreaming. In fact, one of the first times I served as a subject permanently convinced me that true dreaming does not occur in non-REM sleep. In the fall of 1954, I had recruited another medical student who was willing to lose a few nights of sleep to assist me. As the first step in his training, I wanted to demonstrate the miraculous way dreams could be elicited from REM period awakenings. I hastily showed him how to identify rapid eye movements in the emerging polygraph tracings, then got wired for sleep and went to bed.

I was groggy when he first woke me and could remember no dreams. No problem—I had already learned that recall from the very first period of REM sleep was often poor. But after each of the next four awakenings I struggled in vain to find any scrap of a recent dream in my memory. My demonstration of this miraculous phenomenon was beginning to look like a total bust. What was wrong? I am ashamed to say that the sixth time my fellow medical student woke me and I could recall absolutely nothing, I was so embarrassed and upset, I lied. I haltingly produced a phony dream fragment. It was past 5:00 A.M., so I decided to end the travesty. I got out of bed and immediately inspected the polygraph recording. I was overjoyed and incredibly relieved to discover that he had mistaken certain EEG waveforms that occurred in non-REM sleep for rapid eye movement signals. Every awakening had been in non-REM sleep! If anyone wants to claim that subject or experimenter bias plays a role in the REM sleep-dreaming relationship, I could not have been more biased toward recalling a dream, and I was utterly unable to dredge up even a wisp of one.

The next time we tried this experiment, I had given my fellow student much more training. He woke me five times, and I recalled five vivid chapters in that night's book of dreaming. When I inspected the polygraph record, he had hit the target in the bull's eye every time, right in the middle of five successive REM periods.

During REM sleep our bodies become almost completely paralyzed. The nerve signals for movement, which normally travel from the brain to the muscles, are intercepted along the spinal cord and blocked. If this didn't happen, we would physically act out our dreams (which, as I've mentioned, actually happens in some sleep disorders). REM paralysis sometimes is seen at the onset of sleep or in the first few moments immediately after waking from REM sleep. You may have experienced this sensation yourself, just as you're dropping off to sleep. Suddenly you realize you can't move. It can be terribly frightening. Patients experiencing several of these "sleep paralysis" episodes sometimes become so anxious that they rush to the clinic to be examined. We always reassure them that a few attacks of sleep paralysis with no other symptoms are completely normal and innocuous.

REM paralysis isn't absolute: If someone is very motivated to move or has strong feelings in the dream, the paralysis is occasionally overcome. People who are especially disturbed by dreams may jerk their limbs or mumble while asleep. Nightmares commonly produce emotions strong enough to break through REM paralysis, although usually the movement or the emotion wakes the sleeper. In addition, some kinds of movements are not blocked as completely as others. The brief, intense nerve signals that cause the muscles to twitch get through more easily than the longer, less intense signals activated when you make a continuous movement, like swinging your arms.

These phasic signals cause the twitchy movements in dreaming cats and dogs. Twitches during dreaming are also found in humans, although they are less noticeable.

Besides the heart and lungs, another part of the body is not paralyzed during REM sleep: the penis. Normal men always have an erection during REM sleep. When one of my colleagues was asked, for the umpteenth time, where dreams come from, he answered, "I don't know where they come from, but I think that the erect penis serves as the antenna to receive them." This doesn't really violate the rule about paralysis during REM sleep, since erections are not caused by muscle action but by blood engorgement. Since there is usually a REM period right before waking, men often wake up with an erection. In women, other sleep researchers have found that there is increased vaginal blood flow and clitoral engorgement during REM sleep. The increase in blood flow in both men and women during REM sleep is probably an incidental effect of the activation of the part of the autonomic nervous system that controls heart rate and other involuntary body functions.

Penile erection during REM (called nocturnal penile tumescence, or NPT) is sometimes misunderstood, usually because the sleeper or his partner thinks the erection signifies that the dream is about sex. This is not the case. No matter what the dream is about, REM sleep will produce an erection in any man who is not impotent for physical reasons. A patient was referred to me because she was concerned that her husband had an erection every night, and she thought he must be dreaming about sex with another woman. She worried that this was a reflection of a real affair. She was very distressed, but I assured her that, barring any other evidence, she should put her mind at ease. The erection is almost never associated with erotic dream content. Even newborn males have erections during REM sleep. But women don't. Once, through an error in the hospital billing office, over 100 women were billed for an NPT test. When many of these women called to ask about the NPT test on their bill we had to suffer the embarrassment of telling them about the test and our mistake. The worst moment was explaining this to a patient who was a nun.

Many people have watched animals sleep and inferred that they are dreaming. Cats and dogs certainly exhibit unmistakable signs of REM sleep. Imagine a sunny, winter Sunday morning, when the house has been left to the pets. The cat lies on a sofa in a spot of sunlight, eyes closed, deeply asleep but not motionless: Her eyes move back and forth rapidly under the eyelids, her paws twitch rhythmically, and her whiskers move occasionally. Is she dreaming of pouncing on a bird and biting at it? A golden retriever is also dozing off in the kitchen next to the warm oven. Occasionally he emits a small rumble in his throat. Is he dreaming of running after a rabbit, barking in full-throated tribute to the chase? I tend to believe that if all the signs of dreaming are present, dreaming is too. Still, whether animals experience dreams as humans do continues to intrigue people.

Once I did consider talking to an animal about dreams. For a time the building behind the sleep lab housed Koko, a famous female gorilla who had been taught sign language. Here was a chance, I realized, to ask one of our closest biological relatives what she thought about her dreams. The plan would be to watch Koko sleeping until we saw eye movements and then we would wake her and sign "What were you doing?" If she signed "Eating a banana," it would be a reasonable assumption that she had been dreaming about eating a banana.

I found a student who was willing to learn the signs that Koko used to communicate. We visited Koko's pen. My student was introduced to Koko by the woman who headed the project. He began to interact with her in one corner of the enclosure, while we talked briefly in another. After a few moments, I looked over at the student and saw him standing absolutely still, his face ashen, his eyes wide with fear. Koko was unbuckling his pants and trying to get at his penis. Koko's caretaker quickly interceded. Needless to say, the student lost all interest in finding out what a gorilla has to say about dreams, and thus ended my short career studying what gorillas dream about. But Koko and other apes who know sign language have been seen making signs while asleep, as if they were talking in their dreams.

The Reality of Dreams

The philosopher Chuang Tzu, who lived in China around 300 B.C., once remarked on the strange dual reality of the waking and the dreaming worlds: "Once I, Chuang Tzu, dreamed I was a butterfly, a butterfly flying about, feeling that it was enjoying itself. It did not know that it was Chuang. Suddenly I awoke and was myself again, the veritable Chuang. I do not know whether it was then Chuang dreaming that he was a butterfly, or whether I am now a butterfly dreaming that it is Chuang. But between Chuang and a butterfly there must be a difference."

We almost never dream we are someone else, let alone a butterfly. I believe Chuang Tzu was suggesting that there are two realities, however different they may be. Some people say that the dream world is different because of its strangeness. But, according to their own rules of reality, dreams are not so strange. It is only rarely that a dreamer questions the reality of a dream. Almost every event is accepted as real while we are dreaming.

I believe the major characteristic that distinguishes dream from reality is continuity. Our life and events in the real world are smoothly continuous. The dream world lacks this property. Each dream tends to be an isolated event—at best, slightly related to the next. Events within dreams also jump from one setting to another.

Some aspects of what people think about dreaming are the result of imperfect recall. A good example of this is the fact that many people believe we dream in black and white, like an old movie. However, years ago I was able to show that people dreamed in color and could remember the color if they reported dreams immediately upon being awakened from REM periods. Apparently the memory for color faded faster than everything else.

Early in my Stanford career, I wanted to meet the doctor for the Stanford football team but hadn't managed it. I felt highly gratified one day when I saw him sitting in the back of the classroom during a lecture I was giving. The next Saturday I ran into him before a game, introduced myself, and said, "I was really happy to see you taking an interest in sleep research." He looked at me blankly. I said, "You attended my lecture last Tuesday." He took a step back and said, "I was in Chicago on Tuesday." "But I saw you! You couldn't have been." Feeling confused and awkward, I made my apologies and walked away, but I continued to be troubled by the very clear memory of him in my audience. When I started analyzing the memory, I realized that I wasn't very clear on the details. I couldn't remember what I was lecturing about or whether I saw the team doctor at the beginning or the end of the lecture. I finally decided that I must have been dreaming, but for some reason the dream had stayed with me as a seemingly real memory. This experience may be evidence of the real reason we forget most of our dreams, so as not to confuse ourselves. If we remembered every dream clearly, it might become difficult to sort out what really occurred and what was a dream.

You probably do not fully realize the importance of the forgoing supposition. One of the questions I am most frequently asked is "Does everyone dream?" I think we have studied a sufficient number of human beings to give a total and unambiguous yes to that question. Furthermore, equating REM sleep with dreaming, we inhabit the dream world for about two hours every night. Think of the last movie you ever saw. Imagine you were the hero or heroine. You would remember everything quite vividly. If you remembered all your dream experiences from every night, it would put a great burden on your sanity. Many memories from dreams experiences would conflict with the waking world. I truly believe that the wall of memory is a blessed protection. In addition, when we awaken from a vivid dream that we will always remember, recalling it that moment also labels it permanently as a dream. Because we are in bed in the dark, we know it is a dream and we give it this identity.

The eyes offer a window into the brain during REM sleep. The unparalyzed eyes reveal that the brain is reacting to the dream scenes in essentially the same way it would if the dream were real. Once, when we were recording a man in REM sleep, we saw his eyes dart back and forth, left to right and back again in a rhythmic fashion 26 times. This was so unusual that we immediately woke him up and asked what his dream was about. He told us that he had been sitting by the table watching a Ping-Pong game between his brother and a friend, following the ball back and forth while they battled through a long volley. In this instance, we duplicated the event in the real world. We recorded his eye movements while he sat in the same place and watched two players we recruited hit the ball back and forth 26 times. The electrical patterns generated by his movements as he watched were identical with the pattern we had recorded during his sleep. We observed another subject in REM sleep as his eyes were fixed straight ahead, stayed motionless for a number of seconds, and finally made a quick motion up and down. We woke him right away, and he said that he had been sitting in a balcony seat, watching the violinist Isaac Stern perform onstage (eyes fixed straight ahead), until someone stood up in front of him, blocking his view (eyes look up and down). Other sleep researchers interested in the topic have recorded similar results.

Years of experimentation strongly suggest that in REM, the brain is acting very much as it does in waking life, sending out signals to move muscles in response to the scenario that is being played out in the dream. Even though the eyes are not receiving real images from the outside world, the brain orders them to move, to scan a scene that actually exists only in the mind. Signals to the rest of the body, as I've said, are mostly blocked at the spinal cord so that we don't move our limbs. To certain parts of the brain, there is no difference between waking life and dreaming life. When we are dreaming of eating or fighting or thinking, the brain is sending out the same signals it would if we were awake and eating or fighting or thinking.

In a way, all perception is dreaming. The sole difference is that in dreams what we experience is limited only by the brain itself, and not organized and driven by sensory input from the outside world. This idea is summed up nicely by my colleague Stephen LaBarge: "Dreaming is perception unconstrained by sensory input, and perception is dreaming constrained by sensory input."

The Interpretation of Dreams

The idea that dreams are a personal message to the dreamer has a long history. Throughout recorded time, dreams have been mined for their meaning. The ancient Egyptians had dream specialists who interpreted dreams, and Egyptologists have discovered an Egyptian dream dictionary that translates the meaning of dream symbols. The Greeks and Romans felt that dreams contained prophecies about the future, although they thought that not all prophecies were true. They distinguished between "dreams of ivory" (true dreams) and "dreams of horn" (false dreams). Many visions and prophecies in the Bible came to people in dreams. Jacob, who dreamed about climbing ladders and wrestling with angels, is the Bible's first dreamer. His son Joseph was the Bible's first dream interpreter. Even before Freud there were gypsies and folk healers who specialized in interpreting dreams.

Freud brought markedly renewed interest to interpreting dreams, perhaps because he was the first person in modern Western thought to make a systematic psychological study of the subject. As I pointed out in Chapter 2, the Freudian interpretation of dreams involves looking beyond the conscious or manifest content of the dream to find its latent content, which he felt usually involved repressed sexual feelings or other taboo impulses. The "safe" (disguised) release of these impulses of violence, incest, and primitive orality allows people to stay sane, Freud believed. While the idea that dreams are the "safety valve" preventing psychosis is no longer widely accepted by sleep researchers, belief in the significance of dreams has become increasingly common among the lay public.

Years ago in an experiment that was about as primitive as the repressed impulse that we would test, we decided to see what would happen if we substituted food and eating for REM sleep. The idea, as in other studies, was to awaken the sleeper at the very first sign of a developing REM period, thus preventing REM from occurring. If the basic fundamental purpose of REM sleep and dreaming was to discharge primitive oral impulses, we might be able to substitute eating for dreaming by feeding the subject after each REM interruption period. Then, on recovery night, there should be no rebound in amount of REM sleep.

The first subject we tested told us his favorite food was banana cream pie. My wife baked a delicious creamy confection, and I took it to the lab to begin the experiment. Following the usual procedure in REM deprivation studies, I waited until there were several eye movements, then awakened the subject, who reported a very short fragment of a dream about walking down a street in Greenwich Village. He ate his first piece of banana cream pie with great gusto and commented, "What a way to do research!" He went back to sleep, began another REM period about an hour later, recalled another dream fragment when we awoke him, and again he ate his pie with relish. After three awakenings, three minute dreams, and three pieces of pie, the fourth arousal elicited the following dream: "I was having a cup of coffee and a cigarette." He ate his fourth piece of banana cream pie with a little less enthusiasm and commented, "I always have coffee and a cigarette at the *end* of meals." Describing the fifth dream fragment, he said, "I was scraping spaghetti off my plate into a garbage can." He ate his fifth piece of pie with obvious reluctance and left the crust. In the sixth dream fragment he reported, "Dr. Dement, I dreamed I was feeding *you* banana cream pie!"

While I feel there is personal meaning to be found in dreams, possibly even meanings that the conscious mind represses, the interpretations depend very much on the individual and his or her cultural context. Some people try to interpret a dream by looking at "dream books," which are always vague and useless. These nonsense books might tell you, for instance, that a dream of ice represents "frozen emotions." Yet for Eskimos, ice may symbolize the world at large; or for people who live in the desert, it may represent the exotic. Cigars may symbolize a phallus, a capitalist, a nuisance—or, as Freud said, sometimes just a cigar.

Some anthropologists accept the idea that frequent dream objects and actions can have similar meanings to people in the same culture. Some dreams are so common in Western culture that their meaning is taken for granted. For instance, the dream of being naked in public is usually associated with dreamers' fears of being seen for who they really are. Dreams of taking tests or missing lectures are common anxiety dreams. Dreams of trying to get somewhere and being foiled again and again often occur when dreamers have some ambivalence about actually getting somewhere or doing something. Wish-fulfillment dreams might come in the form of a personal visit from a favorite movie star. Usually you wake up from one of these dreams and know exactly what it means. Even if you couldn't articulate it, you would know it held some significance.

And you would be dead wrong, according to another post-Freudian school of thought, which is at the heart of just one of the debates raging at the frontier of neuroscience and psychology.

Meaning vs. Mechanism

A few of today's most prominent sleep scientists have concluded that dreams are not letters to ourselves. They do not reveal our true thoughts and emotions. These folks, whom I have known for years, challenge the seemingly well-established idea that dreams have meaning in our lives. Aided by a range of technologies from EEG machines to PET (positron emission tomography) scans, neuroscientists have made huge advances in mapping the waking brain. Occasionally these techniques have been applied to dream research.

In the early 1970s two prominent Harvard sleep researchers, J. Allan Hobson and Robert McCarley, found that during REM sleep a small area near the brain's base creates strong, regular bursts of nerve signals. These signals travel upward through the brain and spread throughout the cortex, where most of the brain's higher functions take place. The two scientists studied cats but postulated that similar bursts are occurring during REM sleep in all animals, including humans. The two psychiatrists, who are also eminent neurophysiologists and sleep researchers, propose that these bursts are the source of dreams. According to their "activation-synthesis hypothesis," the bursts originating in the area called the pons at the base of the brain "activate" nerve cells throughout the brain, bringing forth images, sensations, and feelings.

Dreams result when the brain does what it does every day in waking life: makes sense of incoming nerve signals. The idea is that the brain takes what is essentially random, meaningless nerve activation and "synthesizes" something that has some meaning and coherence, even if it has to resort to making up its own story. Accordingly, there is no hidden meaning in dreams. Sensations in dreams, the Harvard researchers say, are much like the sensations experienced when scientists painlessly stimulate sections of the brain at random with an electrical probe. When one part of the brain is stimulated, the subject may report hearing music. When another part is randomly probed, the subject remembers a childhood toy. The sensations or memories the subject experiences depend on which nerve cells the probe happened to hit. These scientists propose that the thoughts and memories that emerge in dreams are also the result of random nerve excitation. The superficial content of dreams, they believe, is the whole content; there is no need for finding hidden meanings.

More recently, in 1997 a team led by Dr. Allen Braun of the National Institutes of Health and Dr. Thomas J. Balkin of the Walter Reed Army Institute used PET scans to map the living human brain during REM sleep, with intriguing implications for the peculiar content of dreams. A PET scan is taken after a mildly radioactive glucose has been injected into the brain, rendering blood flow—a measure of nerve activity—visible. In PET scans, the working areas of the brain light up and the passive areas remain dark, whereas the older technology of EEG machines can show only the quantity and quality of brain waves. The PET scans show that during REM sleep, the primary visual cortex, with other areas that compute sensory information, are less active than normal. The frontal lobes—whose functions include short-term memory, planning and executing thoughts and actions, and integrating data from other parts of the brain—are also passive. What remains highly active are the brain's emotional and long-term memory centers. The Walter Reed team has offered this finding as an explanation for why the content of our dreams is laden with emotion and old memories. One major caveat is that PET scans have a very low resolution, and what appears as "passive" may only be 10 to 20 percent less active than what appears as "active."

Many people cannot accept these conclusions. Psychoanalysts, of course, find heretical the idea that dreams are merely a random collage of thoughts and images. But even as Freud and his theories have faded from center stage, there is still a widespread belief that dreams do have some profound messages for us. Many people regularly look to their dreams for insight about their lives, and I won't accuse them of sheer credulity.

I believe that the struggle between neuroscience and psychoanalysis has yielded a false dichotomy. The question is not whether all dreams are pointless or all dreams profound. First of all, we do not know for certain if the same brain-stem process operates during REM sleep in humans. Another possibility is that once the brain stem gets the dream process going, it may, in effect, take on a life of its own within the infinitely more complicated human brain. Finally, some dreams may be without purpose or meaning while others may be quite the opposite.

In addition, we have to distinguish between meaning and purpose. If you were looking up at the clouds and saw a formation that suggested a familiar face, then that face would have meaning for you. The face might make you think of an old friend. It might even change the course of your life, if you then contacted that friend and became close again. However, it would be absurd to say that the cloud purposefully took its shape to give you the experience of seeing the face. In the same way, dreams of a familiar person or a menacing figure can have very personal meaning for you, without having a functional purpose, such as to relieve stress or to express hostility.

I would take my argument even further. What we have learned about the brain since the 1970s suggests that the activation-synthesis theory ought to be modified. Random bursts of nerve activity may be continuously produced in the base of the brain, but the nerve signals' pathways would not be nearly so random by the time they reach the cortex. During the day, as the brain's nerve cells are used, they change their behavior. If they have been stimulated, the cells may become more reactive. If you have been frightened during the day, the nerves that control the startle response and feelings of fear will be more reactive that night. So as these random signals travel through the brain, they are modified and filtered by the brain's current state.

To understand what I mean, it might help to think of a stained glass window. White light, which is a jumble of all colors, enters on one side, but what comes out on the other side has a definite pattern of colors that is often very meaningful. Like the stained glass window (which is a filter for light), the brain acts as a filter that imposes order on the random signals passing through it.

But I can't agree completely with the hypothesis that the brain stitches totally random images together into a story only after dream images and sensations are already created. Rather than dismiss them as completely chance or random, I trace the origin of many of the images and sensations to the state of the brain. And because the state of the brain is created by your experiences, dream images and feelings are real reflections of your experiences.

When I was doing the selective REM sleep-deprivation studies described in Chapter 2, I would watch the emerging sleep recording and awaken and interrupt sleep as soon as I was sure that a REM period had started. Because it took 20 to 30 seconds to be sure, subjects usually could recall a little dream fragment after the awakenings. One subject was a young woman who had recently taken a job making reservations for Trans World Airlines. This was before computers. Mistakes had awful consequences. As she was new to the job, she felt enormous pressure and anxiety. At almost every awakening of the REM deprivation study, she would say, "I was thinking of making reservations and then I was actually on an airplane," but the preoccupation that dominated her abstract thought being raised to the level of dream imagery was quite obvious and her day's preoccupation was clearly the starting point of many of her dream fragments; even though the dream may then have gone in an incredible number of different directions, the intensity of the day's preoccupation may have had a marked influence.

All of this does not close the door on the idea that dreams do present truly unconscious thoughts. Unconscious thoughts have as much opportunity as conscious ones to modify the state of the brain and shape nerve signals passing through from the brain stem. Whether unconscious or not, your experiences of the day, and your life experiences, form the "stained glass" that filters incoming signals—and creates the vivid landscapes of dreams.

I think that is what happened in my smoking dream. Although the overriding significance of this dream was that it changed my behavior, a difficult change that some people cannot accomplish even at the expense of their life and health, there was probably more. As I said, at that time I was smoking a great deal and also worrying about the accumulating evidence that smoking causes cancer. In addition, I felt a lot of internal conflict because I was spending nearly every night away from home in the lab, sleeping during the day and leaving my wife to care for our three young children. My life was, in a way, upside down. I don't think that I repressed these feelings—I was conscious of the problems and worried about them—but I did try to ignore the implications of my smoking and overwork. The neurological activity of the cancer dream dredged up these psychological conflicts and presented them in a way that I couldn't ignore, and led me to resolve the problems in my life.

Current neuroscience also can help explain how some images in a dream can be many things at once—which Freud called condensation. For instance, it is common for people to say about a dream, "I was talking to my father, but he was also Fred, my teacher." Or they might say, "I was holding an apple, but it was also a book, because I began to read it." The truth is that we don't have one neuron that gets activated when an apple is in front of us. When the image of an apple passes from the eyes into the brain, it activates the constellation of neurons that represent the color red, spherical objects, common fruits, and the like.

When initial signals in the brain are not coming from a real apple, but rather from a random generator in the brain stem, it is possible for objects to have qualities that they usually don't. For instance, if the right constellation of nerves is activated, an object could have qualities of a "real" book and a "real" apple, although this is physically impossible (and difficult even to imagine in our waking moments). Such condensation often leads to some confusion when we try to communicate the dream after we wake up.

Thirty years ago I had a very meaningful dream. At the time, my research team was working intensively with an experimental drug that appeared to have profound effects upon the basic sleep processes. About one year into this particular project, I developed a serious suspicion that the experimental compound we had been getting from the manufacturer was not pure, or was even an entirely different compound. Because we had invested so much work, I became extremely uneasy at this prospect. Would a whole year of work be wasted? I decided immediately to get samples of the compound analyzed by mass spectrometry to resolve the uncertainty. But the weekend was approaching, so nothing could be done until the following Monday. I could only wait and hope that I was wrong.

Friday afternoon I went to a party at the home of a friend, a successful artist who was talking about a recent exhibition of his work in Sweden. He related to me that someone at the show asked him if he was Jewish (he is, in fact, a Portuguese Christian), and he responded in jest, "There are absolutely no Jews in Portugal."

That night I had a lengthy, vivid dream that took its theme from the movie *Around the World in 80 Days,* which I had recently seen, and from the day's events. In this dream, I was hunting for the "lost tribe of Portuguese Jews," and I was hot on the trail. I would pursue them over mountains and plains and arrive at the warm ashes of a campfire, only to realize that the lost tribe was still ahead of me. With renewed determination, I followed them across the United States, across the Atlantic Ocean, across Europe and Asia—always arriving, after considerable hardship, a little too late. Eventually I got to Vladivostok, where, upon learning they had sailed for California, I requisitioned a boat and set out to sea.

I was caught in raging storms, and toward the end of the voyage the boat sank. Buffeted by waves, I struggled through the surf and was finally thrown up onto a California beach, totally exhausted and bereft of all worldly possessions. As I crawled up on the sand feeling totally defeated, my head bumped against something. It was a sign-post. I looked up and read the words on the sign: "Ha, ha! We were in California all the time! (Signed) The Portuguese Jews." I awoke with a feeling of overwhelming loss and failure.

With regard to the "meaningfulness" of dreams, my dream clearly depicted the fear that my research team had gone all the way around the world—that is, worked a whole year—and had accomplished absolutely nothing. It reflected the intensity of the work and, at the end, a tremendous sense of loss and waste. But more than this, the dream was a long, coherent, and continuous adventure story—meaningful from start to finish. How could it possibly have occurred as a random process? (As it turned out, my real harrowing, round-the-world trip was not in vain—lab results that Monday showed that the chemical we were using was the right one, it was completely pure, and the research project was fine.)

The most indelible memory from this dream is bumping into the sign at the end. Ever since, whenever I have pictured myself on that beach—bedraggled, discouraged, realizing I had been totally hood-winked—for some reason I find it extremely funny. Over the years it has caused me to chuckle innumerable times.

It is important to point out one thing about this dream and also about my cancer dream. Neither of these nights took place in the sleep laboratory. On both nights, these were the only dreams that I remembered. What about all the other dreams? It may be that when there is a message from the dream world that really needs to get through, we are awakened when an intense emotion overcomes the sleep tendency and we wake up to realize we were dreaming. But we must remember that each night we go through an incredible series of experiences that might as well be the experiences of someone else as far as we are aware of them when we are awake. We must at least feel a sense of awe that some part of us inhabits another world and only occasionally do the worlds meet.

One final aspect of dreaming remains to be considered. Dreams free us from the bonds of the real world. The dream world offers us adventure, entertainment, pleasure, and, all too frequently, terror. It is the realism of the dream world that gives our dream experiences such special value. Most often, in my experience, the value and meaning are better appreciated after we wake up.

For sheer entertainment, an annual high point for me is the one day in my course, "Sleep and Dreams," when students share their favorite dreams. Each dream episode gets better than the previous one, and often the class of several hundred students gasps in amazement or roars with laughter as our traveling microphone is passed from one dream narrator to another. Sometimes I think I would like to devote an entire semester to this exercise.

I hope the future of dream study will yield greater accessibility to our dream world—for our waking selves to have more access to our dreams and for our dreaming selves to have more access to our waking life. For a dream to be experienced as real, it may be that we must not be aware that we are dreaming. But thinking back to my cancer dream, it strikes me that heightened reality within dreams would offer some great learning opportunities. For example, if a person could have the "real" experience of being in a horrible accident caused by drowsy driving, and trying to recover from terrible injuries or burn damage, the experience might forever prevent the dreamer from driving drowsy. I used to wish that Soviet and American leaders and generals would dream about an all-out nuclear exchange and have the experience of slowly dying on a planet bereft of all vestiges of civilization—the so-called nuclear winter. I also have imagined that we might supplement our learning and training in the waking state by studying and practicing in the dream world. And as I've heard Stephen LaBerge remark on more than one occasion, "The dream world may offer our best chance to enjoy truly safe sex."

Since at least the beginning of recorded history, people have looked to dreams for insights about the world. Ultimately, the real importance of thoroughly understanding dreams may be insights into how the brain works, how we perceive, and why we think the way we do. We cannot help but create worlds in our minds, to make sense of whatever neurological signals are buzzing about the brain. We may find that dreaming and being awake have much more in common than we thought and that we live much of our waking lives in a very automatic, dreamlike manner. I think it will be a long time before our expanding knowledge of the brain will reveal every mystery about the meaning of dreams and their relationship to our waking lives. I think it is appropriate to end our discussion of dreams with the words of writer Havelock Ellis: "Dreams are real while they last—can we say more of life?"

Chapter 14

A Little Night Muse: Creativity, Productivity, and Learning

A COMMON JOKE around Stanford is that events in the computer industry "happen in dog years," which means new products and ideas that might take many years to develop in other industries are conceived and produced in about one-fifth that time in booming Silicon Valley. If a company dawdles the least bit in taking advantage of a new idea, it finds that others have outpaced it, or that its key engineers have left to create their own company. I am constantly amazed by the number of new companies created every year and the billions of dollars in capital that flow into Silicon Valley to support this work. Needless to say, it is a place where creativity, productivity, and learning are not just highly valued but essential for survival.

A few years ago I had a patient whose life had completely unraveled. He had been a bright and hardworking executive who had risen to a top job in the computer industry. However, he had been laid off because of poor performance and was being treated for bipolar mood disorder. When I saw him, he was taking lithium and sleep medication at bedtime. He was referred to our clinic because of severe insomnia and blackouts in the daytime. His wife had left him because of his extreme irritability and had obtained custody of his two children. When I arrived at the clinic, I saw him pacing about the waiting room. When I ushered him into my office, he immediately said, "I can't sleep, but I don't think I'm a manic depressive. I just can't sit still. But believe it or not, I fall asleep standing up." Bingo. Restless legs syndrome. He received the diagnosis of bipolar mood disorder about five years previously, and all subsequent clinical efforts had been to find the right medication, not to reevaluate his diagnosis. Although he had been labeled a rising star because of his intelligence, skill, and gift for understanding and analyzing a complex and fast-changing business landscape, his sleep disorder and the associated severe sleep deprivation had caught up with him. He was unable to maintain the performance that was expected.

This executive had an absolutely typical restless legs problem. I stopped all his medications and prescribed one specifically for restless legs. His condition greatly improved overnight. He returned in a week and reported that he had slept through the night six times, and felt reborn. With the return of good sleep, he regained a physical energy he had forgotten, a stamina that helped him stick with hard work. He felt optimistic and motivated to tackle the challenges of the day. Once again he was able to juggle many problems and possibilities in his head at the same time. He felt like a new man, but of course he was just getting back his old self, the one who could use all his faculties to succeed in a demanding business. He quickly found a new job, but we calculated that his undiagnosed restless legs syndrome had cost him at least $500,000 in lost salary.

The computer industry is not the only place where creativity counts, of course. We all want to know how to do more, to solve problems better and faster, to get more out of life while putting our own imprint on what we do. Thousands of consultants tell businesses how to become more efficient or productive, and hundreds of books advise people how to carry over the same concepts to their personal lives. But few convey the idea that healthy sleep and the timing of work are an essential part of achieving the creativity and productivity we crave. Instead, many of us feel we must give up sleep to be more productive, that it is not possible to get enough sleep and be successful. Increasingly, late-night or early-morning hours seem like the only way to extend our productive hours. This routine may yield results in the short term, but in the long run, shortchanging sleep depletes our mental acuity and undermines our potential for sustained achievement.

Along with diet and exercise, healthy sleep provides the essential foundation for the mental and physical health we need to do our best. To that end, here I will explore the effect of sleep, the sleep drive, and clock-dependent alerting on how we learn, how we create, and how we produce.

Night School

Forty years of teaching has provided me a long-term laboratory to study how and when students learn best. My studies and those of my colleagues have allowed me to conclude that sleep debt is the most important factor in the quality or excellence of psychological and cognitive function. When students are sleeping sufficiently, they are alert, interested, ready to soak up knowledge. Among my students who learn to recognize how much sleep debt they have and work to reduce it, the most consistent and excited response is amazement that they no longer fall asleep or get sleepy in class. They can even be wide awake and interested in classes that take place immediately after lunch every day. One student habitually dreaded a 1:20 P.M. class taught by a "very dull" professor. The student would either fall asleep or else spend the entire class struggling to stay awake, not really hearing anything and certainly remembering nothing. After a week or two of sleeping eight hours a night, she had no difficulty at all remaining alert and attentive in class. Strangely, she found that the professor had become "much more interesting."

When we are sleep deprived, cognition is one of the first functions to go. Sleep is a basic biological drive, and strong, unfulfilled drives like hunger, thirst, sex, and sleep have a way of giving us a case of cognitive butterfingers. In both school and work environments, well-slept people are much more engaged, can keep more ideas in their head simultaneously, and can think through new ideas more clearly. The experience of the tired, bored student who, when rested, found her professor's lectures engaging and stimulating is common to many people who finally catch up on sleep. Old interests and hobbies that had long been ignored reassert themselves as involving diversions; new, engaging ideas seem to leap out of newspapers and books. Most important of all, people report again and again that learning doesn't seem so hard when their minds are no longer weighed down by sleep debt. The same thing happens when individuals who have a large sleep debt and excessive sleep tendency caused by a sleep disorder are treated successfully.

Some researchers speculate that the learning process, moving memories into long-term storage, requires actual changes in the connections between neurons and that REM sleep facilitates this activity. Remember that neural growth factors rise during sleep, so REM sleep might be a time when the growth factors and brain activity act together to create the nerve connections needed to put memories in long-term storage. Nobel laureate Francis Crick, codiscoverer of the structure of DNA, proposed that REM sleep is a time when the brain actively discards useless memories, thereby freeing up space for new learning and new information storage. As the Harvard psychiatrist and neurophysiologist Allan Hobson has been quoted in the New York Times, "It seems that memories already in the system are being read out and filed in terms of their emotional salience."

A few experiments even suggest that the process of sleep itself helps the brain form long-term memories and that interfering with sleep hinders this process. The first experiments on sleep and memory were animal studies. Rodents that learned how to navigate a maze or press a lever for a reward had more trouble remembering how to solve these puzzles the next day if they were deprived of REM sleep. In other animal studies conducted by the French researchers, a day spent learning a challenging maze or puzzle resulted in increased REM sleep that night, as if the animals were increasing that sleep to fix the newfound knowledge in their brains.

Human studies of the relationship between sleep and memory have been more complicated and contradictory. Several groups have found that REM sleep increases on nights after people are taught Morse code or some other cognitive skill, and that interfering with REM sleep or denying it completely interferes with memory retention. But other experimenters have found that humans experience no change in their REM sleep after learning a new skill or that depriving people of REM sleep did not affect how much learning they retained.

Other researchers find support for the theory that the brain consolidates memories during sleep by looking at PET scans that measure brain activity during REM sleep, but I remain skeptical. While these scans do show that emotional and long-term memory centers are more active than other cognitive areas during REM sleep, there's a big difference between "activity" and actual memory consolidation.

What all the contradictory evidence points to is less a direct correlation between sleep and memory than an eloquent reflection of just how complex and inscrutable the pathways of human cognition remain. Human memory is much more complex than that of any other species. We remember things through multiple methods and cues. For example, a route along city streets can be remembered according to certain stores or trees, or through a sequence of turns—right, right, straight two blocks, left, right, left. We might recite this to ourselves and remember the sound, the singsong pattern, or even make the words into a song. Each of these techniques helps store the information in a different way, in a different part of the brain. Howard Gardner, a psychologist at the Harvard School of Education, has identified seven types of human intelligence that depend on seven distinct ways of storing and processing information: verbal, mathematical-logical, spatial, physical, musical, interpersonal (understanding relationships between people), and intrapersonal (understanding yourself). While Gardner's model is a helpful development in our understanding of neuroscience, I suspect that even his seven-path map of cognition is a highly simplified form of a much more intricate web.

Given this cognitive complexity, it is no wonder that it is more difficult to test humans for the effects of sleep on learning. For example, some researchers have found that it is easier to retain procedures that require deductive reasoning, such as operating a machine tool or a computer, if the lesson is followed by REM sleep. Spatial learning, tested by flashing shapes quickly in the peripheral visual field, also has been found to be enhanced if REM sleep is allowed afterward. But what these kinds of experiments tell me is that there is no simple relationship between REM and memory; REM is probably involved in some types of memory formation and not others.

REM may be one factor that helps memories "stick," but it is not absolutely required. Here's a dramatic illustration of that hypothesis, one that flew in the face of the once widely held belief that REM sleep was indispensable to long-term memory storage. Israeli sleep scientist Peretz Lavie once found a man who had no REM sleep, a war veteran who had sustained a head wound that left a small piece of shrapnel embedded in the base of his brain. This wound completely wiped out his ability to have REM sleep or to dream. But it did nothing to hinder his ability to learn and remember new skills or experiences. This case proved that although REM sleep may assist memory formation, it isn't the only way new memories can be integrated into the neural memory banks.

It should come as no surprise that I believe that society should make it a priority to study this man in exhaustive detail. Not only could such a case demonstrate conclusively whether REM sleep is vitally necessary for the human organism, it might also confirm or deny a number of theories about the function of REM sleep. If we had a national sleep laboratory, this man could have been referred to the facility and possibly could have undergone continuous observation for whatever length of time it took to convince everyone of the result of the complete loss of REM sleep. In his description of this man, Peretz mentions that he had recovered a tiny amount of REM sleep. Is this a recovery that will continue or not? We don't know.

Whether REM sleep helps us learn and remember has not been proven conclusively. But I think the combination of anecdotal and scientific evidence is very suggestive that the time-honored tradition of cramming late into the night for an overdue assignment, whether a final exam or a professional presentation, can be disastrous.

Years ago many people entertained the wonderful possibility that they could learn in their sleep by using audiotapes that pour information into their ears. You may remember the advertisements: "Why waste that time asleep when you could also be learning a new language or brushing up on American history?" This possibility has been conclusively set to rest. Researchers used EEGs to ensure that the audio information was given only while subjects were actually asleep, and they found absolutely no evidence of learning the next morning. No amount of repetition made any difference. Any other result would have been very puzzling because we now know that the brain shuts itself off from outside stimuli during sleep. Those satisfied customers who feel they have learned something from these tapes were probably picking up information during brief awakenings throughout the night. And if they were woken up by the tape repeatedly in this manner, most likely they were not getting the sleep they needed.

One thing we have learned is that sleep can affect the transfer of information between short-term and long-term memory. When we fall asleep, not only is our sensory awareness of the outside world cut off, but the brain also closes the door between short-term and long-term memory. Short-term memories, such as for phone numbers you have just learned, are stored in short-term memory for a few minutes before they disappear. If you actively reinforce the memory of the number, it can be moved to long-term memory. But memories of events that transpire during the 5 minutes before sleep are stuck in short-term storage and evaporate while we sleep, instead of being transferred to long-term memory. That's the reason someone who is knocked unconscious in an accident usually can't remember what happened right beforehand—the memories vanish before they get the chance to move into long-term storage. When a student snoozes in my class, I never get upset; instead, I often use the occasion to illustrate the impact of sleep on short-term memory. After letting the student sleep for 15 minutes or so, I ask the student in the next seat to wake him, and ask him the last thing he remembers from the lecture. Invariably, he cannot remember what I was talking about in the 5 to 10 minutes before he fell asleep. I go on to explain why. Often, a student cannot even remember coming into the classroom.

The Font of Creativity
The human capacity for learning and understanding is considered a chief characteristic that sets us apart from other animals. But even more distinctively human functions are imagination and creativity. To learn something is to take a piece of the outside world and incorporate it into our lives; but to create is to be a magician, to conjure an idea within ourselves and present it to the world as new.

Truly creative thoughts don't occur in a vacuum. A great deal of preparation is necessary before any significant insight can be achieved, and a lot of follow-up work is required afterward. Creative ideas add a new element to what scientists like to call the domain of knowledge, the collection of all the things known about a subject. To come up with a new business strategy, teaching method, or football play, you must have a firm grasp of your area of knowledge. Creativity, therefore, is dependent on learning and memory, and like these capacities, it can be strongly affected by sleep or lack of sleep.

Psychologists have looked closely at the process creative thinkers use to arrive at their ideas and have found common elements. Besides having mastery of a domain of knowledge, you must possess an intrinsic motivation. And essential to sustaining this motivation is the ability to take pleasure in the creative act. Finally, you need to be able to hold paradoxical ideas in your mind and resolve their seeming contradictions. To make this extralogical leap you must be open to new ideas, question your own assumptions, and examine existing constraints.

Albert Rothenberg of Harvard University has spent many decades studying creativity; and he has found that while there is no single personality type common to creative people, their one shared trait is high motivation. A popular myth about creativity is that insight arrives suddenly and spontaneously, like a bolt of lightning or a visitation from the Muses, that great poets or inventors just go about their daily business until they are struck by a flash of insight. Creative people themselves sometimes foster the idea that creativity occurs spontaneously because it lends a magical quality to the act of creation. But scientists like Rothenberg have demonstrated that almost all creative acts come after long, sustained struggle that requires motivation and perseverance.

A lifetime of sleep research has shown me that motivation is one of the first things to go when sleep is shortchanged. Again and again in experiments I have watched people begin to slack off when they have a large sleep debt, to try less hard to press the buttons at the right times or whatever task is at hand. Before we even notice our sleepiness, we feel a little under the weather, a little less excited about the tasks ahead.

I am a full-fledged lark. At the end of the day I can barely summon the motivation to take a piece of paper from one pile and place it on top of another. Sometimes I just sit in apathetic dullness before making an all-out effort to gather the energy and motivation to simply get up from my chair and go home. With a large sleep debt, the only thing we are really motivated to do is sleep. The effort of staying awake often seems monumental, and there is little energy left for anything but basic survival needs, such as what to have for dinner and how to get it.

After adequate sleep, however, motivation levels rise; we feel much more interested in the things around us and challenges don't seem so overwhelming. Sleep also gives us the sustained mental energy we need to persevere in creative work. While we might be able to rouse our psychological energy in the short term despite being sleep deprived, that energy quickly will give way to overpowering sleepiness. Only by getting adequate restful sleep can we maintain the level of motivation needed for creative work.

Psychologists also find that the most powerful motivator to creativity is the pleasure and exhilaration of the creative act itself. New research shows that intrinsic pleasure is a much more powerful motivator than external rewards, which can sometimes even inhibit motivation if they are too easily provided. Openness to pleasure is an extremely important part of the creative process, and as you recall from my discussion of mood and sleep, our ability to feel pleasure is smothered by a heavy sleep debt.

The creative act takes us beyond the limitations dictated to us by normative reality; we transcend the dross of daily living and discover a source of exhilaration and wonder. Sleep is a potent tonic for the creative process because it helps put us in a receptive state of mind where we feel motivated, are open to new ideas, are able to grasp complex and subtle relationships, and are capable of reaping pleasure from the creative process.

The Late-Night Theater of Dreams

Another aspect of sleep that can provide an important arena for creativity is dreaming. There are innumerable instances in literature, music, and the visual arts in which the artist was inspired by a dream or the solution to a problem appeared in a dream. Perhaps the most famous dream-inspired poem is "Kubla Khan," by Samuel Taylor Coleridge, called the most beautiful and remarkable poem in the English language by one scholar. As soon as he awoke, Coleridge seized his pen and began to write it down. Sadly, he was interrupted by a "gentleman from Porlock" knocking on the door and could not remember the rest of it. What the whole poem might have been can only be imagined. Herman Hilprecht, a professor of Assyrian, dreamed that a priest came to him and revealed the elusive translation of the Stone of Nebuchadnezzer, which turned out to be correct. Robert Louis Stevenson credits his dreams for the plots of many of his stories, such as "The Strange Case of Dr. Jekyll and Mr. Hyde."

There are also many stories of scientists who have solved scientific problems in dreams. A notable example is August Kekule's discovery of the benzene ring, a vitally important chemical structure. In 1865 Kekule and other chemists were puzzled by how the six-carbon-molecule benzene could have only six hydrogen atoms attached, since a chain of carbon that long should have many more sites for hydrogen to bond. One night Kekule fell asleep and dreamed of snakes writhing in the air. Suddenly the snakes looped around and bit their own tails to form loops. When Kekule woke up, he knew he had the answer to the problem: The carbons were not arranged in a chain but in a ring, so that the connected "head" and "tail" offered fewer sites for hydrogen atoms to attach themselves.

Gregor Mendeleev reportedly also got the inspiration for the periodic table of the elements in a dream. Otto Loewi literally dreamed up an experiment with a frog's heart, leading to his discovery that nerve signals were transmitted by chemical impulses and winning him a Nobel prize in physiology/medicine. Albert Szent-Gyorgyi, another Nobel laureate, insisted that his work did not end when he left his laboratory bench: "I go on thinking about my problems all the time, and my brain must continue to think about them when I go to sleep, because I wake up sometimes in the middle of the night with answers to questions that have been puzzling me."

Although dreams have given me many insights into my own life and work, I never have actually solved a scientific problem in a dream. Of course, I must hasten to add that I don't really know. I may have had dreams that if I had remembered them would have won me a Nobel prize.

The golfer Jack Nicklaus once dreamed himself out of a long slump. One day he suddenly got back his championship form, and a reporter asked him what he had done. Nicklaus replied: "I've been trying everything to find out what has been wrong. It was getting to the place where I figured a 76 was a pretty good round. But last Wednesday night I had a dream about my golf swing. I was hitting them pretty good in the dream and all at once I realized I wasn't holding the club the way I've actually been holding it lately. I've been having trouble collapsing my right arm taking the club head away from the ball, but I was doing it perfectly in my sleep. So when I came to the course yesterday morning, I tried it the way I did in my dream and it worked. I shot a 68 yesterday and a 65 today, and believe me it's a lot more fun this way. I feel kind of foolish admitting it, but it really happened in a dream. All I had to do was change my grip just a little."

It is a source of endless speculation why the same brain that was blind to an answer while awake can sometimes see so clearly while dreaming. I think the answer lies in the dreaming brain's ability to ignore many of the norms we live by and to create the unexpected. We walk out of our own bedroom and into the Oval Office, and it doesn't seem surprising at all. What's so strange about shopping for eggs and seeing the "Mona Lisa" in the dairy section if you are dreaming? Dreams open us up to possibilities that we would never think of in daily life.

Dreams are also very good at melding paradoxical elements, an essential element of the creative process. Paradoxical combinations are simply grist for the nightly dream mill. Every dream mixes contradictory elements in ways that are hard to explain logically the next day. You might meet a Hollywood starlet and find out she is your mother; you know simultaneously that you are meeting this person for the first time and that you have known her all your life. Or an object might be simultaneously a book and an orange. It seems impossible to imagine something that smells, tastes, feels, and peels like an orange and yet has paper pages, a cover, binding glue, and printing like a book. We don't even think in those terms in waking life and are often blind to combinations of elements that seem paradoxical. A final point is that often, as in Kekule's dream, the act of creation requires an interpretation by waking consciousness.

A crucial step in making creative use of your dreams is to actively record them immediately upon waking, both in the morning and throughout the night. If you have a problem or a creative goal, try concentrating on it intensively for 30 minutes before bed, then write down your dreams as scrupulously as possible. The British essayist A. C. Benson derived his poem "The Phoenix" entirely from a dream: "I dreamt the whole poem in a dream, and wrote it down in the middle of the night on a scrap of paper at my bedside." The composer Giuseppe Tartini dreamed that the devil picked up a violin and played a tune; when he awoke, he immediately wrote down the tune, which became the basis for the "Devil's Trill Sonata." You may find that a pen and paper or tape recorder at your bedside becomes a tremendous source of new ideas.

I often have my classes experiment with using their dreams to solve problems. The overall results have not been very impressive in terms of dependable and productive approaches to problem solving. Nonetheless, it remains very interesting and occasionally very successful. Let me describe one of my favorite exercises. On three consecutive days, I gave a class of 500 students a problem that required a little creativity. This is one of the problems:

What are the next two letters in this sequence?
O, T, T, F, F . . .

I instructed the students to think about the problem for 15 minutes before bed and to record their dreams upon awakening. Over the three days of the experiment, we got 1,148 responses from 500 students. We found that 87 responses were related to a dream, and if a solution appeared in a dream, we scored it as either correct or incorrect. The correct answer showed up in dreams 9 times, but in 2 of these cases the students actually had figured out the puzzle during the 15 minutes before bed. Here is one of the "solution dreams" by a student:

I was standing in an art gallery looking at the paintings on the wall. As I walked down the hall, I began to count the paintings, one, two, three, four, five. But as I came to the sixth and seventh, the paintings had been ripped from their frames! I stared at the empty frames with a peculiar feeling that some mystery was about to be solved. Suddenly I realized that the sixth and seventh spaces were the solution to the problem!

In other words, the sequence O, T, T, F, F, consists of the letters beginning the words one, two, three, four, five, so the next two letters would be S and S, for six and seven.

Seven out of 1,148 is a low percentage, less than 1 percent. But the fact that some students were able to use their dreams to discover the solution is promising. In addition, most people with an important problem are far more motivated to solve it than these students, who got no reward for getting the right answer. I believe that if people spend a great deal of time thinking about a problem, not just 15 minutes before bed, the percentage of their dreams carrying a solution will be much greater than in my classroom experiment. Who knows how often this method could work if we cultivated it?

Lucid Dreaming

Since most people typically remember only a tiny fraction of their dreams, we can only wonder at the ideas and insights that escape our consciousness each night. An even greater frustration for some of us is our inability to exert any control over the content and course of our dreams, particularly when the dream is very frightening. Who hasn't had the exasperating experience of finding himself in a dream of a wished-for circumstance—whether athletic, social, or sexual— only to have the dream evaporate or diverge in a disappointing direction? If only we could consciously inhabit our dreams and direct their narrative, we could explore any number of intriguing situations.

According to an outstanding dream researcher here at Stanford and others elsewhere, we can. In the late 1970s, a psychology graduate student named Stephen LaBerge approached me to ask if he could use our facilities to study a phenomenon called lucid dreaming. He frequently had experienced the sensation of being conscious of dreaming in the midst of a dream—even directing his actions during dreams—and he wanted to explore this state scientifically. Specifically, Stephen wanted to know if lucid dreaming occurred in REM sleep or whether it might be associated with an entirely different organismic state.

Having never experienced lucid dreaming myself, I was skeptical. But his ideas were intriguing, so I agreed to help him design an experiment to test his claims. LaBerge slept in our lab while hooked up to an electroencephalogram (EEG) machine. Whenever he became conscious that he was dreaming, he would signal us by moving his eyes to look at objects in the dream in a prearranged pattern— left-right, left-right, right-left—that was easily distinguishable from typical rapid eye movements. Once we observed this prearranged pattern of eye movement, we would awaken him and ask him about his dream experience. We also woke him randomly during REM sleep when we didn't see his eye signal, just to make sure he wasn't making up a lucid dream whenever we woke him. All of the lucid dreaming occurred in REM sleep, and in addition, we found a perfect correlation between his eye signals and his reports of what he was doing in his dreams. In 1980 we were able to publish convincing objective evidence for the existence of lucid dreaming, and that it occurs during and only during, REM sleep.

LaBerge has founded the Lucidity Institute (see Appendix) and has continued to study lucid dreaming with intriguing results. It turns out that one in five people have lucid dreams naturally, although most of those are fleeting experiences that occur right before awakening. He finds that a much higher percentage—60 percent—of people can dream lucidly with training and practice, and LaBerge has developed a very successful system for teaching this skill. He outfits his students with a special visor that detects rapid eye movements during sleep and shines a blinking red light on the dreamers' eyelids. The light is bright enough to pass through the eyelid and eventually be noticed by the dreamers, but not so bright as to wake them up. LaBerge trains people to recognize the red light as a cue that they are dreaming. Once they become aware that they are dreaming, they can learn to direct and manipulate their dreams at will. Lucid dreamers report that they can make themselves fly through walls and over houses, that they are able to practice the piano, take vacations to specific locales, and arrange sexual encounters, all while deep in REM sleep. Importantly, lucid dreaming offers us a valuable bridge between the waking world and the dream world, and the possibilities, both for hedonistic and intellectual explorations, are limitless. LaBerge refers to individuals making these explorations as oneironauts.

LaBerge has had quite a bit of success with his training technique, although mastering the ability to dream lucidly requires dedication, and some people are unable to acquire the ability no matter how diligently they train. For anyone interested in exploring this fascinating realm, I recommend reading one of LaBerge's very lucid books on the subject.

Sleeping for Productivity

Most of us want to be more productive in life. How much money we earn and how much recognition we get not infrequently depend on how much work we can accomplish. And, not infrequently, how much work we can accomplish depends upon how much time we spend working.

Many people feel they can, or must, get more work done by sleeping less. It's only a matter of resolve and discipline, they believe. Our culture teems with images of industrious people "burning the midnight oil," sleeping only a few hours a night while finishing a big project. Most modern-day offices seem to be equipped with at least one sleep snob who brags that he gets so much done because he sleeps only five or six hours a night. But how productive are these people, really? And is it a good idea, or even possible, to follow their example? Could we really get more done if we just buckled down and slept less?

The answer is that sleeping less is rarely a good idea, nor is it really possible in the long run. I say "rarely" because there are times when we get less sleep to meet a crisis. If a report absolutely, positively has to be in on a certain day, you may have no choice but to work late at night and get less sleep. If a flood is threatening your home, you may have to fill sandbags most of the night. Having a crying newborn in the house at night doesn't exempt parents from doing a full day's work. But you can get by on greatly reduced sleep only in the short term. And your ability to get by with little sleep will be very much enhanced by going into the crisis with a low sleep debt.

During chronic sleep deprivation performance deteriorates dramatically. Sleepy people are likely to make little mistakes they would never make when well rested. The mind is prone to wander and concentration apt to flag. Students often make the mistake of putting off writing their papers until the last minute and then "pulling all-nighters" to get them done on time. Many times I have heard students describe staring blankly at a page or computer screen for 5 or 10 minutes before "coming to" and remembering what they were doing. One student described the experience of typing the word "the" as "t-e-h," staring at the misspelling a full 60 seconds, erasing it, and then typing again "t-e-h." If you are working with heavy equipment (which includes driving a car), little mistakes can become major, even fatal. Rather than making them more productive, forgoing sleep for the sake of work makes people much less efficient and prone to making mistakes that can require even more work to fix.

Nevertheless, there will always be people who think they can handle the effects of fatigue or believe they can train themselves to get by with less sleep in order to get more work done. All the scientific evidence available indicates that this isn't so. In one study Chuck Czeisler of Harvard University found that when workers rotated 12-hour shifts, switching from the night shift to the day shift or vice versa, their feelings of fatigue rose sharply while both their own perceived productivity and their actual productivity went down. Many other studies the world over have shown the same thing. Every individual needs a specific amount of sleep, and this amount cannot be altered. It's analogous to our body temperature set point. No matter how much our temperature goes up or goes down during the day, it must average 98.6° F when we are healthy. Getting less sleep over many nights only builds up the amount of sleep debt we are carrying. For a time we can fool ourselves into thinking we are adapting to a shorter sleeping time, but eventually the sleep debt catches up with us.

What about those stories of human dynamos who work nearly round the clock? Writers and artists who may have been manic depressive such as Virginia Woolf, Edgar Allan Poe, and Georgia O'Keeffe were extremely energetic and creative in their manic phase but probably accomplished next to nothing when depressed. Others may just be night owls, doing their best work when the rest of the world is asleep and there are fewer distractions. These people tend to do their sleeping during the day. Descartes was well known to stay up late at night and rise late in the mornings, often continuing his work in bed the next day. He fell ill and died after he traveled to Sweden to tutor the king, an early riser who imposed his schedule on the French philosopher.

Then there are the genetically very short sleepers. I have come across one family in which the mother states she has always been a short sleeper since childhood, claiming to need only three hours of sleep per night. As she has aged, she slowly started needing more sleep and now sleeps five hours a night. A few years ago she had a daughter who, once beyond the infant sleep pattern, now also seems to need only a few hours of sleep per night. The girl's parents struggle to make sure one of them can be up during each of the 21 hours in the day when she is awake. The husband, who needs seven or eight hours of sleep per night, is going crazy.

As I pointed out in Chapter 6, no one who is an unusually short sleeper has been studied in a way that absolutely proves the claim beyond a shadow of a doubt. I personally believe that it is extremely important to carry out such studies. Is it really possible that only three hours of sleep per day is entirely adequate in every way, and particularly to be wide awake and alert and energetic the other twenty-one hours. Or, as a few people have claimed, that one hour could possibly fulfill the daily sleep requirement for these individuals? Short sleepers are fairly rare and tend to be highly accomplished, overcommitted people who are too busy to consent to spending time in a sleep lab so we can study them. In every case, these people didn't learn to get less sleep, they were born that way. It is in their genetic makeup, which can't be altered by force of habit or any other method. I occasionally see advertisements for seminars that offer to teach people to sleep less. In my opinion this is not only fraudulent, but dangerous.

Whenever anyone brags about how little they sleep, though, you should remember that people hedge about the number of hours they actually sleep for many reasons, including to show how tough or hardworking they are. Even Thomas Edison, who vilified a full night's sleep as a symptom of moral and physical decay, actually seemed to sleep quite a bit, but he did it for an hour or two at a time many times around the clock. There is a story that Henry Ford, a friend of Edison's, once visited the inventor and was told that Mr. Edison was not to be disturbed because he was napping. "I thought Mr. Edison didn't sleep much," said Ford. "Oh, he doesn't," Edison's assistant said sincerely. "He just naps a lot." I think there may be a little Edison in a lot of us.

The truth is that millions of people who suffer from clinical sleep disorders would literally give their eyeteeth for a good night's sleep. Believe me, I see them every day of the week. That is why it strikes me as so tragic that most people who have access to healthy sleep can be so cavalier about its many gifts. If I could give healthy sleepers a tour of my sleep lab and introduce them to the scores of patients who come there in search of relief, perhaps then they would understand and appreciate the miraculous birthright of sleep.

PART FOUR

The Principles of Healthy Sleep

CONGRATULATIONS! Having read this far, you know more about sleep than do the vast majority of people in the world, and certainly more than most doctors. You may have identified a sleep problem in your own life that you hadn't recognized or understood before. Or perhaps you've realized that someone you care about—your child, spouse, or parent—is suffering from a sleep disorder and may need help urgently. The question now is, what will you do with this newfound knowledge? In this section I want to help you take all you've learned about sleep and put it to work in your own life.

I have been campaigning to change public health and safety policies regarding sleep for decades, but I've shied away from advising people other than my patients about how they personally can address their sleep problems. I think my reticence toward prescriptive advice stems in large part from my disappointment with most how-to health books. Whenever I pick one up in an airport bookstore, I'm struck by the disparity between the miracle cure promised in the title and lack of useful, authoritative advice contained between the covers. In the sleep field, for instance, numerous paperbacks tout insomnia "cures," which consist of rehashed recipes for a good night's sleep, based mostly on folklore and decades-old science. Over the course of my career, I've become increasingly aware of how complex a phenomenon sleep is and how resistant many sleep problems are to simple "one-size-fits-all" solutions. People are individualistic in their sleep habits and sleep needs, so I've been skeptical about the usefulness of generic lifestyle and medical advice.

Something happened in the course of writing this book that completely turned my thinking around. Throughout my career, I've looked to my colleagues in academia and clinical settings to help evaluate my research and thinking on sleep problems. But whenever I wanted to test the usefulness of a principle I was espousing in these pages, I found myself turning to the most candid and constructive audience I knew—my students.

Last year a group of about 20 students calling themselves the Stanford Students for Healthy Sleep began to work with me to put into action the principles they had learned in my course, "Sleep and Dreams." We met once a week to discuss sleep management issues, and I also met with students individually to question in detail their efforts to become healthy sleepers. Their input has proven invaluable to this book, particularly for the principles of healthy sleep set forth in this section. With the help of these students, I've been able to develop and organize what I think is a helpful set of guidelines, culminating in Chapter 20's Sleep Camp, a step-by-step program for integrating the principles of healthy sleep into your daily routine over the course of three weeks. Their positive response to this regimen has given me the confidence to offer it to the general public.

What's been most inspirational to me has been watching these young people take responsibility for their sleep habits and in many cases completely reinvent them. I've witnessed these students achieve a remarkable level of energy and zest for life by learning to manage their sleep. I consider myself an expert on the sleep deprivation that is rampant on college campuses everywhere, so seeing students transform their waking and sleeping lives has been both impressive and personally gratifying to me.

One of the students, Lance D., exemplifies what I am talking about. When I interviewed him about his sleep at the end of the term, he was wide awake, alert, and animated. Lance actually had started reducing his sleep debt in the winter quarter as a student in my course, and during the spring quarter he has maintained a schedule of about seven and a half to eight hours of sleep a night. His formerly pervasive daytime sleepiness is no longer a problem because he has become expert in his own sleep needs and has tailored his sleep habits to serve them. He discussed his circadian rhythms with the relaxed self-confidence of someone who truly knows himself and feels in control of his life. Best of all, he's become motivated to give others the benefit of his experience. In particular, because Lance suffered terribly in high school from poor sleep, he has been telling his story to high school students in the hope that they can avoid what he went through.

Most of the other students in the group report similar feelings of renewed energy and motivation that have accrued by reducing their large sleep debts. They feel more alert and attentive in class and look forward to class assignments that used to fill them with dread (or at least fatigue). No single formula will work for everyone, but these students found that gaining control over their sleepiness was surprisingly simple once they understood the basic principles of sleep.

I've built these last chapters around principal areas for reclaiming healthy sleep. They are all based on a respect for your individual biological clock and a commitment to put your sleep needs at the center, rather than the periphery, of your life. The areas are:

1. Taking stock of your personal sleep needs.
2. Getting help for your sleep problems.
3. Learning to manage sleep crises.
4. Taking age into account.
5. Adopting a sleep-smart lifestyle.

Finally, I've provided a program for putting these ideas into effect, as well as appendices with quick-reference resource guides, so you'll have more information at your fingertips for finding additional help with your sleep problems.

Reclaiming healthy sleep isn't any easier than learning to eat right or stay in good physical condition. It takes discipline and self-knowledge. But my students at Stanford and the citizens of Walla Walla, Washington, have convinced me that healthy sleep is within the grasp of each of us, as long as we care enough to seize it.

Chapter 15

Take Stock of Your
Personal Sleep Needs

THE BEDROCK PIECE of knowledge necessary to build a foundation for healthy sleep is the fact that sleep needs and patterns of sleep and wakefulness are not exactly the same for everyone. Accordingly, the very first and most important step in getting your own sleep house in order and putting principles of healthy sleep to work in your life is self-evaluation. After all, you are the only one who has access to detailed information on your own sleep habits (although you may be surprised by some of your findings once you actually take the trouble to record them). And no one has more motivation than you to locate trouble spots and to reconstruct a solid foundation for healthy sleep.

"Sleep architecture" is a term sleep specialists often use to include the details of a night's sleep: the time needed to fall asleep (sleep latency), sequence of sleep stages and time spent in each stage, total sleep time, and number and length of nighttime awakenings. These are the things we study in the Stanford Sleep Center. As important for you at home is knowing your sleep indebtedness, daytime patterns of alertness and drowsiness, naps, timing and regularity of bedtimes and wake times, sleep disorder symptoms such as snoring or restless legs, and how refreshing you perceive your sleep to be.

In this chapter I will advise you and help you understand your own sleep. Just as a house built to an architectural plan always takes on its own characteristics and idiosyncrasies, even people with similar sleep patterns will have their own signature habits and needs. After completing the following exercises, you should know how much sleep you need on average every day, how much you actually get, what time of day you perform at your peak, and approximately how much sleep debt you are carrying over from one day to the next.

If you conclude that, like most people, you are sleepy during the daytime, I'll help you figure out whether your fatigue is due to self-inflicted sleep deprivation or a clinical sleep disorder or, for that matter, both. Since your own doctor very likely knows less about sleep than you do now, you need to take the initiative in identifying the quality of your sleep and the sources of your problems. If you have determined that you need medical help, I'll share with you what I've learned about seeking effective treatment.

Getting to Know Your Sleep Habits: Keep a Sleep Diary

Managing your sleep is a lot like managing your money or your weight. Just as you would begin a budget or diet with an audit of your actual spending or eating habits, your best starting point is a hard look at your current sleep life. Once again you'll probably see how little we know about our lifestyle until we stop to write it down.

One of the small number of real traditions in sleep research and sleep medicine is the sleep diary, which is also one of the best ways to get a handle on your daily cycles of sleep and wakefulness. In the clinic, patients with serious sleep problems are often asked to keep detailed diaries, including notations of how many minutes they were awake during each nighttime awakening they can remember. For the average moderately sleep-deprived adult, it's not necessary to go to such lengths. A simple notation of when you went to bed, about how long it took to fall asleep, and when you got up will be sufficient. (You should do the same for naps). You can make a mark if you remember waking up at night, and write down the approximate length of the awakening only if it lasts more than 15 minutes, or if there are several. After you have finished reading this book, and you are ready to keep a sleep diary, Figure 15.1 is a good template.

You also should be keeping track of how you feel during the day, using the Stanford Sleepiness Scale. At various times during the day,

Fig. 15.1

SLEEP DIARY

Date _____

Complete after awakening:

Time you went to bed _____

Time you fell asleep _____

Time you woke up _____

Number of times awakened during the night _____

Amount of time awake during the night _____

Total Nighttime Sleep _____

Comments on quality of night's sleep:

_____

Did you feel groggy after getting up in the morning? Yes_____ No _____

If yes, for how long? _____

Complete at the end of the day:

Naps:

Time fell asleep _____

Time awoke _____

Total Nap time _____

Comments on quality of naps:

_____

Using the Stanford Sleepiness scale below, note your alertness during the day:

1) Feeling active, vital, alert, wide awake
2) Functioning at a high level, not at peak
3) Relaxed, not full alertness, responsive
4) A little foggy, not at peak, let down
5) Fogginess, losing interest, slowed down
6) Sleepiness, prefer to be lying down
7) Almost in a reverie, hard to stay awake

6AM		4PM	
8AM		6PM	
10AM		8PM	
NOON		10PM	
2PM		MDNT	

How was your overall sleepiness/alertness today (1-7) ? _____

Other comments on mental and physical:

_____

_____

simply make a notation of the number that best corresponds to how you feel:

Stanford Sleepiness Scale (slightly updated)

1. Feeling active, vital, alert, wide awake
2. Functioning at a high level, not at peak
3. Relaxed, not full alertness, responsive
4. A little foggy, not at peak, let down
5. Tired, losing interest, slowed down
6. Drowsy, prefer to be lying down
7. Almost in a reverie, hard to stay awake

You should make a notation an hour or two after you wake in the morning, during the afternoon dip (usually around 2:00 P.M.), and during the period of early-evening alertness (around 7:00 or 8:00 P.M. for most people). It also would be useful to note how you feel at other random times during the day. (As a class assignment, I sometimes require my students to pay extremely close attention to their alertness by rating themselves every 15 minutes and then, over one whole day, putting all the ratings on a single graph.)

Keeping a sleep diary for at least a week, including the weekend, will give you a good snapshot of your sleep patterns. If you have an irregular sleep schedule, it will be hard to miss on paper. (It might be even more apparent if you graph the information, but that is not necessary.) Examine the times you go to sleep and wake up, and calculate your total nightly sleep times. Look for a drift in your schedule over the weekend. Notice how your scores on the Stanford Sleepiness Scale change over the course of the day and whether there are times of day when the scores are consistently high or low.

Keeping a sleep diary makes all the abstractions about sleep debt and biological clocks concrete. By doing this you will be able to see your daily peaks and troughs in wakefulness and discover what time of day you are performing most efficiently. Even people who think they understand when they feel best and worst during the day sometimes are surprised by the patterns they discover. The only real problem I have observed in asking people to do this is that they often forget to make notations, particularly in the daytime. I would say the best solution is using the alarm on a digital wristwatch. Very inexpensive alarm watches are available, if you don't already have one.

Don't worry if your peaks and valleys in alertness don't closely resemble the standard shifts of biological rhythms. These deviations can be some of the most revealing parts of the sleep diary. When you have a high or low point in sleepiness at an unusual time, ask yourself what was going on in your life at that time that might have contributed to that feeling. For instance, suppose your daily dip in wakefulness is around 5:00 P.M. rather than 1:00 or 2:00. Is the time you fall asleep and wake up also later, such as a 1:00 A.M. bedtime and a 9:00 A.M. wake-up? This pattern could indicate a circadian phase that is shifted compared to the population average. Or perhaps you feel drowsy at 5:00 P.M. because it's the time when work is winding down. All day you are driven by work, so hyped up and aroused that you don't even notice a midday dip in clock-dependent alerting. But when work pressures fall off at 5:00 P.M., your huge sleep debt may really hit you hard in spite of a rise in clock-dependent alerting.

Weekends can produce the same sharp drop-off in stress-related alerting. You may feel extremely sleepy nearly all day Saturday and Sunday and have a strong desire to take a nap, even if you slept in later than usual those mornings. Don't forget that your lethargy is not brought on by "sleeping too much." Your body is sending you a message that you have built up a backlog of sleep debt over the course of the week; it is being revealed now that the arousing pressure of the workday has disappeared.

In Chapter 20 I suggest some other diary entries that can be revealing about the way your lifestyle affects your sleep. For now, you should be able to assemble a good working sketch of your sleep patterns.

To further fill out your sleep blueprint, here are a few other self-diagnostic tests you can run.

Measuring Your Sleep Debt
How much sleep debt are you carrying around? The simplest way to gauge your degree of sleep debt is to measure your daytime sleepiness. To get a rough idea, fill out the following questionnaire, which is part of the Epworth Sleepiness Scale.

How likely are you to doze off or fall asleep in the following situations? Score yourself using the following scale:

0 = would never doze
1 = slight chance of dozing
2 = moderate chance of dozing
3 = high chance of dozing

_____ Sitting and reading
_____ Watching TV
_____ Sitting, inactive in a public place (e.g., a theater or a meeting)
_____ As a passenger in a car for an hour without a break
_____ Lying down to rest in the afternoon when circumstances permit
_____ Sitting and talking to someone
_____ Sitting quietly after a lunch without alcohol
_____ In a car, while stopped for a few minutes in traffic
_____ TOTAL SCORE

Evaluate your total score:
0–5 Slight or no sleep debt
6–10 Moderate sleep debt
11–20 Heavy sleep debt
21–25 Extreme sleep debt

Recall that the best measure of daytime sleepiness and sleep debt is the Multiple Sleep Latency Test (MSLT). Also keep in mind that sleep latency is the measure of how quickly you fall asleep while relaxing in bed in a quiet, dark room. If you are optimally rested you'll stay awake for 15 to 20 minutes or more. When you're seriously sleep deprived or sleep disordered, you'll fall asleep within 5 minutes. These times are modified somewhat by the ebb and flow of your biological clock—the afternoon dip will subtract a few minutes from sleep latency and the early-evening peak will add a few minutes. The MSLT actually measures the combination of sleep debt and clock-dependent alerting, but it does a pretty good job of indicating inherent sleep debt, especially if scores are taken a few different times during the day.

In the sleep laboratory, the MSLT measures the onset of sleep by tracking the moment brain waves change from wakefulness to stage 1 (light sleep). While the electroencephalograph is very precise in measuring the brain's shift into sleep, reasonably accurate versions of this test can be carried out at home.

One method, using a metal spoon, resembles a technique used by Nathaniel Kleitman many years ago, before EEG machines were available. Try lying on a couch or in bed, with your eyes closed, shoes off, wearing comfortable clothes or whatever you usually sleep in. The lights should be low and the curtains drawn. Drape your hand over the edge of the chair, couch, or bed, and lightly hold a metal spoon suspended over a plate on the floor. Check the time, then relax and allow yourself to fall asleep. At the onset of sleep, your muscles will relax enough that the spoon will slip out of your hand and clatter as it strikes the plate. The sound will wake you unless you are very severely sleep deprived. If it doesn't, you need only one test. Check the time again, and calculate how many minutes it took to fall asleep. That number is your sleep latency. The spoon may not fall the very second that sleep onset occurs, but the timing will be close enough to give a rough approximation of what the MSLT would show. The other night I discovered a variant of this approach. I was holding a glass of ice water sort of on my chest while I was lying in bed watching the news. All of a sudden, with a shock, I felt cold water flooding onto and off of my chest. This signal for sleep onset was as sharp and unambiguous as a clattering spoon, but I definitely don't recommend it.

Another home-testing method is to enlist an observer to watch you fall asleep. Choose someone you are comfortable enough to fall asleep in front of. The observer can minimize your self-consciousness by reading a book or doing some other activity while making quick checks every minute or so. Only when you are at last comfortably ensconced in your sleeping position should the observer "start the clock." The observer cannot rely on any single physical marker of the moment signaling the onset of sleep, but he can look for solid clues, such as slow, deep breathing, snoring, or the slight parting of the lips that occurs when the muscles achieve the deep relaxation of sleep. When these signs are present, the observer should wake you and record the time. You may protest that you weren't asleep yet. The first moments of sleep can be deceptively light and, if interrupted immediately, may not even feel like sleep. But most people can tell by looking if someone is pretty close to sleep—if any of the breathing and muscle relaxation signs of sleep are present, you probably are asleep, or close enough to count. On the other hand, it is often hard to see the exact moment when someone else falls asleep so this method will provide a rougher measure than the spoon (or ice water) method.

Assuming you have developed a reasonably accurate assessment of sleep latency, you should recall that the standard MSLT used in laboratories and clinics does not include tests in the evening. The standard test ends with a sleep latency measurement at 6:00 P.M., and many people do only four tests: at 10:00 A.M., noon, 2:00 P.M., and 4:00 P.M. If you could test your sleep latency at all these times, that would be marvelous. If not, I would recommend taking tests at around 10:00, around 12:30, and around 3:00. Or perhaps at 10:00 A.M. and 1:00 P.M., if you can take only two tests per day. Testing at these times would at least give you a sense of how you perform during the morning period of clock-dependent alerting and during the early-afternoon period when alerting is starting to taper off.

The reason for not including an evening test is that the results are often more dependent on age than on level of sleep debt. It would be highly unusual for a young person to be able to fall asleep quickly in the evening, at say 8:00 P.M., although most elderly individuals certainly could. Averaging in an evening test might give a spuriously elevated average score for young people, while doing so for seniors might give a spuriously low score. The lowest score of the day is probably the one that best represents your true sleep latency, because it is likely to be the one that is least affected by clock-dependent alerting. To confirm your findings, test yourself over several days so that no single night's sleep unduly skews the results. Home-testing methods will probably yield an MSLT score somewhat higher than what an EEG machine would detect but are accurate enough to determine your placement on the following scale. The numbers represent how many minutes it took to fall asleep. These scores should be averaged results of many tests.

1 to 5 minutes: Severely sleep deprived, quite possibly due to a sleep disorder like apnea or insomnia. People with untreated narcolepsy score in this range.

5 to 10 minutes: Definitely troublesome. You are likely to feel low energy during dips in the circadian rhythm, or when you are driving or at rest.

10 to 15 minutes: You have a manageable amount of sleep debt, but you could feel some improvement by working it off.

15 to 20 minutes: You have little or no sleep debt, or are taking the test at a time of peak alerting.

If you are still awake at 20 minutes, end the test. You are as alert as you can get.

In some ways, a score of 15 to 20 during a dip in alerting is optimal, because you want a little bit of sleep debt. A little sleep debt makes sleep more efficient; you go to sleep faster and stay asleep longer. If you took more than 20 minutes to fall asleep during your most lethargic period of the day, it very well could take you that long to get to sleep at night. Healthy sleepers with a few hours of sleep debt might have a sleep efficiency of 89 to 95 percent, meaning that they were awake 5 to 11 percent of the time they were in bed. Someone with insomnia might have a sleep efficiency of 60 to 85 percent. If you eliminate sleep debt completely, your sleep efficiency can fall far enough to feel like insomnia.

Daily Sleep Need

The most basic and important bit of sleep self-knowledge is how much total sleep you need on the average in each 24-hour period to keep sleep load and alertness in optimal balance. Remember that just as a thermostat keeps a room at a constant temperature, your own sleep homeostat works to make you fulfill your daily sleep quota. You accumulate sleep debt at a certain rate and have to pay it off by sleeping a certain amount each day. You may be a naturally short sleeper, needing fewer than eight hours a night to achieve this equilibrium, or a long sleeper, needing more.

To determine your personal sleep requirement you need to find out how much sleep it takes to keep your sleep tendency constant over several days. Here is how you do it. Most people have a vague notion of their sleep need, so that figure should be the starting point. For the purpose of this example, let's say you think you need eight hours of sleep. Start by picking a bedtime when you think you can fall asleep easily, let's say 11:00 P.M. Assuming it will take you about 15 minutes to fall asleep, you should set your alarm for 7:15. Follow this pattern for a few days, and pay close attention to how you feel during the day, especially during lulls on the job, after lunch, or while driving. How sleepy are you during these times? (To quantify this feeling you could use the Stanford Sleepiness Scale.) Keep track of your tendency to fall asleep while watching TV or reading a book. Do the home MSLT during your midafternoon dip and see if the scores stay the same or become higher or lower over a few days.

If you begin to notice that you are more tired and more liable to become drowsy with the same amount of sleep at night, then you are getting less sleep than you need. Add 30 minutes to your sleep time, and keep monitoring. If your tendency to become drowsy and fall asleep declines, you are paying off your sleep debt (although you may still have a substantial one). If your tendency to become drowsy and fall asleep stays the same, then the amount you are sleeping each night *is* the amount of sleep you need, or very close to it.

Another approach has the advantage of eliminating sleep debt at the same time you establish your sleep need. This is what I try to do in an organized way in Chapter 20. It's best to try this on vacation or during any other two-week period when you have a flexible schedule. Pick a reasonable bedtime that you can stick with every night over the whole two weeks and then put away the alarm clock. The next morning don't try to wake up at a certain hour, just let your brain find its own reveille. If you wake up naturally at your usual time, let yourself go back to sleep and sleep in as long as you can. It helps to block out any light and noise from the bedroom. Repeat this routine each night. You are likely to sleep quite late the first few days as you make payments on your sleep debt, but after a while your sleep time should settle into a steady state, probably somewhere in the range of seven to nine hours. If you add up your hours of "extra sleep," this is approximately the sleep debt you were carrying. Once you are sleeping essentially the same amount each night, you have identified the amount of sleep that you need. A clearer, but for most people less-practical method is to do what subjects did in the Wehr study introduced in Chapter 4: Put yourself in a dark, quiet room every night and sleep as long as you can.

Don't forget that you may rather suddenly have sleep problems if your sleep debt reaches a level that is too low—that is, a level that is insufficient to help you get to sleep quickly when you go to bed.

Obviously, your responsibilities make it difficult to sleep late. If you are a morning person, it is likely that your strongest period of clock-dependent alerting occurs at this time and will wake you up more or less at the same time each day. I know that I am a morning person, and whenever I am sufficiently sleep deprived to be concerned about it I always deal with my concern by going to bed early.

Whether it is more difficult to go to bed early or to sleep late depends on your personal situation. I know that on weekends when you do not have the excuse of having to get up early for a job, it is difficult to leave guests or a party or your spouse to go to bed at 7:00 P.M. But if we who know about sleep don't make the courageous stand to lie down and sleep when we need it, who will? So learn to have the gumption to go to bed early to catch up on sleep debt you have been carrying from one day to the next.

If you are a morning person, you probably won't need to do much winding down to get to bed early. But if you do feel tension and stress, you might do things that foster sleepiness at least two hours before your early bedtime; the conventional wisdom is take a hot bath, read a boring book, watch TV (only if it makes you sleepy—otherwise switch the set off early in the evening), or do something else calming to redirect your mind away from the stress and arousal of the day. The key is to learn how you can best accomplish the goal of getting extra sleep by any means necessary, whether by getting to bed early or sleeping late—or both, if you have an aptitude for it. Obviously, if you sleep in the same room as someone else, you may have to compromise in order to accommodate his or her sleep needs too.

My favorite method of determining whether I am maintaining a reasonable sleep "diet" is to keep track of my episodes of heavy eyelids and struggling to stay awake, and the circumstances in which they take place. I am now so sensitive to these events that I know exactly how often they tend to happen. I am convinced that most people do not know this about themselves, but I am also convinced that everyone can learn.

In conclusion, all people can learn to monitor themselves and improve their sleep, but they must want to be more alert and energetic. One student with whom I interacted felt that the reduction in social interactions was worse than being sleepy. My hope, as we go forward, is that it is never an either/or situation and that everyone can—by understanding and managing their own schedules—come close to getting adequate sleep and enjoying life. It is amazing to me that some people do not seem to mind being sleepy most of the day, do not seem to mind being deprived of the zest of operating at the peak of their creativity and the peak power of their mind, to do things, to see things, to understand and create.

Chapter 16

Facing Up to Your Sleep Problems

Deal with "Emergencies" First

SOME PEOPLE who read this will be completely disabled by a sleep disorder, or even at death's door. Others will realize that this grim description fits a spouse or family member. We have learned that the majority of people whose sleep disorder began years ago have been languishing undiagnosed in or out of the health care system and getting progressively sicker and sicker.

Currently we are seeing dramatic evidence of this in our studies in Walla Walla, Washington, and Moscow, Idaho. For example, earlier I mentioned that severe cases of obstructive sleep apnea can stop a sleeping patient's breathing for more than 45–100 times an hour. In over 1,000 sleep tests in these two towns, 80 percent of those tested had progressed to this very high degree of severity. That means that the large majority of people with apnea had a severe case.

This lack of awareness was designated a health emergency in 1992 by the National Commission on Sleep Disorders Research. In its report to the U.S. Congress, the commission stated, "The absence of awareness about sleep disorders is so pervasive and complete, it can be changed only by a strong federal initiative." The commission instructed the Congress to "remedy this situation without delay."

Unfortunately, the Congress did not respond to its own commission. Today, therefore, the primary responsibility to do something must fall to individuals and their families. For those who are very sick, addressing their sleep problem in the future will probably be too late. They must act now.

The only good news, though grim, is that when sleep disorders have progressed to extreme severity, anyone possessing the most rudimentary knowledge, can immediately make the correct diagnosis. The most prevalent chronic sleep disorders are obstructive sleep apnea, restless legs syndrome, problems with the biological clock, and the primary insomnias—all of which are associated with easily recognizable symptoms.

Not long ago I was on a question-and-answer radio show. One concerned caller described flagrantly obvious, very severe sleep apnea in her six-year-old daughter. "You have an emergency on your hands!" I blurted out. "Wait," my host interrupted. "We're not talking about ambulances and sirens." "I don't mean that kind of emergency," I replied, "but something should be done right away."

By "emergency," I mean there should be no delay in addressing the problem, because a catastrophe can happen at any time. The overall danger from all sleep disorders is an accident due to fatigue. For sleep apnea, there is also the danger of a fatal arrhythmia, heart attack, or stroke. Let me illustrate this by recounting still-vivid memories from years ago of two relatively young doctors who came to the Stanford Sleep Disorders Clinic soon after it opened in 1970. Both were family practitioners.

The first physician was 41 years old, moderately obese, snored loudly, and knew his severe fatigue was not normal. His sleep test showed very severe obstructive sleep apnea. When he learned that the only effective treatment (at that time) was a permanent hole in the throat to open the airway (chronic tracheostomy), he simply could not accept it. He decided that he would lose weight and see what happened. We asked him to return in two months. Just about four weeks later I was reading the local paper and was greatly shocked to see his obituary. No cause of death was mentioned. I called the grief-stricken family and found the young doctor had died in his sleep, and it was thought to have been the result of a heart attack.

The second physician, 40 years of age, had actually fallen asleep hovering over a female patient while using a stethoscope to listen to her heart. The patient, to put it mildly, was startled and very upset when his head came to rest on her naked breast. This physician's sleep test showed more than 50 episodes of halted breathing per hour during sleep and very serious heartbeat irregularities that put him at high risk for cardiac arrest. By this time I had become absolutely convinced that refusing treatment was essentially a death warrant. I confronted the young doctor and told him it was either tracheostomy or death. He accepted the surgical procedure.

After the operation this physician was reborn. Today he can look back on an additional quarter century of healthy, productive life. He has never wanted to give up the tracheostomy for a nasal continuous positive airway pressure (CPAP) machine or other surgical approaches. Since tracheostomy is the most effective treatment that gives effortless normal breathing every night, he may well live with the hole in his throat until he is 100 years old.

Today, scientific studies have revealed that huge numbers of individuals who have untreated severe obstructive sleep apnea. Untold numbers have died prematurely through the ages. My sense of horror is only worsened when I realize that this situation still exists. Premature death, catastrophic illness, or accident is the lot for most, while the few who receive treatment can look forward to healthy decades added to their life span. (We did our best, but many of our early patients refused tracheostomy and joined the millions of people who had died prematurely.)

Making a Self-Diagnosis

I believe it is safe to say that the single symptom most frequently found in all severe sleep disorders is daytime fatigue. I should reemphasize that people who feel fatigued complain of lack of motivation, apathy, and irritability, and rarely complain of excessive sleepiness. They usually say they are worn out, exhausted, or depressed. Such people don't know that a sleep disorder is a possible cause of the fatigue, and usually think they must have some other medical problem instead. Only unambiguous, recurring drowsiness—requiring a real effort to stay awake throughout the day—finally causes people to admit they are excessively sleepy.

Doctors tend to make the same mistake. Although sleep specialists have known for years that fatigue is very often excessive sleepiness due to a sleep disorder, primary physicians invariably look elsewhere for explanations. When they cannot unambiguously identify the source of the fatigue, the problem often gets labeled chronic fatigue syndrome or depression. In marked contrast, the results of our primary care project strongly indicate that when fatigue is the patient's major complaint, a sleep disorder is the culprit in more than half the cases. If you or anyone you know is plagued by chronic fatigue, I urge you to explore the possibility that a sleep disorder is the cause. For my part, I always assume that fatigue is obstructive sleep apnea until proven otherwise.

I usually assess patients' or anyone's level of sleepiness by first asking "Are you generally wide awake, energetic, and highly motivated all day long?" If they answer yes, it is very unlikely that they have a serious or persistent sleep problem. If such individuals are also cheerful, optimistic, or happy, a sleep problem is even less likely. Those who say they are not at this optimal level of alertness and energy are candidates for a sleep disorder and should be questioned further. You know from the studies I have mentioned earlier that individuals who deny feeling sleepy can score less than 5 on a clinical MSLT. Keep in mind that denying daytime sleepiness is not the same as claiming to be wide awake, and energetic all day long.

If you snore, in addition to being very tired during the daytime, then you could have either obstructive sleep apnea or upper airway resistance syndrome. Either problem can be treated effectively. If you are among the 30 percent of the population who sleep alone and are not sure if you snore, consider apnea a likely explanation if you are fatigued, substantially overweight, and accustomed to waking up with a sore throat and/or headache. You should definitely investigate further if you have any possibility of apnea and have high blood pressure or any cardiovascular problem—doing so could save your life.

One simple way to tell if you snore or stop breathing at night is to place a tape recorder near your pillow and set it to record while you sleep. If you have the equipment, videotaping is even better. If you become convinced you may have sleep apnea, do something! If you are among the 70 percent of the population who sleep with someone, ask your bed partner to observe your breathing when you are asleep.

Periodic limb movement disorder in its extreme form should be infuriatingly obvious to anyone sharing your bed. Restless legs syndrome is absolutely obvious to anyone once they know that the disorder is characterized by uncomfortable, tingly, achy, or creepy, crawly feelings in legs when they lie down. Nonetheless, nearly all victims remain undiagnosed because neither they nor their physicians are aware their disorder exists or is so very common.

The foregoing are among the most common sleep disorders, but if you come to suspect that you may be suffering from any of the dozens of others, consult the list of disorders and symptoms listed in Appendix B. If your symptoms seem to match any of those thumbnail descriptions, take matters into your own hands. Get help.

The Patients Who Never Were

Even when people are told or suspect they may have a sleep disorder, they themselves can be the major barrier to successful treatment. I know from my studies in both Walla Walla and Moscow that more often than not, people do nothing about even very serious sleep disorders. Most of those who have been informed they may have a serious sleep disorder and are advised to make an appointment with their doctor do not. I've had the same problem with the parents and relatives of my students who realize that a family member is seriously ill. Obstructive sleep apnea victims simply refuse to accept the possibility that they are dangerously ill, even in the face of convincing evidence.

Two or three years ago we worked with a group of patient volunteers to set up a booth at the San Mateo County Fair. We had dramatic posters, pamphlets, questionnaires, and constantly running videotapes. When fairgoers who filled out a brief questionnaire clearly had serious problems, including fatigue-related disability, cardiovascular disease, dramatically loud snoring, and witnessed pauses in breathing, we would urgently advise them to consult their physician. We would give them a brochure describing obstructive sleep apnea and its treatment, a list of sleep disorders centers in the San Francisco Bay area, and a very urgent recommendation to ask their primary physician for a referral. With their permission, we recorded their names and addresses so we could watch for them to show up, particularly those judged the most severely ill. As far as I know, of the approximately 300 persons who we were certain had obstructive sleep apnea, not one availed himself of qualified assistance. Why didn't any of them show up?

I got a more detailed glimpse of how much people can resist treatment in the case of a Stanford student, Sarah C., who worked several summers in the Stanford Sleep Disorders Clinic and learned all about obstructive sleep apnea. When Sarah went home to rural New Mexico for the holidays, she listened to her father while he slept and heard him snore and stop breathing many times. She told him what was wrong and tried to convince him to do something. Because of the fear that someone with severe obstructive sleep apnea will suddenly die, or have a heart attack or a stroke, or an auto accident, the motivation to push a loved one into seeking help is very intense. Sarah pressed her father very hard, but he would not listen and finally said she could come home only if she never mentioned the topic again.

Meanwhile her father had to stop driving his car because of his increasing fatigue and sleepiness. This greatly increased his isolation and further diminished the quality of his life. Even with this loss, he resisted treatment. Fortunately, his meanness to his daughter motivated his son to get involved. The son lives in Kansas and is a registered nurse. He traveled to New Mexico and spent a night with his father. He carefully counted and timed all the apneic episodes, and videotaped his father asleep for about an hour. He was able to say to his father the next morning, "Dad, you stopped breathing 400 times, and each episode lasted for over a minute. You turned purple and I can prove it. You've got to get to a sleep specialist." Playing the videotape and watching himself strangle finally did it. The father obtained expert help in a sleep center. The diagnosis was confirmed and treatment was initiated. The change was miraculous. He woke up, his daytime alertness returned, and he is driving again.

If people with such a severe sleep disorder tend to deny the problem or delay treatment, those who have less severe cases deny or delay even more. In my opinion, when sleep disorders symptoms are only partially disabling, and the victims are not truly desperate, the single biggest problem is that people do not believe their symptoms justify seeking medical help.

In a recent National Sleep Foundation survey, 75 percent of the subset who responded that they were obtaining enough sleep also said they regularly experienced daytime sleepiness and fatigue. Apparently they considered daytime fatigue to be normal. If our sleep is healthy, we should not be tired and sleepy in the daytime.

These and other studies have convinced me that most people think it is normal to be tired all the time. In one of our primary care sites, three-quarters of all patients interviewed admitted to varying degrees of trouble sleeping, but none had mentioned the difficulty to a doctor. Included among the silent sufferers were 30 percent of all patients in this site whose trouble sleeping was severe enough to have daytime consequences, interfering with work and other activities.

One of the most poignant examples of denial was recounted to me by our on-site assistant in the Moscow clinic. A young man had a doctor's appointment to have a wart removed from the bottom of his foot. Our assistant, who knew him and knew he had recently started a contracting business, asked how it was going. To her surprise, as the young contractor told her about the severe stress of managing his new business he began to cry. He told the assistant that the stress was giving him severe insomnia. Unable to sleep night after night, he was too tired to do his work, which increased the stress and worry. The vicious cycle of stress and insomnia had led him to the brink of bankruptcy. The conversation ended when he was called into the doctor's office. After the appointment, our assistant and the doctor compared notes. Incredibly, the young man had not mentioned his insomnia to the doctor, even though the doctor had asked if he wanted to discuss any other medical problems after the wart was removed.

This man is typical of many people who don't realize that a doctor might help, or are embarrassed or otherwise reluctant to talk about sleep problems. There are several reasons for this. One is that men in particular are afflicted by a senseless macho resistance to seeking help. In the case of sleep apnea, it is usually a wife who pushes her husband to see the doctor, and the husband who resists acknowledging that anything is wrong with him. For some reason men also have more trouble than women do in accepting the mechanics of apnea treatment. A huge hose attached to your nose and a machine blowing air into it seem very unpleasant and something to be avoided if at all possible. Surgery seems worse.

Second, if the only result of the disorder is fatigue, many people simply don't recognize their fatigue or acknowledge that it is a symptom of something larger—rather, they simply accept it as normal. And even when they admit to fatigue, they may come up with any number of justifications, such as "It's just a part of growing older." The fatigue also may play a major role in immobilizing patients and preventing them from seeking help.

Third, many sleep problems are not directly experienced; people who snore have never heard themselves snore, and they never realize they have stopped breathing; those with periodic limb movements aren't awake to see the legs kicking or stretching.

Last, patients worry they won't be taken seriously or that their doctor will think they are neurotic. All it takes is for one doctor to respond to a complaint of insomnia or restless legs with skepticism and the patient may never mention the problem again.

As a society we've made great inroads in destigmatizing such illnesses as epilepsy, eating disorders, and mental illness. I can only hope that attitudes about sleep disorders are next in line. I am very happy that some high-profile people, such as New York Congressman John LaFalce, and Georgia Senator Max Cleland, have gone public with their sleep apnea conditions. If other well-known public figures would do the same, it would make a big difference.

Getting Help from Doctors

Unfortunately, getting medical help for sleep problems is likely to be a lot more difficult than dealing with other health problems. Medical schools currently spend an embarrassingly small amount of time, or none at all, educating future doctors about sleep. During family practice and internal medicine residencies, very little attention is devoted to sleep disorders. When in active practice, there is no easy way to obtain adequate training in sleep disorders. The number of sleep specialists qualified to provide training through continuing medical education classes is far too small to reach the vast primary care community. As a result, primary care physicians are not knowledgeable about sleep disorders, even though sleep disorders affect half their patients. Physicians are also likely to suffer from the same misconceptions about sleep that plague the lay public. Finally, physicians themselves have sleep disorders that they do not correctly diagnose.

The primary care physician at the front line of medical care is the first to identify a health problem, evaluate its seriousness, treat the patient, or refer the patient to a specialist. While the vast majority of these crucial health professionals do their best, without knowledge about sleep disorders they are not able to keep their patients from getting sicker and sicker.

This lack of knowledge means that victims of severe restless legs syndrome are misdiagnosed with various psychiatric disorders and treated with strong tranquilizers. Obstructive sleep apnea patients are often treated for "misdiagnosed" depression. Children with sleep disorders are commonly diagnosed as having attention deficit disorder. I am acquainted with a man who worked in the top levels of the National Security Council until he began to fail at work because of severe apnea. He got labeled as having treatment-resistant depression until one physician finally said, "If the eight medications you are taking aren't helping at all, it can't be depression." Once patients receive the wrong diagnosis, they may never receive the correct one. For example, once an unrecognized sleep apnea patient develops heart disease, for example, the consequence of the sleep disorder becomes the focus of treatment instead of the original problem—the sleep disorder itself.

Last year I sent a proposal to a small foundation requesting funds to promote apnea awareness. Shortly thereafter, the president of the foundation called me in a panic. "Your material exactly describes my son's condition! He had his second heart attack last month, and he's only 43 years old." I referred his son to nearby sleep specialist, who carried out the standard overnight test to diagnose apnea. Sure enough, the test revealed that the man's son stopped breathing 85 times every hour that he slept, which represents extremely severe obstructive sleep apnea. His blood pressure was very high, and as noted he had suffered two previous heart attacks. Although he had been in the care of several doctors and had been treated for years for his high blood pressure and his heart condition, none of the doctors even considered the possibility of sleep apnea.

His apnea is now being successfully treated, and his blood pressure has fallen. I'm sure he would have died within a couple years or sooner if his father hadn't read my grant proposal. But someone's life shouldn't hang by such a slender thread. Any of the doctors who treated him could have recognized his apnea. Even though this man lived in a large metropolitan area with ready access to specialists, his true medical condition was completely overlooked. This story has a postscript. As the family became more aware of the nature and symptoms of apnea, they realized that a daughter was also seriously ill. She too was successfully treated.

Cases like this have haunted me for years. Ever since I realized over 35 years ago that almost all victims of narcolepsy were not being diagnosed and treated, I have been a passionate patients' advocate. The more I learn, the more I realize that I am continually underestimating the scope of this national health crisis.

For those who doubt this is the case, I have some hard data to prove the point. In the middle of the 1980s I became curious about where our Stanford Sleep Center patients were coming from. We analyzed our records and discovered that only about 2 percent of our patients were referred by primary care physicians. I was slightly surprised by the low percentage, but I realized I could no longer ignore the educational problem. I hasten to add that back then it was still possible for large numbers of patients to come directly to our sleep clinic. The majority of our patients were being referred by respiratory specialists and ear-nose-and-throat surgeons, with a smattering from other specialists.

While I was chairman of the National Commission on Sleep Disorders Research, the absence of primary care referrals to our clinic came into sharper focus. One of the commission's first tasks was to look at all available data and make a reasonable estimate of the prevalence of several sleep disorders. We had enough survey and anecdotal information to make very rough estimates about the incidence of apnea and insomnia. In addition, I wanted to learn more about the level of awareness about sleep disorders among primary care physicians in particular and the medical community in general.

By this time computers and computerized databases had evolved to the point where they could be readily accessed. Accordingly, I called clinic administrators all over the country, identified myself as chairman of the sleep disorders research commission, and requested a search of their clinical database for all of their diagnoses of sleep disorders. (In these databases, all illnesses are assigned standard international diagnostic codes, which include numbers for sleep disorder diagnoses.)

As the search mounted into the millions of patients, the results were absolutely astounding and shocking. I have already talked about some of our finding with regard to insomnia in Chapter 6. After scanning more than 10 million patient records, we found a grand total of only 73 diagnostic codes for obstructive sleep apnea and 7 for narcolepsy. No other specific sleep disorder diagnosis was found. It might as well have been a big fat zero.

The other commissioners simply could not believe these results. I responded by sending research assistants to conduct on-site examination of individual patient records. Individual records are the color-coded manila folders that you may have seen filling the shelves at your doctor's office. Page by page, my team examined the records of well over 10,000 patients in primary care clinics, mostly in the San Francisco Bay area, and did not find even one specific sleep disorder diagnosis.

These two sets of data convinced me that, for all intents and purposes, somewhere between 95 and 99 percent of all sleep disorder sufferers in 1991, and today in 1998, remain undiagnosed and untreated or misdiagnosed and mistreated. That is millions and millions of people. We have solidly confirmed this conclusion in our continuing on-site studies of primary care medical practice.

Understanding the Doctor's Dilemma

I want to do what I can to help you get the treatment you need by giving you some practical advice about talking to your doctor about your sleep problems, finding a sleep specialist if your doctor can't help you, and getting insurance companies to pay for up-to-date and effective treatments. It won't be easy.

It is important to try to understand the logistical and psychological barriers doctors face in treating sleep problems and then devise strategies for overcoming any resistance. There are several key reasons why primary care and other doctors lack the inclination or time to deal with sleep problems. First and foremost, as I have said, is lack of education. Second, physicians often believe that sleep disorders are not serious or life-threatening. "Sleep apnea is not a fatal disorder," they may claim. While it is true that few people actually die during a nighttime apnea attack, the disorder leads directly to many fatal events such as heart attacks, strokes, and accidents. Likewise, many doctors subscribe to the misguided notion that insomnia is a neurotic complaint that causes no lasting harm.

Last, there is the issue of available time. My colleagues and I have conducted observations on the duration of direct doctor/patient contact. Typically doctors spend between four and five minutes with patients—long enough only to deal with the specific problem for which the appointment was made. It is certainly not enough time to evaluate a patient's sleep patterns and problems.

I believe most primary care doctors are truly concerned about their patients and willing to take extra time with someone when they feel it is necessary. But doctors are also human; they are paid according to the number of patients they see and procedures they do. More patients are always out in the waiting room. The financial incentive is to treat patients quickly and get them out the door. If your doctor spends a lot of time talking with you about your general health during a visit, hang on to that doctor: This breed is getting more and more rare every day.

Adding to time constraints are physicians' natural desire to solve problems quickly and decisively. Doctors are a very goal-oriented group of people; they like to identify a problem, provide the solution, and move on. Consciously or unconsciously, they shy away from grappling with a problem like insomnia, which may take a long time to diagnose accurately and may not have a clear solution. Doctors deal with signs of alcoholism in an analogous manner. In one study, young doctors were asked what they would do if a patient walked into the office with the smell of alcohol on his breath and a broken toe. Nearly all of them responded, "Fix the toe." The doctors knew that the patient probably had an alcohol problem and likely would end up breaking his toe again and again until the alcoholism was addressed. But treating alcoholism is much more difficult—it takes a lot of time, requires an emotionally difficult confrontation with patients about their alcohol problem, and there is good possibility that in the end the problem will not be solved. It is far easier to fix the toe, declare victory, and move on to the next case. So for a doctor faced with a case of hypertension, which is a classic symptom of sleep apnea, prescribing a pill may be a more attractive option than inquiring into the patient's sleep history.

There are some chronic insomniacs that even sleep specialists want to avoid. My favorite example of this type of patient is Mildred B. I was told a woman was lying on the steps of the hospital and refusing to move until Dr. Dement would see her. Since this was 20 years ago, when it could be easily done, and she had traveled all the way from Michigan to see me, I decided to admit her to the hospital. When I saw her in her room she talked on and on about her various problems, the consequences of her incredibly severe insomnia, and her sorry state. She had so many complaints that I could not keep track, so I said, "Write your complaints down in prioritized order. I will not come back until you have done this." Apparently it required 24 hours because she did not call until the next day.

The list numbered well over 30 complaints. The 3 that bothered her most were: (1) incapacitating insomnia, (2) severe palpitations, and (3) itching ears. It turned out that she had drug-dependency insomnia and responded very positively to controlled withdrawal of medication. I found that the palpitations were associated with postural hypotension which responded very well to the use of support hose. However, I could find no reason for her itching ears. I discharged her from the hospital as significantly improved. She returned to Michigan and initiated a malpractice lawsuit because I had not solved all 30 complaints.

Because this tiny minority of insomniacs go from doctor to doctor, and have probably interacted with quite a few, I suspect they have done a disproportionate amount of damage to the credibility of insomnia in general. Any doctor who had previously dealt with Mildred B. would surely be gun-shy about caring for insomnia patients. However, I hasten to add that sleep specialists are fully qualified to deal with difficult insomnia patients and almost always can cure or improve their condition.

Each of the reasons for doctors' neglect of sleep problems is compounded by managed care. As of 1998, 160 million Americans belonged to a health management organization (HMO), with more patients and physicians enlisting every day. Physicians in managed care systems are pressured to cram an ever greater number of patients into each hour. In some systems doctors are "capitated"—told they cannot give more than a certain amount of care to a patient per year, or their pay will be cut. The upshot of this system is that at a certain point, every time physicians try a new treatment or refer a patient to a specialist, they lose money. Even without capitation, insurers discourage or deny outright referrals to other doctors. In this kind of through-the-looking-glass medical environment, patients with insomnia or apnea are unlikely ever to be seen by the doctor who will do them the most good. I am not arguing to abolish managed care; that would be like spitting into the wind. But it's patently illogical for any medical care system to give sleep disorders short shrift, when all our outcome data to date show that lives and dollars are saved down the line when these disorders are detected and treated early.

It might seem ridiculous to have to negotiate with your doctor to get the most advanced treatments for your sleep disorders, but pragmatism is the rule of thumb. When dealing with your HMO, it is best to get a referral to a sleep center from your current physician; otherwise you can simply refer yourself. Every week the staff of the Stanford Sleep Clinic sees people who have made appointments for themselves or come in without a referral. This is easiest to do if you are not part of an HMO and have a type of health insurance that can be used with any doctor.

If you are a member of an HMO, you probably will be required to get a referral from your primary care physician. Since there are only about 1000 board-certified sleep specialists in the United States, not many physician networks include a sleep specialist. Insurers can be extremely resistant to referring patients to specialists outside the system. If you work for a large company, the human resources department may be a helpful advocate on your behalf with the insurer. Sometimes the key to getting the help you need is knowing the right complaint, such as telling your doctor that you are afraid of falling asleep while driving. When seeking medical help for sleep disorders, there are some points you should keep in mind.

Tactics and Talking Points

The medical system's failure to treat sleep disorders is an obstacle no patient should have to overcome. But in the real world, patients face precisely this challenge. Empowering patients to demand treatment from their doctors is one obvious remedy. But merely encouraging patients to be assertive is simplistic.

I was reminded of this by a recent personal experience. I had scheduled an emergency haircut appointment because I wanted to be presentable for an appearance on a local television show. The hairstylist was chopping away when I happened to glance in the mirror and realize that she was doing exactly the opposite of what I had requested. I could hardly believe it, because the last time I had received the "exact" haircut I wanted. I relate this seemingly trivial crisis because I found I had great difficulty bringing myself to stand up to my own hairdresser. It was almost easier for me to glower silently and feel self-conscious about a bad haircut than to confront her. I was a little surprised at my timidity, but it occurred to me that if I didn't have the gumption to challenge my hairdresser when I thought she was ignoring my directions, how could I possibly expect patients to challenge their physicians effectively, particularly primary care physicians who are usually in a hurry?

My failure of will at the hairdresser's was a humorous insight into my psychology, but it drove home the importance of learning techniques for working effectively with anyone in authority. The risk of not confronting my hairdresser was only the possibility of a bad haircut. But the consequence for patients who don't assert their concerns about sleep problems to their physician can be very serious.

Here are the points to keep in mind when talking with doctors about sleep:

- *Point 1: Make an appointment specifically to talk about your sleep problem.* I can't emphasize how important this is. Don't go see the doctor about itchy skin and then bring up your sleep problem at the end of the visit. Doctors generally are very task-oriented people. Most allow a certain amount of time to solve the problem, and then they are on to the next patient. If you bring up the problem at the end of the visit, the physician may not have enough time to give you a full hearing. Don't take that chance. By setting an appointment specifically for the sleep problem, you are letting the physician know you take it seriously and expect him or her to take it seriously too.

- *Point 2: Don't be afraid to bring in material you have read to support your complaint.* You already have learned a great deal about sleep by reading this book. Don't be shy about using this information.

Show this book to your doctor as well as anything else you can gather from other sources. If you think you have apnea, insomnia, restless legs, or some other disorder, pick up information from the appropriate sleep disorders associations or patient support groups and bring it to your appointment. Web sites of organizations that have good information about sleep disorders are listed in Appendix C. Doctors try to keep abreast of new developments in medicine, but they cannot be aware of everything that's being published around the world.

• *Point 3: Remember that doctors are people.* They care a great deal about their patients and are justifiably proud of the years of medical training that they have gone through. On the other hand, they probably have not received the training they should have about treating sleep problems. They may have their own prejudices about sleep disorders or may resist treating people for some of the same reasons patients resist treatment.

So when talking about sleep problems to a doctor, you need to walk a fine line between assertiveness and collaboration. You shouldn't go in demanding sleeping pills or a continuous positive airway pressure (CPAP) machine for your apnea. To quote John Grauke, one of the Moscow doctors involved in the primary care project: "Doctors like to apply their knowledge and skill to solving a problem. We like to think we are more than just short-order cooks."

If you start the visit by insisting on a certain solution, you may get into a confrontation from which it is not easy to disengage. The trick is to be neither argumentative nor totally compliant. With the information gleaned from this book you might already have a pretty good idea of what you need. The best tactic is to present your problem in a neutral manner and let the doctor question you and suggest an approach. Then you can present what you think might be a good solution. You might say, "That approach seems good, but I have read that just a couple nights of sleeping pills can help me get through this tough period without any danger of addiction or rebound insomnia. Could we try that?" Doctors might be willing to compromise or negotiate further if they are not put on the defensive.

- *Point 4: Be persistent.* If you don't feel a doctor has answered your concerns, ask again. If you leave the doctor's office with issues still unresolved, make another appointment and bring them up again. I learned from a salesman that the number-one rule in sales is persistence. The same rule applies to medical consumers, except that you are trying to get someone to pay attention instead of money.

  A recent study of elderly patient care published in the British medical journal *Lancet* showed, not surprisingly, that doctors disliked treating patients who were demanding, preferring the more compliant types. Yet those doctors also tended to make more mistakes treating compliant patients or didn't treat them as aggressively. The demanding patients ended up getting better care and living longer. When compliant patients did worse, the doctors blamed it on the patients' age rather than their prescribed treatments.

- *Point 5: Lay the groundwork now for future problem-solving.* Even if your problem seems as mild as insomnia a few times a year, mention that you are reading a book on sleep medicine and ask your doctor if he or she sees many patients with sleep disorders. Doctors should be detecting at least a few cases of sleep apnea and insomnia every year. If they really are on top of the field, they should spot apnea in about 10 percent of their patients.

  If you have occasional bouts of insomnia, mention that when an episode occurs, you would like to be able to get one or two nights' worth of sleeping pills on short notice. One good arrangement is to call your doctor when you have a particularly stressful day coming up and are worried about sleeping the night before, so the doctor can call in a prescription to the pharmacy. At times, I employ another option with patients I know well: I prescribe a small supply of sleeping medication, perhaps 30 tablets, for the patient to use very occasionally as needed over the course of a whole year. If the patient depletes the supply in a shorter period of time by taking a pill every night—still a very safe level of medication—I require another appointment with the patient to discuss the situation before prescribing any more medication.

- *Point 6: Know when and how to find a specialist.* My fervent hope is that someday people will need to see a sleep specialist mainly for rare, complex, or treatment-resistant sleep disorders, because primary care physicians will be qualified to treat most cases of insomnia, restless legs syndrome, straightforward sleep apnea, and other common disorders. Every medical group and hospital should have a knowledgeable nurse or nurse practitioner on staff who will be able to spend a fair amount of time working with patients on various insomnia-fighting techniques or getting the right fit and pressure on a CPAP mask. Until that day arrives, the reality is that you may need to see a specialist for the many kinds of sleep disorders that primary care physicians are unable to treat. If you have a good relationship with your primary care doctor, discuss your case with him or her first. But if you aren't getting results, don't get into a battle over treatment with your doctor. Suggest that he or she refer you to a sleep specialist. Every accredited sleep disorders center in the country is listed by geographic location in Appendix A. Take that list with you to your appointment.

What Can You Expect?

I wish I could provide a lot of encouragement, tell people about the positive response they will get from their doctors if they approach them sensibly. But my experience has contradicted that hope. Most often physicians who are not sleep specialists will downplay or even deny a sleep problem. After making extraordinary efforts to convince your doctor to help you, you may end up no closer to getting crucial treatment.

I can only say to concerned victims and family members: Do whatever is necessary, don't give up no matter what obstacles are in your path. If your spouse or child had cancer, you would find a way to get the necessary treatment even if you had to pay out of your own pocket. If your sleep disorder is life threatening and nothing you do is working, by all means pay the money and get a proper diagnosis. Once a diagnosis is made, it is easier to convince primary care physicians to take the problem seriously and easier to induce insurance companies and HMOs to pay for treatment.

To get a proper evaluation, you will need to go to a specialist. At this time few primary care practitioners can perform an apnea test.

Theoretically they could, and insurance companies probably would be delighted to have them do it, but most physicians are not prepared to take the time to learn a new technology that requires both diagnostic and interpretive skills. The last time I checked, only 25 primary care physicians *nationwide* had obtained the necessary education and training to be certified as a sleep specialist by the American Board of Sleep Medicine (ABSM). In order to qualify for the ABSM examination, the physician must have an M.D. degree, must have completed a residency program, and must demonstrate proficiency in administering and interpreting various diagnostic tests for sleep disorders. Most sleep specialists are affiliated with a sleep clinic or a sleep center within a hospital.

I will very briefly tell you what to expect when you go to a sleep clinic. The staff will give you an initial interview and questionnaire to get an idea of your problem and decide on your best course of treatment. At Stanford, the interview runs about two hours. Then the staff does a physical and neurological exam to make sure they haven't missed any physical problems that didn't come up in your medical history. Sometimes the initial exam will be enough to make a diagnosis, but about 80 percent of the time the sleep clinic physicians decide to keep people overnight and monitor their sleep. On the arranged night you check into the clinic, get dressed in pajamas and gown, and then get wired up with sensors to your chest, head, and legs. They'll also hook you up to a tube that measures air pressure in your throat. Your sleep is then monitored from a nearby control room, largely by computers that record data from the sensors. In the morning, the sleep specialist physician will analyze your polysomnograph and recommend therapies that you or your own doctor can carry out.

But this brief description gives short shrift to the most outstanding feature of coming to the sleep clinic. For most patients, this is the first time in their lives that their problems with sleep are completely accepted and understood. Everyone patients interact with is respectful and sympathetic. Everything patients say is taken seriously and responded to. For many people this is a new experience after years of frustration and steadily increasing distress.

Regardless of the nature or source of your sleep problem, you should never feel bashful about seeking medical help. The fundamental principle that should guide everyone is this: We are not healthy unless our sleep is healthy. Everyone is entitled to healthy sleep, and in most cases, the knowledge and treatments that will transform unhealthy sleep into healthy sleep are available.

Chapter 17

Learn to Manage Your Sleep Crises

WHEN A changing situation reaches a decisive turning point, the moment is termed a "crisis." Before antibiotics there were dramatic portrayals of individuals with pneumonia reaching a crisis point, where they either died or got well. Some people may think the term "crisis" a little overdramatic for sleep-related situations, but I do not. It is certainly a life-or-death crisis when a driver is beginning to nod and struggle to keep his eyes open. Another variation of a sleep crisis would be an unexpected summons to stay up all night for a critical task or emergency. Doctors are infamous for being on call or on duty for long hours. Railroad engineers are essentially on call all the time; though their work hours are regulated by federal transportation rules, those rules do not ensure that engineers get adequate sleep when not on the job. Finally, a sleep disorder may have worsened to a crisis (a sleep disorder emergency), to the point where serious damage to health, family, or safety is so likely that the victim must do something immediately.

When the moment of crisis arrives, actions taken can make things either better or worse. Therefore, it is important for you to learn the correct strategies to manage sleep crises with a minimum of collateral damage to your health, work, and family commitments. As in any crisis, the keys to getting through a sleep crisis are knowledge, preparation, and intelligent use of the tools at your disposal. Potential crises include typical sleep-unfriendly conventions of modern life such as long drives, jet travel, shift work, and emergencies.

I cannot emphasize often enough that if you are driving or doing some other potentially dangerous activity, and you feel sleep tugging your eyelids down, you absolutely must stop. This is the number-one life-and-death sleep crisis. You are seconds from tragedy and should hear a warning alarm blaring in your head. You should feel and act as you would if you heard a police siren and saw flashing lights right behind you: You pull over immediately. No job, no vacation, no goal, is worth endangering your life—or the lives of others.

Understanding

The first and foremost key to handling any sleep crisis is to possess the basic sleep knowledge and understanding that this book provides. You must know your own sleep needs and your best times of day for action or sleep. You now know that you may feel fine when you start out on a long road trip in the morning but drowsy in the early afternoon. You understand that if you take an afternoon break for a few hours, you will start feeling better as clock-dependent alerting once again pushes your fatigue aside. If you understand beyond the shadow of a doubt that sleep debt is additive, you know that getting extra sleep one night before a crisis situation may not sufficiently reduce your sleep debt so that the situation is not still fraught with danger. You will avoid alcohol in a crisis because you know it multiplies the effects of sleep debt, and even a very small amount of alcohol that otherwise might do nothing can precipitate fatal fatigue.

Finally, although you can learn the general rules about sleep, there are important individual and age-related differences about which sleep researchers still know little. Consider two normal adults, whose peak alertness and performance typically occur in the evening, both of whom have stayed up all night. One might feel wide awake and alert during the following evening, regardless of severe fatigue earlier in the day, while the other individual may experience no evening relief of fatigue at all. Although they carry exactly the same sleep debt, staying up all night might affect them very differently. One might be too tired and unmotivated to do anything, and the other might feel only slightly impaired. Learn your own personal sleep and rhythm talents by referring to the self-evaluation in Chapter 15.

In the future, I fervently hope that this learning process will begin in the home, continue through the school years, be refined in college, and easily applied throughout life. Today very few people clearly understand their own sleep needs. I encourage you to compare notes with your spouse, family members, friends, anyone who shares your interest. If you are working, or when you are traveling with a group, pay attention to the behavior and mood of the other members of the group to see if individual differences are apparent.

I have been asked by audiences countless times what is a dangerous sleep debt and how big can a sleep debt get? Before I address this question, I would like to say that we can now explain certain puzzling individual differences by evoking the concept of sleep debt. For example, if someone tells me that he cannot take a nap in the afternoon because then he cannot fall asleep at night, I suspect his sleep debt is so low that he requires the uninterrupted (no nap) buildup of sleep debt over the entire day to have a strong sleep tendency at bedtime. Conversely, a person who has no trouble falling asleep at the usual bedtime if she has an afternoon nap probably has a much larger sleep debt. Someone who can enjoy a bottle of wine at lunch and not be a zombie all afternoon probably has a lower sleep debt than those of us who are drowsy all afternoon with one glass.

Recall the study described in Chapter 3, in which for 5 weeks subjects maintained a daily schedule of 14 hours in bed in the dark followed by 10 hours awake in the daylight. When the subjects woke up on the last morning of the five-week study, they probably had the lowest sleep debt that a normal human being could achieve. We can assume that their total sleep debt when they went to bed each night of the final week was only that day's accumulation because they had slept off all their carryover sleep debt. We can figure out a specific number to the mean sleep debt the subjects brought into the experiment: It is the grand total of all sleep more than 8 hours and 15 minutes per day for the entire 14-hours-in-bed period, or about 25 hours per subject.

We can then conclude that a carryover sleep debt in the ballpark of 25 hours does not cause severe or even obvious impairment in healthy young adults. However, we must conclude that the subjects were somewhat impaired coming into the study, because of the substantial improvement in mood and energy they experienced, presumably due to getting rid of 25 hours of carryover sleep debt.

I think we now know enough to throw out some reasonably accurate figures, but this area should be the target of much more research. I propose that healthy young adults need a 10- to 20-hour carryover sleep debt, plus the sleep debt created by being awake 15–16 hours during each day, to sleep efficiently during the nocturnal 8–9 hours in bed. I also think that by attaining 8–9 hours of sleep every night, the daily need for sleep is completely fulfilled. No additional sleep debt will accumulate. On the other hand, if 10 to 20 additional hours are added to the sleep debt, due to inadequate sleep, I think that daytime function will be clearly and obviously impaired. I suggest that starting the waking day with 50 hours of carryover sleep debt will be the upper limit the average healthy adult can stand. Beyond this, any reasonable level of function will be impossible. People at this level of sleep debt are in the twilight zone of sleepiness, and their lives are fraught with extreme danger.

Although questions about the best amount of sleep debt have barely been addressed by formal scientific research, by following the guidelines presented in this book, individuals can learn these things on their own. In the same way you learn how much you can eat without feeling uncomfortable and how fast you can run 100 yards, you can learn your own sleep needs, sleep debt tolerances, and the strength of your clock-dependent alerting.

A few days ago, I was an after-dinner guest at one of Stanford's dormitories, and about 50 students gathered in the lounge to hear my remarks. I started by asking, "How many of you feel a little tired right now?" (It was 7:00 P.M.) Most of the hands went up. Then I asked, "How many of you felt much more tired earlier this afternoon, or after lunch?" Every hand went up. Then I said, "How many of you expect to feel better later this evening, maybe around 10?" And again, most of the hands went up. Then I said, "Do you realize how amazing this is? This afternoon you were very tired and sleepy, you have had no sleep, and yet later this evening, you expect to feel less sleepy, and many of you will do homework at that time, socialize, or whatever. But you won't be thinking about going to bed. How can you get less sleepy with no sleep? Does anyone have a guess?" Only one hand went up. So I said, "Tell us your explanation." The student replied, "Well, it's something you just get used to. We do this every day, and it becomes a habit." Not a single student in the audience knew the true explanation for their evening alertness, or their afternoon tiredness for that matter. These students are prime examples of all the millions who are likely to get into a sleep crisis and to mishandle it when it occurs.

The paramount piece of knowledge that everyone must master is that drowsiness can become sleep in an instant. Without warning. Once your eyelids start feeling heavy, you are only a few seconds from sleep. An analogy that comes to mind has to do with the cliffs overlooking the Pacific Ocean 30 miles west of Stanford. Every once in a while people ignore the warning signs and walk along the cliff edge. They think they can keep from going over by staying a step or two back from the edge and carefully watching their footing. But then, without warning, the soil gives out from under their feet and they plunge to the rocks below. Likewise, too many people are tempted to think they know exactly when they are in danger of falling asleep and that they can safely skirt the abyss. But when wakefulness suddenly slides out from underneath them, they are powerless to save themselves.

No one wants to die or be horribly injured or brain damaged because of drowsy driving. The feeling of drowsiness is the warning sign at the edge of the cliff. Feeling drowsy is red alert!

Prevention

You can prevent many sleep difficulties from becoming crises through prudent preparation. The simplest way to protect yourself is to keep your sleep debt low in the first place. Then, if you lose sleep before a meeting or vacation, it won't hit you nearly as hard. If you know you are going to have a difficult stretch in a week or two, work on lowering your sleep debt by getting extra sleep in advance. Some people think of getting more sleep in advance as "banking" sleep, but technically you can't save sleep because sleep debt can't be lower than zero. When you get extra sleep you will still have some sleep debt, but it will be lower than your usual amount. Keeping your baseline sleep debt low can make the difference between being sharp enough to function in a crisis and being too fuzzy-headed to think, between feeling just a little less energetic and feeling really awful.

Finally, decide when, how, and where you will sleep during the difficult period coming up. Make a plan—just as, if you're the coach of a basketball team, you'd plan to rest some starting players during the third quarter to make sure they're not totally tapped out during the final minutes of the game. Then make a contingency plan in event the first plan falls through. Don't just assume you can push yourself through the crisis and keep yourself alert and productive simply because you're facing an important deadline.

I must admit that I have never in my entire life heard anyone say, as part of getting ready for a trip to Europe or a drive across the country, "I am going to bed extra early," or "I am going to sleep late for the next several days." Nonetheless, doing so can be amazingly effective. I have tried on several occasions to suggest this approach when I knew someone was off to far-distant lands, particularly for a demanding task or high-level event.

A complete strategy should also include a plan to cope with the aftermath of the crisis if you can't avoid it. Find a cot or get a motel room instead of driving home after working a double shift. Set aside extra time on the weekend to recover from a sleepless week. Arrange for a relative or baby-sitter to watch the kids, and then get some sleep. Don't be fooled into thinking that you can get through the day following an all-nighter just because you've met your deadline.

Napping

Napping is by far the most important and effective tool for coping with sleep crises. Adult napping should not have a bad connotation. Many people feel that napping is only for children, the sick, the lazy, and the elderly. The phrase "caught napping" reflects people's belief that, for healthy adults, napping is the most blatant manifestation of sloth. My fellow sleep specialists and I are campaigning to rehabilitate napping and demonstrate that taking naps is an excellent and respectable strategy for sleep management. Naps can make you smarter, faster, and safer than you would be without them. They should be widely recognized as a powerful tool in battling fatigue, and the person who chooses to nap should be regarded as heroic.

While the number of people who nap every day is relatively low, several national polls, including the very recent (1998) omnibus poll carried out by the National Sleep Foundation, report that only 20 percent of adults never nap. Over the years the percentages of Stanford's undergraduates who say they never nap has been consistently less than 10 percent; last year the figure was 7.6 percent. I, and I hope most of my colleagues, know that people can nap in the daytime only when they have a sufficiently large sleep debt and the biological clock is not strongly alerting the brain. I have noted already that in one study prepubertal children (ages 10 to 12) had absolutely no desire whatsoever to nap and, in fact, were completely unable to do so when they tried.

There is no official definition of what constitutes a nap. In my mind, a sleep period longer than four hours should not be called a nap, and if the sleep episode is less than five minutes, I would prefer to call it a microsleep. Only daytime sleep should be called napping. Moreover, I would prefer to call a sleep episode a nap only if an individual intended to sleep. This is a gray however. For example, many of the passengers I see sleeping on the plane and students sleeping in the library surely did not make a clear decision that they would sleep, but they would probably say they were napping.

From the point of view of managing the sleep and alertness in your life, naps can be roughly categorized as follows: the emergency nap that is used to cope with drowsiness in hazardous situations; the preventive nap, taken, for example, when an individual has to stay up all night, or a nap in the afternoon to be more alert at a dinner party or the opera; and finally, the habitual nap. Some habitual nappers take a nap every day at more or less the same time, usually after lunch. Other habitual nappers consistently nap whenever they feel they should.

Some formidable historical figures understood the power of planned napping. Winston Churchill took naps during the day so he could work late into the night, a skill that was useful during the Battle of Britain. President Lyndon Johnson was a dedicated napper. He actually donned his pajamas in the middle of the day and slept for 30 minutes, which gave him the stamina to work longer hours.

Regular napping is a completely natural answer to a biological call. The opponent process model allows us to understand the midday dip in alertness as a slight lull between the morning period of clock-dependent alerting and the evening period. Accordingly, our minds and bodies are more inclined to sleep after lunch and during midafternoon than during any other daytime period. Napping in the evening is generally a bad idea, because once your midday dip in alertness is past, the nap won't be as efficient and you may not be able to nap at all.

Daily naps can be an excellent strategy for students who study late but have early-morning classes, or for people who work in the evening, also known as the swing shift, but have to get up early to get their kids off to school. Daily napping in the early afternoon used to be common in many tropical and Mediterranean countries; midday sleep is a good way to escape the day's worst heat and enable people to utilize the cooler evening hours more efficiently. The practice of napping tends to fade away once a country adopts a modern economy. When I was in Madrid a few years ago, I looked everywhere for signs of the siesta but found none.

On that same trip, I was the keynote speaker assigned to kick off the symposium, with a lecture at 8:00 A.M. The day before the symposium we were all invited to a party that was to begin at midnight. I could hardly believe my ears. I had no intention of participating in such foolishness, but I was worried about offending my host if I refused the invitation. It was at this meeting that I conceived the excuse that I have used on innumerable occasions ever since: "I have devoted my whole life to the study of sleep and to advocating adequate sleep for all human beings. If I do not stand up for these principles, if I do not put sleep first, who will?" As it turned out, my talk was delayed until 10:00 A.M.—which was apparently no surprise to any of the locals. Even if I had known that my lecture would start later, I would not have attended the party for the simple reason that I would not have enjoyed staying up so much beyond my usual bedtime.

We at Stanford and researchers elsewhere have shown in laboratory experiments that selective, strategic naps can improve performance and measurably decrease subsequent sleep tendency. Generally, the longer the nap, the greater the benefit. Furthermore, the benefits seem to be long–lasting. We found that a 45-minute nap improved alertness for 6 hours after the nap. Other investigators have found improvement in alertness for 10 hours after a 1-hour nap.

Laboratory studies and anecdotes raise the question of how naps affect people in the real world. An inspired study on naps in an operational setting was done as part of Mark Rosekind's NASA study discussed earlier. Flight crews flying a four-leg transpacific route racked up a fair amount of sleep debt over three or four days of flight. The result was an increased number of microsleeps during the last 90 minutes of the flight, including some in the 10 minutes during the plane's approach and landing. Microsleeps were most common at the end of flights, during night flights, and throughout the last leg of the four-leg route.

For me, the most important findings of this study emerged from an experimental program of planned naps in the cockpit. The NASA research team gave flight crews a planned 40-minute rest period during each flight. The crew's average sleep latency (the time it took them to fall asleep) was 5.6 minutes, and they got an average of 25.8 minutes of sleep. During other flights, the crews got no rest. The huge difference between the level of alertness and performance in the two conditions was startling. On the napping flights, crews had an average 16 percent improvement in reaction times and a 34 percent decrease in lapses in awareness during the flight. During the no-rest flights the crews racked up a combined total of 120 microsleeps during the last 90 minutes of flights (the descent and landing phase), including 22 during the last 30 minutes. In contrast, the crews that napped recorded 34 microsleeps during the last 90 minutes of flight, including zero microsleeps during the last 30 minutes.

Since the NASA report came out, British Airways, Air New Zealand, Lufthansa, Swissair, and Finnair have implemented planned rest periods on their long-haul flights. Other airlines are looking at such plans. Regrettably, in the United States pilots are still relegated to napping "off the record." Although pilot naps, unintended or otherwise, already occur on American flights (according to Mark Rosekind), it has proven politically impossible to pass regulations allowing them; there is still the unfortunate perception that permitting pilots to sleep in the cockpit is dangerous—even with a fully awake co-pilot—despite the studies that show planned napping to be safer than not napping.

This is one of the most preposterous and illogical policy decisions of all time. While Mark was doing these studies, he regaled me with innumerable horror stories of cockpit sleeping that he had heard from pilots. In one, the pilot fell asleep and awoke with a start to find that his copilot and navigator were also asleep. Although it was mid-flight, he was concerned enough to summon the senior flight attendant and order her to stand guard. Again, he lost the battle against sleep. Once more he awoke with a start, and turned to chastise the flight attendant for allowing him to fall asleep—but found she was asleep herself. Every airline passenger who flies is concerned about safety. Clearly, the decision makers are not well enough informed to appreciate the significance of the research, and an uninformed public will not protest such a counterproductive failure to act.

David Dinges, Mike Bonnet, and others have taken the lead in studying "prophylactic naps" as a preventive measure before a long period of sleep deprivation. Dinges and others have found that a single nap of 30 minutes prior to staying up all night can prevent significant loss of performance throughout the night. In the two most extensive laboratory studies, prophylactic naps of 60 to 120 minutes greatly improved performance during a subsequent 24-hour-period of sleep loss.

Coffee and tea are by far the most widely used tools for combatting fatigue currently, and I have no reservations about using them to get a boost. I've talked before about the ways you can manage your caffeine use to get the most benefit. What most people don't realize, however, is that naps and caffeine can be additive. Michael Bonnet of the Dayton Veterans Affairs Medical Center in Ohio found that a 4-hour nap, from 4:00 P.M. to 8:00 P.M., combined with 200 milligrams of caffeine (two strong cups of coffee) at 1:30 A.M. and another two cups at 7:30 P.M. kept performance and alertness at daytime levels throughout the night.

An interesting aspect of the napping studies is that naps improve objective performance more than subjective performance. In other words, even though subjects often don't feel any better after the nap and don't believe that their performance has improved, objective measurements prove that it has. Just as we are not very good at perceiving how badly we are affected by sleep deprivation, we don't seem to be very good at perceiving the benefits of a nap. The cause of this misperception may be the sleep inertia that lasts for 15 minutes or so after a nap, when some people feel groggy and performance is poor. Anyone who feels sleep inertia has to count on spending this quarter hour adjusting to wakefulness after a nap. I like to have coffee right after a nap, to help pull me out of the sleep inertia and get me going again.

On the other hand, some people claim to be immediately refreshed by a 5- or 10-minute nap. This is very difficult to explain in terms of our current knowledge. However, I am a believer. I remember one such nap vividly because it happened fairly recently and I treated it as a personal experiment. I was driving my daughter to the Great America amusement park 15 to 20 miles away. I had turned off the freeway and was only two or three blocks from the parking lot when a strong wave of drowsiness struck me. In a few seconds, my eyelids became very heavy and I had to struggle to keep them open. Although I slowed the car, I was sure I could make the short distance to the parking lot, so I did not stop. Immediately after I was parked, I told my daughter I absolutely had to take a nap or I wouldn't be able to function. As I leaned the seat back, I said, "Look at the clock so you will know how long I slept." I closed my eyes and probably fell asleep very quickly. I awoke spontaneously and looked at the clock. I had been asleep for just a little over 3 minutes. I did not remember the beginning time myself, but my daughter did. I did not feel completely revitalized, but my eyelids were no longer heavy. My drowsiness was definitely gone and did not recur at any time during the remainder of the day. Three minutes of sleep shouldn't be this restorative but apparently can be.

In addition, I have similar experiences fairly frequently on planes. I am usually heading back to Stanford on a late-afternoon flight, during which I plan to work or read, but my eyelids get heavy, and I can't. I lean the seat back, and suddenly I am aware I have been asleep. It is never longer than 10 minutes, and sometimes I feel it couldn't have been much more than a minute or two. Yet I am almost always refreshed and easily able to resume working or reading. I sometimes think the sitting posture might make a difference in the effect of a brief nap, but as far as I know such a possibility has never been studied.

The whole subject of napping needs a lot more research, but it is already clear that people can use naps to manage sleep debt and improve performance. There is no shame in planned napping—to the contrary, people should be proud of a decision to take an emergency or preventive nap when driving a car or operating heavy machinery and people's lives are at stake. Some segments of the transportation industry are just beginning to get an idea of how planned napping can improve safety. A few other businesses are adopting the pioneering view that napping actually can help promote productivity. Silicon Valley companies like IDG Publishing (the publishers of *MacWorld* magazine) provide a nap room for employees. In the software industry, where long hours hacking computer code are the rule, napping at work is seen as a way to get employees to stay on the job longer and get more done. Jake Wideman, the editor of *Publish* magazine, expresses the logic of napping succinctly: "I can either spend the late-afternoon hours drowsy at my desk, or go take a short nap and be productive." Unfortunately, I doubt that most businesses will follow this example. Eventually naps may be seen as some sort of executive perk, but generally I imagine they will be restricted to jobs (such as in the computer industry and agriculture) that require weeks-long bursts of work to finish a product on time or get in the harvest. For the "typical" 9:00 to 5:00 job (which is becoming less typical than it used to be), napping should probably be restricted to an emergency measure. If you regularly need a nap at work, you probably are not getting enough sleep at home.

I often feel that if I am sleepy but not actually struggling to stay awake, there is a good chance that I won't fall asleep if I try to nap. However, I have learned that if I am patient, I usually can. But picking a good time for a nap is important. If sleep debt is low I won't be able to take a daytime nap outside of the mid-afternoon dip. Some people have trouble napping in the late afternoon because they feel sleepy during the afternoon, but put off their nap until later, when clock-dependent alerting is typically on the rise. As far as possible, an intended nap should be scheduled at the right time and in the right environment. In my own case, I have lots of little finicky things about my position, how I must feel, how many pillows, and so on. I also like to have a distraction, such as an unexciting radio program just loud enough to hear so that it will distract me from my immediate concerns. To sum up, successful nappers are as confident that they can nap as they are that they can drive a car. In my opinion, anyone can nap when he or she is very drowsy, unless the person's stress level is unusually high. However, often we need to nap at other levels of sleepiness, so it is well worthwhile to work on napping skills.

Self-Monitoring—The Eyes Have It

Years ago, when we first developed the Multiple Sleep Latency Test, we found very high correlations between the longest sleep latencies (people took a long time to fall asleep) and levels 1 and 2 on the Stanford Sleepiness Scale, and similarly, between the shortest sleep latencies (people fell asleep quickly) and ratings 6 and 7. (Ratings in the middle—scores from 3 to 5—were not very good at predicting sleep latencies, however.) In the study of predicting falling asleep at the beginning of Chapter 9, the data showed that the number-one predictor of sleep occurring in the two-minute period was when the subjects clicked on the icon for "eyes," meaning that they were aware of closed or partially closed eyelids, or the eyes unintentionally going out of focus. Head-nodding and trouble thinking also had some predictive power. Remember, however, clicking on these icons predicted sleep onset pretty well, but even if they noted these signs of sleepiness, the subjects weren't very good at connecting those signs to the overall likelihood of falling asleep. This fact suggested to me that people could be taught that these behavioral signals and greatly improve their ability to predict when they were in danger of falling asleep.

I have learned that by far the most reliable signal of impending sleep for me is heavy eyelids. If I have to struggle to hold my eyes open during a meeting or while reading, I know that it is useless to continue. Recently I have explicitly designated the first sign of any difficulty keeping my eyes open as the signal to get off the road. I *never* ignore it. In the prediction study, every volunteer was by definition sleep deprived, and they all acknowledged being tired or sleepy. What we observed with simultaneous videotaping and electroencephalogram monitoring was that when the eyelids drooped, a microsleep occurred. If the eyes closed, generally the subject stayed asleep for the remainder of the two-minute interval.

I have decided that we cannot apply the word "sleepy" to the entire subjective range from not quite wide awake to the moment of sleep itself. In my own lexicon, I never use the word "drowsy" merely because I do not feel at peak alertness. If I am somewhat sleep deprived and change from an active situation to a sedentary situation, the feeling of sleepiness increases gradually. Eventually there comes a moment when my eyelids want to close and a conscious effort is required to keep them open. For me this moment is very clear. I use the term "drowsy" or "feeling drowsy" specifically to indicate the period of time when there is a very strong urge to sleep and sleep is imminent. The word "sleepy" should be used to designate a broader range of feeling, say anytime that one is not fully alert. I admit that I settled on these definitions before doing a lot of lexicological research, but when I finally did look in *Webster's Unabridged Dictionary* I was pleased to find that the two words are not synonymous. Webster's defines the word "sleepy" as "having an inclination to sleep," and "drowsy" is defined as "ready to fall asleep, or half asleep."

Most people usually become aware of their drowsiness when some sort of conscious effort is required to remain awake. Again, depending on the size of the sleep debt and the time of day and the situation, the interval between the onset of drowsiness and the moment of sleep can be as brief as a few seconds. Although I am confident about my own ability to detect my own drowsiness, can other people detect their own drowsiness?

In the past three years I have passed out questionnaires to nearly every audience I have been in front of, asking which physical signs define drowsiness. Usually I provide a checklist, but sometimes just a blank sheet of paper. I have collected several thousand of these forms, and well over 80 percent of respondents associate drowsiness with sensations involving the eyes: heavy eyelids, difficulty keeping the eyes open, difficulty focusing, a feeling of heaviness in the eyelids. A distant second are head-nodding and difficulty concentrating.

The other question I ask is: Do you always feel drowsy before you fall asleep? Only a small percentage say no, (and I think this can be accounted for by retrograde amnesia).

When a truck driver falls asleep and awakes immediately with a startle, there is no question about the clarity of the signal, even if he does not have an accident. I would now say that if a driver would use feeling drowsy as the signal to stop driving, instead of falling asleep, the risk of a crash would be greatly reduced, and the reduction in time on the road would be negligible. I am certain the signs of imminent sleep can be learned and perhaps should be part of commercial drivers' training. I would further speculate that the reluctance to heed the more general admonition of "If you're tired, don't drive; if you're fatigued, don't drive; if you're drowsy, don't drive" indicates that these feelings may not be sufficiently unambiguous.

The point of all this is that for my undergraduate students, who are all at high risk for falling asleep at the wheel, I have created and promulgated a mantra: Drowsiness is red alert! Drowsiness is an emergency and calls for an emergency nap. When you are in a dangerous situation and the eyelids start to close, you may be at death's door. Since driving is the situation in which most people by far will face extremely dangerous drowsiness, I would like to go into the subject at greater length.

Surviving Driving

For people who drive long distances on the job, live far from relatives, or take car vacations to distant resorts, road trips are a fact of life. But increasingly, the typical commuter also contends with a long, tiring drive twice daily—average one-way commute times in major metropolitan areas are approaching 50 minutes. Driving is monotonous, it's not very challenging mentally, and it doesn't involve much physical effort. All of these factors relax drivers, diminish psychological alerting, and uncover the sleep debt lurking in the brain. Driving provides a terrible combination of increased risk of falling asleep and thus increased risk of injury or death.

If you are planning a long drive, think about how your sleep debt is going to affect you. Prepare for your trip by reducing your sleep debt, and if possible plan to drive while your circadian clock is making you most alert. If your peak is during the night, of course, you need to factor in the added danger of driving in the darkness, particularly if your night vision is not that great. Most of all, resolve beforehand that you will not continue to drive if you start feeling drowsy.

To reiterate the life-saving message I feel you must take away from this book: The subjective feeling of sleepiness is due to a combination of underlying sleep debt, the degree of alerting provided by the biological clock, and the amount of stimulation provided by the world around us. A high sleep debt and low clock-dependent alerting become extremely dangerous in monotonous situations. Depending on the phase of your clock-dependent alerting, a very large sleep debt can make you dangerously drowsy even during a peak in alerting. The only way to be sure that you will remain alert during a long drive is to have a low sleep debt and to drive during periods of peak alerting.

If, despite all your planning, you find yourself feeling drowsy on the road and have no one else to take over the driving, you must immediately find a safe place to take a nap. Coffee can help keep you stay alert if your sleep debt is low, but at high debt levels there is no substitute for sleep. As I've said before, a nap doesn't have to be long to have a big impact on your alertness. A 15- to 30-minute nap can move you back from the edge of the abyss. If you can nap until you awaken naturally, that is even better.

When told they must get off the road and take a nap if drowsy, many people have indicated that they feel uncomfortable and vulnerable taking a nap in a rest area, especially at night, or parking on the side of the highway. As urgent as it is to get out of harm's way when drowsiness hits, we must be realistic. If my eyelids were dragging down, and there was no obvious place to get off the highway, I would pull over as far to the side as I could and get out of the car. I would run around the car, pinch myself, jump up and down, splash water on my face—anything to reverse the drowsiness, even if only for a few minutes. Then I would get back into the car and drive until drowsiness returned. If there was still no place to park and nap, I would repeat the exercise. To stay alive, you must be exquisitely sensitive to your own feelings of drowsiness—you must know when sleep is imminent.

A study from the United Kingdom suggests a new twist in a strategic combination of coffee and a nap. Louise Reyner and Jim Horne from the University of Loughborough put volunteers in a driving simulator during the usual afternoon dip in alertness. At one point the volunteers spent two hours in the driving simulator with no rest and no coffee. Another time they had coffee but no nap. A third time they had coffee with 150 milligrams of caffeine (about two cups), followed by a 30-minute nap before their two hours in the simulator. Caffeine alone significantly reduced the number of incidents in which drivers drifted out of their lane on the simulator, but caffeine plus a nap reduced incidents much more dramatically—by almost a factor of four. This is just one study, done in a simulator instead of on the road, but its conclusions are intriguing. Because individuals have different amounts of sleep debt and vary in their reactions to caffeine, you will have to do your own experiments to find what combination works best for you.

The beauty of the Loughborough method is the synergy of drinking coffee before taking a nap. Consider the alternatives. With coffee alone, there is a 15- to 30-minute window of time before the caffeine takes effect; during this period you will continue to be dangerously drowsy. With a nap alone, there may be a 15-minute period of sleep inertia after you wake where you feel just as sleepy—if not more so—than before the nap. (Driving during the period of sleep inertia is also dangerous.) And if you drink coffee after the nap, the sleep inertia and precaffeine window occur at the same time—again, not a good condition for driving. As long as you are not extremely reactive to caffeine, coffee before a nap won't keep you from falling asleep, and you can wake fairly easily after 15 to 30 minutes as the coffee kicks in.

Even the synergy of naps and caffeine is no match for a huge sleep debt combined with monotonous activity. I can't emphasize enough that if your sleep debt is high, the only real overall solution is to lower it. Remember, it is sleep debt that causes your drowsiness, not the monotony of driving. If you have any flexibility in your schedule and find yourself unbearably drowsy, consider taking a four-hour nap or checking into a motel to get a full night of sleep. Better yet, work at reducing your total sleep debt in the week leading up to the road trip. Reducing all or most of your sleep debt will render you far less likely to feel drowsy, even while driving monotonous roads for long hours. A lower sleep debt also will make naps and caffeine much more effective.

Staying alert in a crisis takes far more than just a can-do attitude or a determination to tough it out. Mark Rosekind is perpetually chagrined that although pilots almost never admit personally to having problems with fatigue, they can usually tell some horror story about a pilot friend who got into terrible trouble through a fatigue-induced mistake. I have heard many stories of heartwrenching tragedy of falling asleep at the wheel, but there is one that could have been personally devastating to me. My wife fell asleep in 1974 while driving home from Oregon with our three beloved children in the back of the car without seat belts. The car drifted off the road at a pretty high speed, she said. Thank God the gravel noise woke her and she was able to keep from crashing into a deep ravine. But it scared her so much that she never tempted fate again. It usually takes only a single personal brush with death to convince people that they are courting disaster when they continue to drive while drowsy. They never do it again. The problem is that many people don't live to learn from their experience.

Jetting to Hell

When people traveled no faster than horse or sailboat over long distances, they changed time zones too gradually to create much of a lag between their body's clock and the motion of the sun. As transportation has speeded up, unforeseen problems for passengers have been created. Once we could travel faster than the biological clock could be reset, the circadian rhythm got out of synchrony with the local rising and falling of the sun.

Plane and jet travel gave birth to a peculiar twentieth-century malady commonly known as jet lag. In a nutshell, jet lag is feeling sleepy when everyone else is wide awake and having insomnia when everyone else is sleeping. About half of people experiencing jet lag also feel nauseated, and nearly all feel hungry at odd hours or not hungry at mealtimes. People with jet lag are distracted and fuzzy-headed, so out of sync with their normal body rhythms that they can feel as if they were sick with a flu virus.

In spite of this, businesspeople will fly across time zones to conduct meetings on which millions of dollars—and even their careers—are riding, without taking the time to prepare themselves and alleviate the symptoms of jet lag. I've heard that Lyndon Johnson solved this problem by staying on Washington time on a trip he took to Asia. His aides protested when Johnson proposed a meeting at 10:00 P.M. local time, which was 9:00 A.M. Washington time. Johnson reportedly replied, "If they want to see the President of the United States, they can goddamn meet with me when I want." Unfortunately, the rest of us don't have that sort of clout, so we have to figure out how to function by the local timetable.

The truth of the matter is that you don't have to be the President of the United States to go some distance in scheduling things to your own advantage. When traveling east, one should schedule work late in the day; when traveling west, work should come early in the day. Years ago, one of the pioneers in biological rhythms research, Franz Halberg, scheduled appointments with me at 6:00 A.M., which was 8:00 A.M. where he lived. Initially I was taken aback by his presumption, but I soon realized that this was an excellent strategy for him, enabling him to conduct his business at his peak—and as I grew older and became more larkish, for me as well.

On average, the body needs about one day for every time zone crossed in order to adjust to jet lag. So for a trip from New York to London, which is five time zones away, it takes at least five days for the body's temperature and hormonal rhythms to adjust to the new time. Yet everyone doesn't feel the symptoms of jet lag for five days. Some people actually feel better in a day or two, while others feel lousy for a week. Susceptibility to the symptoms of jet lag is determined partly by the peculiarities of an individual's circadian cycle and partly by the amount of his or her sleep debt at the time of travel.

There is no question that it is usually easier to adjust when flying west than when flying east. People used to say this was because our "natural" circadian rhythm is closer to 25 hours to 24. Consequently, getting to bed later (flying west) works with our natural rhythm and getting to bed earlier (flying east) works against it. But now that we know that our natural circadian rhythm is pretty close to 24 hours, we can see that it is easier to fly westward at least partly because it is easier to stay awake when clock-dependent alerting is in decline than to go to sleep when the clock-dependent alerting is strong.

For people like me who habitually go to bed early and get up early, however, traveling three or four time zones to the east is easy. Flying west is what's hard for me. For example, at home I try to be in bed by 9:00 P.M., but no matter how late I go to sleep, I always wake up at 4:00 A.M. So if I fly west to Tokyo, which is seven time zones earlier, I feel I should be going to bed at 2:00 P.M. Tokyo time. Waking is even more disorienting, because my body clock's 4:00 A.M. wake time is 9:00 P.M. in Tokyo. I wake just as everyone else is getting ready for bed. The opposite is true when I fly to New York. I can always manage to get to sleep before midnight New York time, which is 9:00 P.M. California time. If I wake up at 7:00 A.M., which is my usual 4:00 A.M. waking-up time at Stanford, I will have fulfilled my sleep requirement. If I return immediately to California, I will not have to reset my clock at either end.

Strategies for Dealing with Jet Lag

Most frequent travelers have tried a system to beat jet lag, but no one beats jet lag completely. I won't make any promises for a miracle jet-lag cure, because there is no practical way to instantly adapt to a new time zone. But there are some things you can do to make flying easier. The first principle is the same as it is for all sleep crises: understanding. Knowledge about sleep debt, biological alerting, and light's effect on the biological clock is critical for understanding how you can best manage your jet lag.

Remember that the mismatch between our internal clock and the external (local) clock is the cause of jet lag. Accordingly, the first step is to calculate when your strong clock-dependent alerting will be occurring in the new time zone. For instance, the time difference between New York and Paris is six hours. If people fly from New York to Paris and arrive in the early evening, their biological clock will tell them that it is early afternoon. Our travelers may even feel a little bit tired, because their midafternoon dip in alerting is just happening. They have dinner and go to bed at 10:00 P.M. but can't stay asleep. Why? They are trying to sleep just as their biological clocks are swinging into the strong evening alerting period. Let's assume our travelers have biological alerting that is very strong from 6:00 P.M. to midnight at home. This "forbidden zone," when sleep is almost impossible, now extends from midnight to 6:00 A.M. in Paris, which is why they may fall asleep briefly in the hotel room but wake shortly afterward and are unable to go to sleep for hours.

I would strongly recommend that these travelers plan to stay up, tour Paris, and see the sights at night. Paris at night may be even more beautiful than Paris in the daytime. They should go to bed in the early morning, and plan to sleep until after lunch. Getting out immediately into the bright light of early afternoon could help advance the circadian clock, which is good to do if travelers plan to spend more than a day or two in the new time zone.

Business travelers making the U.S. to Europe trip should try to schedule afternoon and evening meetings so that they are alert. If this is not possible, and travelers want to be at peak alertness in the morning, they should take a sleeping pill or attempt to advance their biological clock a few hours in the days before the trip. The number-one fact in dealing with jet lag is the duration of the stay in the new time zone. If the visit is only one or two days, it makes no sense to reset your clock, since you will only have to reset it again when you go home, if you have any success in the first place.

Let's say, on the other hand, that our travelers arrive in Paris at 8:00 A.M. Now their biological alerting is falling rapidly, since it is 2:00 A.M. in New York. If they have a lot of sleep debt, they will feel terrible throughout the whole morning. In the afternoon they may feel a little better, because their morning alerting starts to kick in around noon in Paris (6:00 A.M. New York time). But morning alerting is fairly weak, and by this time they have accumulated an even larger sleep debt, so they will still feel terrible. The ultimate irony is that by the time evening rolls around and they allow themselves to sleep, they can't stay asleep for long because the evening alerting is just coming into play.

The second factor people need to consider is how much sleep debt they are carrying when they begin the trip. At first it might seem that before people fly, they would want to lower their sleep debt, as with driving. But we have found that a low sleep debt actually will lead to more middle-of-the-night awakenings, fracturing sleep and lengthening the effects of jet lag. A large sleep debt can help people stay asleep longer when they do want to sleep. So if travelers are arriving in Paris in the evening, they may want to have a lot of sleep debt to help them sleep that night. If they are arriving in the morning, they may want to have a slightly lower sleep debt so that they can make it through the day, or they may take a short nap in the late morning or midday.

People who know about sleep debt and clock-dependent alerting can prepare knowledgeably for travel. Most discussions of jet lag don't adequately address before-flight preparation. Many advisors recommend changing your watch to the new local time immediately upon boarding the plane, so that you start thinking on the new schedule. But why not change your watch a day before you depart (or two days for long trips), so that you can start adapting even sooner. This may be tricky if you have appointments on the days before you leave, but some quick calculations should enable you to begin the adjustment process while honoring your commitments in the old time zone. I also try to eat meals, go to bed, and get up an hour closer to my local destination time during the 24 hours before I leave. All of these techniques help shift my thinking to the new time and my body to the new rhythm.

There are three ways to reset the biological clock: exposure to bright light, ingestion of melatonin, and physical activity. To work effectively, these interventions must be scheduled at the proper time, as I described in Chapter 4. There are, however, individual differences in how people react to each of these methods. Readers who intend to follow some of the recommendations for travelers and shift workers should understand their own sensitivity and what to expect.

If you are trying to shift your clock forward (flying east), spend some time in direct sunlight as soon as the sun comes up. To shift your clock back (flying west), sleep late in the morning and get out in the sun in the late afternoon. About 20 years ago I spent a week in Hawaii, where the time was three hours earlier than at my California home. By this time in my life, I had become a lark and my biological clock had drifted to waking me up at between 3:00 and 3:30 A.M. at home, but it was vital that I function in the evening on that trip. The first morning I woke up at about 6:15 A.M., which was 9:15 Stanford time. I took care to get bright light that evening, watching the sunset, and the next morning I woke up at about 6:45. Each day there was about a 30-minute shift of my wakeup time, with at least two hours of bright light exposure around sunset. If I wanted to shift the clock even faster, I could have put a special bright light in my room and exposed myself to it even a little later in the day. Melatonin should be taken late in the day to advance the clock, or in the morning to delay the clock.

Whether you decide to nap or stay awake during the flight depends on whether you want to be awake or falling asleep when you arrive. For example, someone flying from San Francisco to New York with an evening arrival should avoid naps during the flight in order to be good and tired from traveling and ready for an earlier-than-usual bedtime. On the trip home, the person should take a nap on the plane so he or she can stay up later and adjust to Pacific Standard Time again.

A few points about sleeping on airplanes. Airline seats are terrible for sleeping, as most people know. There is no lower back support, the leg room is cramped, and it's hard to keep the head from rolling around. Furthermore, the upright angle of the seats is exactly the angle that we've found is best for depriving people of sleep. (I've heard that this is the angle recommended for chairs used in torture.) Obviously, leaning the chair back as far as possible will help. More important is to place a pillow, blanket, or sweater under the small of the back to provide lumbar support. A good pillow for your head is helpful, but an inflatable neck ring, which keeps the head from rolling in all directions, may be much more useful.

Many people use sleeping pills on planes to great advantage, especially during red-eye flights or long international flights. Make sure you've already used the pills several times and are familiar with their effects before taking them on a flight, so you'll be fully alert in time for arrival. Don't take a pill if you must change planes in the middle of the flight.

Some "experts" advise you to stick to the local schedule once you arrive at your destination, but I think this is too simplistic an approach. If you find it too grueling to do everything the locals are doing on their schedule, go ahead and take a nap—although it is best to make the nap coincide with your dip in clock-dependent alerting. Plan on spending some of your first night awake. Your goal should be to try to do things on the local schedule, but don't torture yourself over it. Plan on getting adequate sleep over the 24-hour period, and use the principles you've learned about clock-dependent alerting and sleep debt to help you through until your clock can adjust.

The option I like best is deliberately planning not to reset my internal clock at all. This is what I did when I recently traveled to Italy for one day—my purpose was to give a keynote lecture at the annual meeting of the Italian Sleep Disorders Association. Midnight at Stanford is 9:00 A.M. in Italy. The trip, door to door, was about 17 hours. I departed Stanford at 7:00 A.M., changed planes in Washington, D.C., and arrived at the Milan airport at 7:40 A.M., which would be 10:40 P.M. in my head. I slept about an hour in the limousine from the airport, and when I arrived at my hotel, I immediately went to bed and slept about four to five more hours. I had requested that my lecture be scheduled in the late afternoon, so I was at my peak when I delivered it, and wide awake and alert at the subsequent banquet in honor of the speakers.

I returned to the hotel at 11:00 P.M., which would be 2:00 P.M. at Stanford. I worked until 3:00 A.M., which would be 6:00 P.M. at Stanford. I broke a sleeping pill in half, took it, and had no trouble falling asleep because I was not fighting strong clock-dependent alerting, and I was somewhat more sleep deprived than usual. I also packed so it would take no time to leave in the morning. I slept solidly till 10:00 A.M. and caught another hour of sleep in the limousine. When the plane took off at noon, Italian time, it was pretty close to my regular wake-up time, and I had nine wonderfully productive hours of work before the plane landed in Washington, D.C. I continued working at the airport until my flight time of 5:00 P.M. EST, and arrived at the San Francisco airport at 7:30 P.M., with plenty of time to get to bed at 9:00 P.M. Pacific Standard Time. By careful scheduling and making no effort at all to shift my clock, I was back in sync the instant I arrived in Stanford.

You should shift your clock to be in sync with local time if your stay is long enough to make it reasonable and worthwhile. If you were traveling to a time zone that is eight or nine hours away from your home and staying there only a week, the effort to be completely in sync would be hardly worth it. Depending on the various demands and constraints, partial shifting might be a good solution.

My skills in jet lag management were put to a highly visible test in 1986 when I was approached by the coach of the Stanford football team. That season the regular Stanford vs. University of Arizona football game was scheduled to be played in Tokyo, Japan, in what was called the Coca-Cola Bowl. The team was to leave San Francisco for Tokyo on a Wednesday morning; the game would be played four days later, on Sunday. The coach asked if I could help the team avoid the effects of jet lag. The unspoken implication was that this would ensure a win.

To be honest, I was torn. The year before I had participated in Mark Rosekind's study to counteract jet lag in airline pilots with some success, but the danger of being responsible—heaven forbid— for a loss by the Stanford football team in such a high-profile game caused me some trepidation. On the other hand, my professional reputation was at stake. Feeling I had no choice, I devised a schedule that would let the football team members shift their biological clocks a little each day. I attended one of the team meetings prior to a regular Sunday evening postgame review to discuss the procedure. Figure 17.1 shows the recommended schedule.

Since the players arrived in Japan several days before the game, there was no need to start shifting their biological clocks until the day of departure. I told the team that once they arrived in Tokyo on Thursday, everyone, including the coaches, would have to be in bed and falling asleep by 7:00 P.M. Tokyo time, which was 2:00 A.M. in California. They were to stay up late according to their biological clocks but go to bed early by Tokyo time. On Friday morning they got up at 4:00 P.M. Tokyo time—giving them nine hours of sleep that night to pay back some sleep debt accumulated by staying up so late California time. Friday night they were to be in bed by 9:00 P.M. We shifted these times forward by two more hours on Saturday, waking the team at 6:00 A.M. (for another nine hours of sleep) and getting them to bed at 11:00 P.M., which was their usual time back home. They then got up at the normal 7:00 A.M. on Sunday morning, alert and ready for the game. This schedule meant that the players would miss the nightclubs in the Ginza district but catch a beautiful sunrise. I warned them that once they started on this course, a failure to comply 100 percent actually could leave them worse off.

Two days before the team left for Tokyo, I heard a rumor that the Arizona football team also had retained a sleep expert. As there are only a minuscule number of such experts in the country (and none in Tucson), I could not imagine who it might be. But apparently this unnamed expert had advised Arizona simply to "tough it out"—to adopt the Tokyo schedule immediately and hope their biological clocks would adjust in time for the game. Thus the international battle of the football teams became, for me, the battle of the sleep experts.

The game was broadcast on cable television in California, so I was able to watch it at 8:00 P.M. California time. The advantage that our special jet-lag schedule was supposed to give the Stanford team was not apparent for most of the game, but in the fourth quarter, senior tailback Kevin Scott returned a kickoff 88 yards for the winning touchdown. One of the players, I was later told, exclaimed, "Now

Fig. 17.1

Jet-Lag Recommendation
The Stanford Football Team Coca-Cola Bowl

Tues. 11/25	Asleep	11:00pm	
Wed. 11/26	Wake Up	7:00am	
	Bus Departs	7:30 am	
	Leave SFO	10:00 am	
	(avoid dehydration on plane)		
	A brief (1 hr) nap before 3pm PST recommended.		
	No napping after 3pm PST (8am Tokyo time).		

		Tokyo Time	S.F. Time(PST)
Thurs. 11/27	Arrive Tokyo	1:40pm	8:40pm
	Bus Departs	3:00pm	10:00pm
	*Outdoor light as much as possible		
	Arrive Hotel	4:30pm	11:30pm
	Meal	6-6:30pm	1-1:30am
	Asleep	7:00pm	2:00am
Fri. 11/28	Awake	4:00am	11:00 am
	*Outdoor light as much as possible		
	Asleep	9:00pm	4:00am
Sat. 11/29	Awake	6:00am	Your body is now adjusted to Tokyo Time
	Asleep	11:00pm	6:00am
Sun. 11/30	Awake	8:00am	3:00pm
	GAME	1:00pm	8:00pm

Dehydration Techniques
- Drink plenty of fluids on plane (no caffeine)
- Walk around frequently on plane, ankle flexing 5 mins per 2 hrs

Sleep Techniques
- Follow the recommended schedule and avoid naps
- Keep the room completely dark during scheduled sleep times
- Relax in the final hour before bedtime

Diet
- Avoid caffeine, tea, chocolate, coffee, colas
- Avoid spicy food before bedtime

there's the edge Dr. Dement gave us!" Stanford won the game 29 to 24.

Obviously this result isn't what we would call "statistically significant," but the players felt the schedule helped them. The whole experience was a thrill for me, and for several years I loved recounting my tale of the battle of the sleep experts at every opportunity. This habit took an awkward turn at a professional meeting in Washington, D.C., a year later. I was telling my story to a colleague, loudly and with great dramatic embellishment, and I ended on a triumphant note: "I still can't imagine who that Arizona sleep expert could be, but whoever he is, he's a dope."

A voice beside me said: "*I* was the Arizona sleep expert." I turned to find the voice was that of another friend and colleague, Timothy Monk, who works at the University of Pittsburgh. I had insulted someone whom I thought was 2,500 miles away, only to find him right beside me. So I listened, with some embarrassment, while Tim explained why he had advised the team to tough it out. "Since I couldn't get to Arizona personally to motivate the team to comply with an elaborate adjustment schedule, I was afraid they wouldn't stick to it." Under the circumstances, he may well have been right.

In the fall of 1989 I got another chance to play sleep expert for a football team. Jim Fassell, whom I got to know pretty well when he was the offensive coordinator at Stanford during the Coca-Cola Bowl era, had moved on to become the head coach for the University of Utah. He asked me what I would recommend for his team when they played the University of Hawaii, four time zones to the west. Brimming with the confidence of my undefeated record, I recommended a similar schedule. Since the Utah team's practice field had lights, they were able to practice later and begin shifting their clocks before their departure. I wasn't able to see the game, but I read in the newspaper that Utah lost, 50 to 38. I called Jim to ask what had happened. He assured me that the team had no problem with jet lag, just with their defense. Nonetheless, my career football record of one win and one loss is not likely to impress anyone. On the other hand, Jim is now head coach of the New York Giants.

Shift Work

Before World War II, few people worked at night except for night watchmen, hotel clerks, and bakers. After Pearl Harbor, extraordinarily high production goals dictated that factory workers churn out war materiel 24 hours a day, in three shifts of eight hours apiece. These shifts are still called the day shift (8:00 A.M. to 4:00 P.M.), the evening or "swing" shift (4:00 P.M. to 12:00 A.M.), and the night or "graveyard" shift (12:00 A.M. to 8:00 A.M.). Workers are rotated in order to spread the undesirable shifts evenly.

Changing from one work shift to another is disorienting in the same way as jet lag. When workers change shifts, it is as if they had flown eight time zones away, such as going from Denver to Tokyo, or San Francisco to London. When the biological clock is not alerting the brain, the sleep debt pushes it toward sleep. The biological clock is at its lowest ebb in the middle of the night, and people are more prone to distractions, lack of focus, poor memory, bad mood, and slow reaction times. Mistakes result. Nearly every major industrial accident in recent decades has occurred after midnight, in the early hours of the morning: the *Exxon Valdez* grounding, the Chernobyl and Three-Mile Island nuclear accidents, the Bhopal chemical plant disaster.

Theoretically, it should be possible for people to adapt to working at night and sleeping during the day, just as we can adapt to a new time zone after a few days. But workers don't ever completely adapt; night workers revert to a daytime schedule on weekends and vacations when, let's face it, people want to see their kids, spend time with their spouses, pursue outdoor activities, have a life. The only way they can do this is to break their nocturnal cycle, usually just when they are getting used to it. Studies show that shift workers commonly get two hours less sleep when their sleep time is during the day as opposed to during the night.

This brings up the second major problem with shift work. Due to shift rotation, workers never become fully adjusted to any single schedule. The brain is often fighting to go to sleep when work demands are being made and resisting sleep when bedtime arrives. The most common rotation schedule in the United States is one week per shift, followed by a "counterclockwise" change to the previous period (night shift to evening shift, evening to day, or day to night shift). This is the worst possible combination; a week is just long enough to become acclimated to a schedule, and it is more difficult to make a counterclockwise change than a clockwise one. I must also point out that a counterclockwise rotation is analogous to flying in an eastward direction. Just as workers are beginning to acclimate to a shift after one week, another eight-hour phase shift is imposed on their biological clock. And that phase shift is in the more difficult direction, demanding alertness just when clock-dependent alerting is lowest. For instance, going from the day shift to the evening shift is not a problem—starting at 4:00 P.M. and working until midnight only means staying up a little later than you normally would. But moving from the day shift back to the graveyard shift demands that workers start work just as clock-dependent alerting is descending to its weakest point in the day.

Chuck Czeisler has done a great deal of consulting on shift work for various businesses as well as for police and fire departments. For one company in Utah, he recommended a change from a one-week counterclockwise shift rotation to a three-week clockwise rotation (day to evening, evening to night, and night to day). The three-week periods gave workers a week to make the adjustment to the new schedule and two weeks to maintain it. When it came time to rotate, it was to the later shift, which is easier to adapt to. More than 70 percent of the workers preferred the new schedule, and there were fewer complaints of sleep and various other health problems. The company reported a 20 to 30 percent increase in productivity and lower absentee rates.

Time and Tide

Last year I saw my friend Jim Maas on the *Oprah Winfrey* show promoting his own book *Power Sleep*. One of the other guests was a woman whose story I knew quite well. Her husband was a maintenance worker whose company had required him to work more than 40 consecutive hours during an emergency. When he finally finished and drove home it was midafternoon—the time of lowest daytime alerting. He fell asleep at the wheel, went off the road, turned over several times, and sustained a very severe traumatic brain injury. The couple had two young daughters. I met his wife, Kathy, about a year after the accident at a symposium on safety in Seattle, Washington. An intelligent, attractive woman, she was as distressed as anyone I had ever seen. I learned that she had just been informed by doctors that she could not expect further recovery in her husband, and although his mobility was not impaired, he would remain a kind of lobotomized zombie for the remainder of his days. His daughter (now age 17) and Kathy described the impact on their family and their lives. How unnecessary! The company should have sent this man home in a taxi and provided him taxi fare for the return trip. This tragedy could have been avoided for a $50 cab fare.

I am worried that there is a similar time bomb ticking away in my own field, sleep disorders medicine. Sooner or later, if we are careless, an all-night polysomnographic technician driving home in the morning will fall asleep at the wheel, with tragic consequences. I recently talked at a regional meeting of the Association of Polysomnographic Technologists about this issue and was dismayed to hear that most sleep centers do not address it with the vigor and effectiveness it deserves.

I believe that driving drowsy has exactly the same risk and tragic consequences as driving drunk (although people have not been trained to recognize when they are too drowsy to drive, as they have been educated to recognize when they have drunk too much). Often people do not know they are sleep deprived and are surprised when a strong wave of drowsiness strikes while they are behind the wheel. Just as frequently, people know they are sleep deprived but drive anyway because at the moment they do not feel drowsy. The only hope for saving lives is if people recognize that drowsiness is an extreme danger signal. Furthermore, if we know a friend or a guest or a colleague is at risk for falling asleep at the wheel, we should not let them drive. Friends don't let friends drive drowsy.

The more knowledge that is accumulated about the interplay between the alerting action of the biological clock and sleep-inducing activity of sleep debt, the more I am in awe of the exquisitely beautiful system we have for waking us up and putting us to sleep. Managing your sleep crises comes down to understanding the subtle but powerful interaction between sleep debt and arousal. The opponent process model itself is simple, but its implications are not always obvious. For instance, most people don't understand that the biological clock is strongest in the evening, not in the morning. Likewise, if your sleep debt is high and clock-dependent alerting is low, the loudest music won't keep you awake while driving. You can't necessarily adapt to any new schedule by just toughing it out, and individuals vary widely in their ability to adapt to change.

In order to put the principles of the opponent process model to work during sleep crises, you have to evaluate the role of sleep debt and alerting in your own life—no simple formula works for everyone. I hope that the expertise you've gained by reading this book and examining your own life will give you the tools and the confidence to take a prudent and flexible approach to managing your sleep crises as they arise.

Chapter 18

Take Age into Account

OVER THE life cycle our bodies grow and then decline. There is also a pattern in the life cycle of sleep and wakefulness, a series of changes that take place throughout life. As I mentioned infant sleep patterns are different from childhood sleep patterns, and childhood sleep patterns are different from teenage sleep, adult sleep, and sleep in older people. We are just beginning to understand how the biological clock and the homeostatic sleep processes change over the life cycle.

I think that understanding the big picture on the lifelong evolution of our sleep cycles is a must for all of us who have assumed responsibility for our own health. It is even more important if we are responsible for infants, children, adolescents, our aging parents and others. Children should be taught the fundamental principles of healthy sleep as soon as they are able to understand them.

I also hope that people will utilize their knowledge about sleep as they themselves age. If we are old enough to understand sleep and to be sensitive to the way we feel, we can start applying the principles of managing sleep debt and clock-dependent alerting. If you are a young reader and you have owlish tendencies, there will come a time sooner or later when you will notice that this is changing; you will notice you get up more easily in the morning and can't stay up as late at night. Almost no one has paid close enough attention to describe how quickly this change occurs, but it may take place in less than a decade. A recent study reported by David Dinges found that the change from owl to lark may come as early as age 30, and most individuals between 30 and 50 have made this transition. For the 10 to 20 percent of young adults who are already larks or larkish, we have very little idea about how they change as they get older.

Each stage of life tends to have different sleep requirements, different pitfalls, and different pathologies. But just because age-related sleep problems are "natural" doesn't mean they can't be managed. The discipline of sleep disorders medicine can improve the quality of your life no less dramatically than other medical breakthroughs have rescued us from age-specific scourges such as measles or clogged arteries. The goal of sleep medicine is not to "trick" Mother Nature but to give her her due—a good night's sleep, regardless of age.

Although many of the sleep disorders I have described in this book can hit at almost any time of life (and the treatments are much the same no matter the age of the patient), certain sleep problems have a definite age preference. Sleep in children and the aging presents its own special challenges, and it is important to understand how to address them. And while our sleep patterns have consolidated somewhat in young adulthood, we're often under more time pressure in our 20s and 30s than in any other stage of life, pressure that erodes and fragments sleep to an alarming degree. When the stressful demands of work, family, and child rearing converge with full force, the impact on sleep can be devastating. One of the biggest disruptions of sleep in adults is the sleep problems and patterns in their infants and children.

If you don't have children, you may think that childhood sleep issues are irrelevant to your sleep life. Think again. If you really want to understand the underlying mechanisms of adult sleep, the best place to start is by observing the template of childhood sleep. In many ways, the patterns we observe in children are blueprints of adult sleep, writ large. Children are very alert in the day, and at night they tend to sleep very deeply and are hard to awaken, especially at the beginning of the night. A child's strong clock-dependent alerting throughout the day and a strong homeostatic sleep drive through the night are graphic illustrations of adults' daily cycles of sleep and wakefulness. Sadly, age tends to erode the happy extremes of childhood waking and sleeping cycles. Childhood can also be the time when the basic habits of sleep hygiene are formed—whether we view sleep as a lifestyle priority and a source of pleasure, or whether we go to bed only as a grudging concession to the crushing weight of sleep load. Psychologically, most of us are all children when it comes to wanting to stay up past our biological bedtime.

Rock-a-bye Baby

As you recall, infant sleep cycles are adrift for the first months of life. Babies sleep about 8 fragmented hours at night and nap roughly four times during the day, totaling about 16–20 hours of sleep over the 24-hour period. Parents of newborns are said to lose 2 hours of sleep per night until the baby is around 5 months old, which decreases to 1 lost hour per night during ages 5 to 24 months. Sleep and nap times shift steadily from day to day, so that parents might find themselves up at midnight one night and at 3:00 A.M. the next.

Although the biological clock plays a subtle role in infants' sleep patterns, the strongest factor by far is their homeostatic sleep drive. Infants build up a strong sleep debt over just a few hours, then pay it back right away with a nap. They keep this pattern through all 24 hours of the day. Slowly, sleep times begin to coalesce into a nighttime block and a morning and afternoon nap time. Once that consolidation begins to occur (usually, but not always, by the eighth week), you may be able to encourage that pattern by keeping the baby's room dark at night and exposing him or her to bright light in the morning. We have never really done experiments on this, but we can tell that time cues are beginning to exert an influence on sleep and wake times. It might be a good idea to keep a sleep log of your baby's sleep to better observe the emerging patterns.

Many parents are completely unprepared to cope with a baby who does not sleep well, who wakes up much more often than normal during the night and cries. Some infants begin to sleep through the night almost immediately, and others do not do so for many months. I mentioned the mysterious phenomenon of colicky babies earlier. I do not believe that we have proof that colic is a cause of crying, screaming, and repeated arousal, but, whatever the cause, these babies are an extraordinary challenge to parental equanimity.

There are only so many times a night that a baby can be calmed

through nursing or a bottle, and inevitably the parents lose a dangerous amount of sleep. Over the first year of a baby's life, parents each
lose an estimated 350 hours of sleep at night (although we guess from
what we currently know about sleep debt that they have to make up
much of that lost sleep by napping, getting to bed earlier, and the
increased sleep efficiency brought on by heavy sleep debt). Though
the evidence is scant, the National Commission on Sleep Disorders
Research concluded that infant abuse and infanticide often occurs
when parents are at the end of their rope and lose their temper,
shaking or even hitting a helpless infant because it will not stop
crying. Even the best of us could fall victim to such a momentary
loss of control, so I have long recommended that preparation for
parenthood include a consideration of strategies for parents to cope
with their own loss of sleep as well as wakeful babies.

Toddlers and Young Children
We tend to think of sleep disturbances as primarily an adult afflic-
tion, but with young children sleep problems may be the rule rather
than the exception. Sleep problems in these early years are so common, in fact, that people tend to think of them not as sleep disorders
but as normal manifestations of childhood. Children resist going to
bed, stall, become cranky when tired, have nightmares and night
terrors, and wake up at odd hours demanding food or comfort or
crying with growing pains. But with proper sleep hygiene and bedtime routines, these problems can be mitigated and will usually re-
cede on their own as the years pass, giving way to that magical time
from around 7 or 8 to 12 when children get what may be the best
sleep and wakefulness of their lifetime.

   The difference between sleep problems in young children and
adults is that with children it is not the child who complains, but the
parent. Sleep-deprived parents of sleepless children quickly reach a
peak of frustration as they deal with their child's difficulties. I know
very well from personal experience the intense emotions that desperate parents feel as they try to balance their own sleep demands and
the demands of a child crying in bed. Add to the mix a conflict
between two parents about how to handle the problem, and you have
a combustible mixture. There are few familial situations worse than
being groggily awake at 3:00 A.M. and arguing with a spouse about

whether it is better to get up and comfort a crying toddler or to let the child cry herself to sleep.

The Pediatric Pioneer

Until 20 years ago the sleep problems of toddlers and young children received almost no serious attention from pediatricians. The most basic question—how to handle a child who awakes and cries repeatedly throughout the night in search of parental comfort—was more a subject of folk wisdom than science. The early advice in child care books tended to fall into one of two camps: either "Let the child cry—you're spoiling him by comforting him constantly," or "You should always comfort a crying child—it's essential for his well-being."

One pediatrician who wanted to go beyond this dichotomy was Richard Ferber of the Boston Children's Hospital. In the late 1970s Ferber was just getting started in his medical practice and wanted to investigate sleep problems in children. At the time, there was little research on sleep beyond the infant stage; sleep problems in toddlers and young children (besides bedwetting) weren't even on the radar screen. During the 1970s, the Stanford Sleep Disorders Clinic was Mecca for physicians interested in sleep disorders; Dick Ferber was one of the first pediatricians to visit our program. Ferber and I talked about his interest, and I encouraged him heartily. "Please pursue this area," I told him. "You will be a pioneer." After Ferber published his book, I was pleased that he credited my encouragement for giving him the confidence to proceed.

Ferber's book, *Solve Your Child's Sleep Problems,* which is the closest thing so far to a sleep best seller, offers parents a step-by-step method for dealing with the most common predicaments. His technique for training infants and young children to put themselves back to sleep after nighttime awakenings has become known as the Ferber method. It's based on the premise that getting yourself back to sleep is not something you know automatically but is something everybody learns. All people wake up many times each night, scan their surroundings, and go back to sleep without remembering the awakening. When infants wake up and scan their environment, though, they can be frightened to find that their parent is no longer in the room, or that their blankets have fallen off and they don't know how to get them on. This wakes them up fully, allowing them to become more alarmed.

To make his point a little more understandable to adults, Ferber asks how you might react if you woke up in the middle of the night and your pillow was gone. If it was close by, you might tuck it under your head and go back to sleep without remembering the incident. But what if you reached around and it wasn't there at all? What if it wasn't even on the floor next to your bed, and you got up and turned on the light to look, but couldn't find it anywhere in the room? This would be very strange, and you might be angry, frustrated, and bewildered. You might think someone was playing a joke on you. It would be hard to get back to sleep after something like that. To infants and toddlers, the night can be just as strange, and problems that seem simple to us are bewildering and frightening to them. Besides, they've learned that the problem gets fixed if they let out a wail.

By about six months of age, most children are physically mature enough to sleep through the night without feedings—and emotionally ready to learn to put themselves back to sleep without physical comfort from their parents. Ferber feels that parents often help perpetuate their child's nighttime awakenings by their well-meaning ministrations. He believes that the best thing parents can do for their children is help them learn how to get back to sleep on their own by slowly weaning them from parental intervention.

Ferber's method uses behavioral conditioning to teach children what the rest of us do automatically. When a child wakes up and cries, Ferber advises the parent to go into the room and verbally reassure the child—but not feed or physically comfort him. After speaking calmly, the parent should then leave the child's room, even if he is still crying, and let him put himself back to sleep. If the child is still crying 5 minutes later, the parent should return and repeat the verbal reassurance. The next time the parent waits 10 minutes before going back into the room. The time after that, the parent waits 15 minutes before comforting the child. The maximum wait for the first night remains 15 minutes for each successive visit to the child's bedroom.

Each night after that, the amount of time for the first wait, and the maximum time to wait, increases by five minutes. So the second night, the parents wait 10 minutes, then 15 minutes the next time, 20 minutes the next time and every time after that. After a couple of nights of this admittedly taxing regimen, the child usually stops expecting the parents to appear with open arms and learns to put himself back to sleep.

Some critics of this method feel that it is barbaric and cruel to "Ferberize" your child. I endorse Ferber's method, because it helps most infants make the transition to consolidated sleep with the least amount of stress for both child and parent—the typical "Ferberization" takes only two or three nights. I understand parents' distress at listening to their child cry, but it's a huge relief when a child is able to return to sleep. Unfortunately, we need to *learn* to allow ourselves to fall back to sleep, and the sooner we acquire this life skill, the sooner we can enjoy a consolidated night's sleep. Also, the parents' need to return to normal nighttime sleep should not be dismissed. If parents are up every two hours with a baby, they won't be much use to themselves or to that child in the daytime.

Of course, the Ferber method does not work for all children. Some will cry and keep crying no matter how long you wait. In those cases, I recommend that the parents wait a month and try again when the child may be better prepared, physically and emotionally, to sleep through the night.

The Childhood Sleep Drive

We can really see and appreciate the power of sleep in children once they pass the stage of having trouble going to bed and getting to sleep. When kids are awake, they're fully alert and adamantly opposed to sleeping. When kids are ready to sleep, there is little anyone can do to stop them. And sometimes it is almost impossible to wake a sleeping child. When my young grandchildren would visit from the eastern time zone for a few days, their clock remained in Columbus, Ohio. Their 9:00 P.M. bedtime would coincide with our 6:00 P.M. dinnertime. On one visit recently my middle grandson fell facedown in his turkey, mashed potatoes, and gravy—sound asleep. Seeing a perfect opportunity to illustrate the strength of the sleep drive in children, I grabbed my camera to take some pictures, but my daughter indignantly stopped me. Another time she came running into the house yelling "Asleep at the wheel, asleep at the wheel!" More curious than concerned, I rushed outside to find a grandson nodding off at the wheel of his pint-sized, battery-powered toy car as it circled the driveway. That time I did manage to get some great pictures made into slides, I show them to my class every year to illustrate the power of sleep.

Both of the opposing processes, homeostatic sleep drive and clock-dependent alerting, are very strong in children. The strength of the sleep drive contributes to the problems of night terrors and sleep-walking, because the kind of stimuli that normally would trigger full wakefulness cannot completely overcome the powerful sleep tendency. Yet the equally strong clock-dependent alerting rarely allows older children to experience daytime sleepiness. A typical pattern is for a five-year-old child to sail through the day under the influence of strong clock dependent alerting, full of zest, then often getting wilder or more emotional as the strong alerting and strong sleep drive battle near the end of the day, and sinking swiftly into sleep once in bed. Many were the times I have put my children or grandchildren to bed despite their fierce protests, only to witness them fall soundly asleep literally within a minute. Kids can keep themselves awake a little longer by running around the house or playing outside, but once they lie down and relax, usually there is nothing they can do to resist the embrace of sleep. Some of my fondest memories of childhood are the times when I closed my eyes at night for what seemed like an instant, only to open them and find that it was morning. This was sleep at its most robust, undisturbed by remembered arousals.

Just as the starting point for addressing adult sleep is to understand how much sleep we need, it is important to understand children's sleep need. As I explained in Chapter 5, not only does sleep need change over the years, but different children (like adults) have different sleep needs. You and the child will only end up frustrated if you try to make him get 10 hours of sleep if he needs only 8. To figure out a child's daily sleep, follow the technique I described for grownups in Chapter 15.

Once you understand how much sleep your child needs, the most important strategy for improving his or her sleep is to set a daily routine and stick to it. Between the ages of 5 months and 5 years, the social cues imposed by parents become the primary factor in children's sleep patterns. The last feeding or snack, the story in bed, the brushing of the teeth—these activities teach children when to go to sleep. Often they will fight the imposition of this routine. Around ages 9 to 18 months, children may delay bedtime because they are experiencing separation anxiety, and many 3-year-olds battle with parents over bedtimes and rituals. In the face of this resistance, it's important that parents be firm and consistent in setting good sleep habits. As children get older they learn to accept bedtimes more easily.

The bedroom environment is also a factor in good sleep hygiene for children. Make sure the temperature in the room is neither too hot nor too cold—around 65 degrees is ideal. The curtains should be heavy enough to prevent light cues at unwanted times, such as the very early sunrises and late sunsets in midsummer. But a pitch-black room is not necessarily optimal either. Dim artificial light, from a night-light or a cracked door leading to a hallway light, might be a comfort to a child, particularly after a bad dream.

After poor sleep hygiene, occasional nightmares are the most common sleep problem for young children. The nightmare is a genuine, conscious, frightening experience, and your child must be comforted and reassured just as you would do with a waking, daytime scare. I will be stating the obvious when I say that doing this will in no way encourage your child to have nightmares. The occurrence of frequent nightmares is a rare but usually serious problem. Children who have frequent nightmares will resist going to bed, and when they awaken at night, they will resist going to sleep. Remember, the very young child may not be able to tell the difference between a dream and reality. Elsewhere (chapter 13) I briefly touched on the issue of the very young child learning that a dream event isn't a real event. This issue is much sharper in the case of nightmares.

Barry Krakow and colleagues from the University of New Mexico School of Medicine recently have done experiments showing that mental rehearsal of happier versions of nightmares during the day can lessen both the fear of nightmares and their scariness when they occur at night. Children in the experiments closed their eyes and remembered nightmares, but then consciously imagined better outcomes. Krakow reported that kids were genuinely surprised by how easily they overcame their disturbing dreams. Furthermore, it seems that this technique can work for both children and adults.

I'd like to make one other point about parents and their children's sleep that is often overshadowed by the crisis management approach of just getting through the night. I believe that instructing our children about the basics of sleep hygiene and safeguarding their healthy sleep is one of our most important parental obligations—on a par with our need to supervise any other childhood health issue. Most of us are vigilant about making sure our kids are inoculated against infectious diseases, have sound nutrition and good dental hygiene. Healthy sleep is just as important to a child's well-being, and good sleep habits learned in childhood are a gift of health children carry with them throughout life. Wise parents teach their children the basics of healthy sleep in an age-appropriate fashion—not as rote rules that invite rebellion, but as reasoned principles that children can appreciate as being in their best interests.

No reader should be surprised that I am intensely fascinated by the question of what age children can accurately judge when they are and aren't sleepy and/or drowsy. I have a memory of occasionally feeling very sleepy in the early afternoon when I was in the third or fourth grade. I don't think I said, "Gee, am I sleepy." It was more like something was wrong, and it was very unpleasant. When our sleep camp research team actually restricted sleep to four hours for a single night in 8-, 9-, and 10-year-olds, even though their scores on the Multiple Sleep Latency Test changed dramatically, their self-ratings of sleepiness did not. If we want to be successful in instructing our children about the basics of adequate sleep, they must be sensitive to their own levels of daytime alertness. I don't know if children should be deliberately sleep deprived enough to understand the difference. I would hope they could learn it mainly through verbal instruction, such as teaching them to recognize their heavy eyelids or emotional volatility.

I believe that a substantial portion of children's behavioral and learning problems during the day can be traced to not getting enough sleep. This becomes especially clear when children are in school. Many children of elementary school age are allowed to stay up well past 9:00 P.M., and sometimes until midnight, by indulgent parents. Kids are the ones who pay the price in classrooms the next day; their attention span and ability to absorb new information are seriously impaired. As Philadelphia school principal Madeline Cartwright found, when earlier bedtimes are restored there is less acting out in school, less aggression, and more attention paid in class.

I always hear people attribute episodes of irritability and crying in young Sally or David to not getting enough sleep, there has never been a thorough investigation of how much the lack of sleep has to do with children's behavior problems. I have tried on many occasions to keep track of the sleep of my grandchildren, particularly since they tend to have a bit of jet lag when they travel three hours to the West to visit me. But keeping track of an entire day's worth of mood swings, crying episodes, and fights, and quantifying all this in a way that can be correlated with the amount of sleep at night, requires a full-scale research project. Just as it is unwise to overlook the role of sleep, it is not a good idea to attribute all children's problems to not getting enough sleep. For example, a child with attention deficit hyperactivity disorder (ADHD) may behave as if he is getting too little sleep—and sleep-deprived children may act as if they have ADHD. Parents should certainly have a pretty good idea of what is enough sleep for their young children so they can know when to fault lack of sleep and when not to.

As I rhapsodized in chapter 5, sleep in children from 8 to 12 years old is usually wonderful and fosters days of zest and joy. If the children have learned good bedtime habits and don't have a chronic problem like bedwetting, sleep in these years can be the strongest and most solid sleep of their lives.

Sleep in the Teen Years

Parents should continue their role as teachers and enforcers of healthy sleep habits through the teenage years. Unfortunately, these days they seldom do. Teens are typically allowed more latitude to set their own bedtime hours as they get older. They are caught between two schedules: the one determined primarily by their biological clock and the one required by society. By the time teenagers reach high school, their sleep time is encroached upon from both ends: They are required to rise an hour or two earlier to make the earlier start times of most high schools, and they are pressured to stay up later than ever to study or maintain a respectable social life. As I explained earlier, a later bedtime is actually more in tune with the phase-delay shift common in teens' biological clocks, a delay that causes them to feel very alert even late at night. Rising before dawn for school, however, is a miserable affair because of the phase delay of the teenage biological clock. Compounding this evil is the fact that teens still need nearly as much sleep as when they were younger— about 9.5 hours a night. Ten-year-olds need about 10 hours sleep, and usually get it. But with society's imposition of an adult schedule, even the most straitlaced teens can easily end up with 6 hours of sleep on most nights—a whole 3 to 4 hours fewer than they need.

The result is that teens are universally sleep deprived. When the school bus arrives at 6:30 A.M., the body is awake, but the brain is barely so. Once when I was giving a talk at a local high school, a girl came in late, sat down, put her head on her desk, and went to sleep. I didn't say anything about it during the class, but afterward I asked another student if she did this all the time. "Oh, yeah," he said, "and Miss Jones wouldn't even let [and here he named four or five other kids] come to class today because she knew why they would fall asleep and embarrass her." Subsequent observations showed that this was not an anomaly. When I and other members of the National Commission on Sleep Disorders Research visited some high schools in Charleston, West Virginia, we peeked into a number of classrooms and saw up to 30 percent of the students with their eyes closed and their heads down on the desk.

Addressing the teen sleep crunch is tricky due to late-night alerting. Teens also tend to schedule their time so fully—after-school sports, drama, homework, jobs, socializing—that there seems little room for reorganizing their priorities. One technique may be to allow time for short naps in the afternoon, right after school. Another possibility is to use light therapy: Bright lights in the early morning, then dim lights and sunglasses in the evenings, so that the biological clock gets ready for sleep sooner. I might also recommend turning off the TV, loud or stimulating music on the stereo, video games, or other electronic amusements after 9:00 P.M., in addition to cutting down on other social stimulation. Any family with a VCR can tape favorite shows and watch them at a better time, with the added bonus of being able to fast-forward through commercials. The rule of thumb is that exciting or stimulating activities should be avoided. If television or other activities act as a pacifier or block out stressful thoughts, they may be a good idea shortly before bed. Finally, make sure your teenagers understand the impact of caffeinated drinks on sleep, particularly if their night life includes coffee, and make the case for drinking only decaf at night.

There is only so much creative scheduling you can do, however. Ultimately, for the most time-strapped, sleep-deprived teens, something has got to go: More sleep time means less time for other things. I feel very strongly that the first thing to go should be an after-school job. For high school students, after-school jobs probably do more to undermine healthy sleep and damage school performance than anything else they do. A 1998 report by the U.S. Department of Education on high school students' performance in math and science worldwide found that 55 percent of American teenagers work at paid jobs three or more hours daily, compared to 18 percent of teenagers in 20 other countries including Canada, Australia, South Africa, Russia, and numerous European countries. Also in Charleston, West Virginia, we found that 88 percent of high school students had evening and nighttime jobs on school nights. Many spent more time on the job than in school. The commission found that working outside of school is associated with less sleep time, more falling asleep in class, and more oversleeping. And why do teens work? Surveys show that they do so rarely to save for college, to supplement family income, or even to gain job skills. Teens are working to pay for personal luxuries and entertainment. A lot of people feel that students should have jobs to "teach responsibility," but after-school jobs show an irresponsible attitude toward school and health habits on the part of both adults and students. But allowing or encouraging after-school jobs is actually an irresponsible attitude toward school and health habits on the part of parents and other adults. It is harder to indict the students whose judgment may be immature and who find it hard to resist peer pressure. I am not sure about other parts of the country, but in my home state of California, public education is considered to be in crisis. When and if reform takes place, knowledge about the principles of healthy sleep and optimal daytime alertness, which can foster learning, positive mood and motivation, must be part of it.

For high school students who want to be accepted into a good college, and are highly driven to achieve excellent grades and to excel in extracurricular activities, the high school years can be very stressful—particularly when severe sleep deprivation is part of the mix. Many undergraduate students tell me that high school was by far their worst time. Even though in college it is just as difficult to fall asleep early as it was in high school, there is more flexibility to get extra sleep or to schedule classes later in the day.

In my opinion, teenage sleep is truly a big issue that we must examine further. We must know how much of what we consider the negative aspects of adolescence—rebellion, violence, drug abuse, dropping out—are caused by or exaggerated by sleep deprivation. Then, perhaps, we will have the means to do something to reduce these serious problems.

A Woman's Childbearing Years

The ebb and flow of hormones cue our bodies and minds to move in and out of sleep over the course of the day. Women have another hormonal cycle over the course of the month. It may not be news to many women that the menstrual cycle can independently affect sleep, but for sleep scientists it has been a relatively recent discovery. In 1975 Christian Guilleminault and I were the first to document yet another sleep disorder. This was a case in which a young woman became incredibly sleepy around the time of menstruation. Every month she would sleep for 14 hours or more out of every 24 for about a week.

A landmark national survey of American women's sleep was carried out in 1998 by the National Sleep Foundation. The poll revealed a host of sleep problems that are particular to women. Fifty percent of women report that bloating disturbs their sleep during their menstrual flow; and 25 percent report disturbed sleep the week prior to the beginning of their period. Overall, 71 percent of women reported sleep disturbance in association with cramping, bloating, headaches, and tender breasts during the menstrual flow while 43 percent reported such factors during the premenstrual week. This representative sample of American women seemed to refute the older idea that most of the problems are premenstrual. On the other hand, 68 percent of all menstruating women felt sleepiest during the week before their period compared to the rest of the month.

We still don't understand how the sleep and menstrual cycles interact with each other and why there can be totally opposite effects in different women during the same phase of the menstrual cycle. However, research on women with premenstrual syndrome is now giving us a window into some of the possible interactions between the sleep and menstrual cycles. "Premenstrual syndrome" is the term used for a collection of symptoms that affect many women in the days leading up to menstruation, including headache, emotional fragility, inability to concentrate, breast tenderness, water retention, and for some, sleep disturbances. Although Hippocrates described the symptoms of premenstrual syndrome about 3,000 years ago, modern medicine has taken some time to research the problem seriously. At last premenstrual syndrome is receiving the attention it deserves in scientific circles. In 1994 psychiatrists and other mental health professionals classified its psychiatric symptoms as premenstrual dysphoric disorder (PMDD).

Despite this increased scientific interest, however, no one yet knows what causes PMDD or how to cure it, although some newer antidepressants seem to help somewhat. Researchers have shown that PMDD often improves with light therapy or sleep deprivation. Some interesting changes in sleep-related hormones also show up in many women with PMDD: Prolactin levels tend to be higher at night, and the secretion of thyroid-stimulating hormone is shifted in the circadian cycle. Melatonin secretion is blunted in general, and bright light doesn't affect melatonin levels the way it usually does. This information leads some researchers to suggest that PMDD might affect the biological clock itself. If that is the case, then the similarity between the symptoms of PMDD and a bad case of jet lag may be more than a coincidence.

Pregnancy commonly changes how women sleep. In the National Sleep Foundation poll, 79 percent of women reported that their sleep is more disturbed during pregnancy than when they were not pregnant. Sleep recordings have been carried out in small, nonrepresentative samples of pregnant women. Some investigators claim that slow-wave sleep is significantly elevated; other studies indicate that REM sleep increases somewhat in the early stages of pregnancy. The National Sleep Foundation poll reports that 36 percent of women suffer more from daytime sleepiness during pregnancy than at other times. I was surprised at this result. I had become firmly convinced that only the first trimester of pregnancy is a period of hypersomnia. In retrospect, I had been overly impressed by several cases a long time ago.

My wife was incredibly sleepy during her early months of pregnancy. I was an intern at the time, and was given tickets to the then-shocking Broadway hit *Who's Afraid of Virginia Woolf?* Though I was on the edge of my seat throughout, my wife was mostly asleep. Soon thereafter, curiosity prompted me to ask a friend who usually slept about six hours a night to keep a sleep diary during her pregnancy. Her daily sleep time increased by an average of two and a half hours in the first trimester and then declined.

There are probably marked individual variations in sleep-related responses to pregnancy, but judging from the National Sleep Foundation poll, one would have to call pregnancy a sleep disorder. In addition to hormonal and other effects, sleep is disturbed in the third trimester by the difficulty of finding a comfortable position and the frequent need to urinate in the middle of the night. In order for pregnant working women to make up this lost sleep, they should not only be allowed but encouraged to nap. Strategically placed pillows to support the stomach more comfortably sometimes can aid sleep, and a full body pillow does the job best. I have seen some pregnant women at the beach scooping out a contoured spot in the sand and sleeping there quite happily.

Although sleep can be severely disrupted during the reproductive years, the end of that period brings its own problems. My heart goes out to the women I talk with who have severe insomnia during menopause. Hot flashes—a feeling like that of being in a microwave oven—can occur many times a night and severely disrupt sleep. There is some evidence that estrogen replacement therapy might improve sleep in the short term, but a more recent study suggested that in the long term hormone replacement therapy might actually make sleep worse. When the sleep disturbance is severe and daytime performance is affected, I would prescribe a safe and effective sleep medication. When the problem is less severe, the first approach might be napping, or perhaps earlier bedtimes or sleeping late to make up for sleep lost during nights of hot flashes. It is my impression that some women have much more sleep disturbance during menopause than others but no systemic observations have been done.

Because I am a compassionate person, and because making the public aware is my mission, I have been tempted to editorialize, it seems, on almost every page, mostly to call for more research, more education, or more implementation. The reader will have no idea how much of this urge I have suppressed. Now it is impossible to do so. I hope that every woman who reads this book will rise up and demand that the sleep problems related to childbearing and women generally be recognized as part of the male neglect of women's health problems. Thank God for the NSF poll. The official classification system of the American Sleep Disorders Association has a category called "possible sleep disorders." These are defined as sleep disorders for which insufficent or inadequate information is available to substantiate their unequivocal existence. Included in this category are menstrual-associated sleep disorder and pregnancy-associated sleep disorder. Nowhere could you find a problem associated with menopause. Although all of these problems are very common as documented by the NSF poll, female victims apparently do not get past their obstetricians to sleep specialists. Elsewhere I have spoken of the tremendous need to educate primary care physicians. Obstetricians are in large part primary care doctors, and it is absolutely clear that they must be part of this process.

Middle Age and Beyond

An important part of growing old gracefully is learning to accept the physical changes that we all experience. Our skin loses elasticity, wounds don't heal as quickly, and muscle aches occur more frequently. Gray hair starts appearing in our 30s or 40s. Our midsections expand and our agility and quickness decline. Recently I overheard someone in his mid-30s telling friends about this phenomenon: "I played basketball for the first time in years yesterday, and it felt like someone slipped about 20 pounds of weights in my pants when I wasn't looking." That's just the beginning, I thought.

We are also stuck with certain facts about our own sleep patterns as we age. Between 50 and 90 percent of people over age 65 get irregular sleep. In the very old, the changes are obvious. Summing up her extensive studies of sleep, Sonia Ancoli-Israel found, "The typical nursing home patient is not continuously awake nor continuously asleep for more than an hour during the entire day." In life's last act the swings of clock-dependent alerting become so diminished that alerting is almost entirely gone. Some people have commented that this deconsolidation of sleep in the very old is a fitting return to infantlike sleep. However, the sleep of young children is famously deep, and they dazzle us with their bright wakefulness.

As a rule, it is a wrenching decision to have to send an older person, usually a parent, to a nursing home. But severe mental and/ or physical deterioration often force the decision. I do not believe we arrive at this point as the result of very gradual, indiscernible changes. Some of the most energetic and wide-awake people I have ever known were in their 70s, 80s, and even 90s. Then there seemed to be a relatively sudden change in their ability to stay alert. My mother entered a retirement home when she was 96, and at first she remained energetic and alert, though somewhat frail. Then in the year before her hundredth birthday, there was then a discernible decline and she had to be transferred to the affiliated nursing home. Toward the end of her days, she was almost always asleep when I visited her and, she had great difficulty sustaining wakefulness. We need to do much more research to explore whether this type of change is due to a rapid age-related failure of clock-dependent alerting.

In synchrony with other early signs of aging, we experience intimations of elderly sleep in our 40s and 50s, some people experience it as early as their 30s. There is no question that sleep gets lighter and more fragmented as we age. Falling asleep and staying asleep are more difficult. Nighttime awakenings last longer and are more disruptive—how many children or teenagers note the time when they wake up in the middle of the night? As we age sleep also becomes less efficient (less sleep for more time in bed). We now have objective scientific evidence that homeostatic sleep drive weakens with age, and we begin needing a little less sleep than in earlier adulthood. I estimate that sleep need declines by 30 minutes to an hour over the course of our adult life. In elderly people, sleep problems are pretty evenly divided between the sexes: Women tend to have more problems with insomnia, and men have a higher incidence of apnea, snoring, and other medical conditions that worsen sleep.

From middle age onward, the central problem we sleep scientists must confront is to sort out how we are affected individually by a combination of age-related changes: increased sleep deprivation, the onset of one or other sleep disorders, and a possible deterioration of the homeostatic sleep drive (and/or clock-dependent alerting). It is my hypothesis that most people have strong clock-dependent alerting well into very advanced years. In other words, the very sketchy evidence available suggests to me that the homeostatic sleep drive weakens earlier than clock-dependent alerting.

Fortunately, the changes in sleep are usually as gradual as the unfolding of the years, granting us time to adapt. If you tend to wake up often at night, or wake up too early in the morning, it can be disconcerting for a while. But if you manage to organize your sleep so that you don't feel especially drowsy in the day, waking up at night need not be upsetting. You can learn to expect it a few times a night or to expect an earlier wake-up time than when you were younger. These changes are less demoralizing if you focus not on how well you slept at night but how alert you feel during the day. I used to pride myself on being a night owl, working late nights in the sleep lab and being very productive. When my circadian cycle shifted, though, I began trying to do important work in the very early morning. I have learned to treasure these quiet morning hours before others get up and the phones start ringing.

If you feel tired during the day, however, that is another story. It doesn't have to be that way. One of the saddest wastes in our society is the idea that seniors cannot escape being tired and worn out. Excessive daytime sleepiness is not an inevitable corollary of aging. Rather, it is usually a sign of an emerging age-related sleep problem that may not be immediately apparent. Sleep apnea and upper airway respiratory disorder become more and more common as people age, so snoring at night and daytime fatigue may be warning signs of respiratory problems that disrupt sleep. Repetitive limb movements, which also become more common with age, can disrupt sleep surreptitiously. These disorders are usually caught by a spouse who shares the same bed and is awakened by the loud snoring or kicking legs. And these sleep disorders are very treatable.

Frequent insomnia, especially early-morning awakening, is also more common as people age, and depression is sometimes the cause.

Many times depression is misdiagnosed in the elderly because the confusion, memory problems, and behavioral changes that accompany it are thought to be part of a senile dementia. In middle-aged adults, a feeling of daytime slothfulness and lack of energy or drive also can be signs of depression that people might assume is just part of getting older and more cynical about the world. Most cases of depression are also very treatable.

The Later Years
No one should passively accept a higher level of daytime sleepiness with age, even if sleep disorders have been ruled out as the cause. Researchers in geriatrics have demonstrated that for elderly people, exercise improves bone density, heart function, and the general feeling of well-being. A number of studies also have shown that exercise during the day improves sleep: People who exercise have fewer awakenings, fall asleep faster, and spend more time in deep sleep. To get that exercise you may not be able to go out and join a pick-up basketball game or run 10 miles like you used to—usually you must be more careful to stretch, do low-impact exercise, and build up slowly to the heaviest part of the workout. Exercise doesn't have to be excessive; even a 15-minute walk will help. The rewards of exercise for physical health and mood are just as high in old age; we simply need to be smarter and more cautious than in our youth about the kinds of activities we try.

Sleep is also improved by psychological arousal during the day, because it helps us stay up long enough to build up sufficient sleep debt, making sleep more efficient and facilitating relaxation at the end of the day. Remember that some sleep debt is necessary for good sleep. Anything that fights the flattening of the circadian rhythm helps, such as spending time outdoors during the day to soak up some light therapy. It is particularly beneficial to remain socially active or to seek out exciting activities in old age. If your life is dull, you'll tend to sleep longer (when you can), go to bed earlier, and take more naps than you need during the day.

Not that naps are always bad. If naps are scheduled into the day as a part of your normal sleep pattern, and you take care not to rid yourself of too much sleep debt, a short nap—even 15 minutes of shut-eye—can improve alertness without decreasing the day's total sleep debt much at all. In other words, short naps can keep you feeling good without keeping you from falling asleep at night.

The underlying message is that as you get older, your sleep health, like other aspects of your health, requires more attention and work. You can't just assume any longer that you will fall asleep at the end of the day and sleep well. As you get older you have to watch what you eat and get the right kind of exercise. You also have to manage your sleep. This means planning how you accumulate and pay off sleep debt—sleeping enough to enjoy a vital day, but not sleeping so much that it is hard to fall asleep at night.

Medicating the Sleep Cycles of Aging

Very often insomnia in elderly people is a symptom of chronic medical conditions such as arthritis, aches and pains, congestive heart failure, depression, or Parkinson's disease. Insomnia also can be a side effect of the medications used to treat these conditions—for example, some anticholesterol drugs or antidepressants. While drug treatments for these conditions are not a barrier to concurrent drug treatment for insomnia, due to the possibility of adverse interactions I usually advise against sleeping pills as a first line of treatment for insomnia in older folks. Rather, the first step should be to treat the nonsleep condition, or adjust the timing, dosage, or type of medication, and see if these measures improve sleep. Only after these factors and sleep hygiene have been addressed should sleeping pills be considered. At that point, however, some sort of medication may well be necessary to improve sleep.

If long-term use of sleeping pills by elderly patients is to be considered seriously, the medication must be chosen carefully. A primary hazard is the potential for developing tolerance and rebound insomnia. Only the hypnotics Ambien and Halcion have passed adequate double-blind, controlled clinical trials to verify safety and efficacy in elderly patients. These drugs do not induce tolerance or cause rebound insomnia when used in the proper doses, so their long-term use is no more problematic than prolonged use of heart medication, or daily insulin by diabetics.

Whatever sleep medication is prescribed should be short-acting, such as Ambien, because daytime carry-over sedation would be as bad as the sleep problem. I recall a study in which the medication being tested significantly improved sleep at night, but in the daytime the Multiple Sleep Latency Test showed a deterioration in alertness roughly equivalent to two nights of complete sleep loss. There is also greater risk of falls if elderly people rise in the middle of the night to use the bathroom while affected by sleeping pills. Even without medication, nighttime falls are a leading cause of broken hips in older people. Ultimately improved melatonin pills and other similar drugs of the future may better synchronize elderly biological clocks with the cycles of night and day. We know that melatonin production in the body wanes as we age, so melatonin replacement therapy may one day be as common as estrogen replacement therapy. I also think that we should be looking at restoring the alerting processes of the biological clock. Stimulants may provide a safe means of replacing clock-dependent alerting if the brain isn't doing the job anymore. I think it's an exciting possibility that alert wakefulness might be prolonged a few more years by the judicious use of stimulants. In my mother's last years, I pondered requesting her doctor to do the unthinkable and prescribe a modest dose of Ritalin, but I never reached a decision.

It is a truism that aging is a lifelong process; just as growing old no longer means giving up on overall health, it shouldn't mean giving up on sleep. It simply raises the stakes for understanding the capabilities and limitations of our bodies.

Chapter 19

Adopt a Sleep-Smart Lifestyle

THERE IS A story I sometimes hear about "cargo cults" in the South Pacific. It seems that when Westerners went to Melanesia, especially during World War II, the natives noticed that soldiers would go into a radio shack and call for more supplies. Some days later a ship or airplane would come with goods. The natives themselves started to build similar shacks with bamboo "antennas," and built "airstrips" for planes to land on, in the hope that new cargo would arrive on the island. This story is often used as an example of how trying to achieve a goal through ritualistic behavior can be futile if one doesn't understand the underlying reason that certain behaviors have certain effects.

In the recent past, quite a few how-to-sleep-better books have been published. They all contain tips for better sleep. The largest number that I have seen in such a book is 75 tips. Most of the pamphlets that are scattered around have a standard 10 tips, all of which are very rational and well established. They are mostly strategies and behaviors that any informed person would almost certainly adopt without undue urging. These tips are generally fine, but they shouldn't necessarily be followed as dogma. Everybody has different sleep needs and preferences. For example, one of the most obvious tips is to avoid coffee and other caffeinated beverages in the hours before bedtime. Yet if you say this, there are always a few people who say "Coffee doesn't keep me awake." These are probably the same people who say "I can sleep anywhere."

Any suggestions or tips for better sleep should be regarded as options. Instead of following a recommendation blindly, you should be able to use the principles I have taught you to understand why the recommendation should work and to decide whether it will work in your particular circumstance. For example, one of the standard tips for better sleep is: "Be regular. Go to bed at the same time every night and get up at the same time every morning." For some people, this is not optimal or even possible. When an exam is scheduled for the next day or a report is due, studying and writing take time. Students or executives might plan to lose a certain amount of sleep during the week and make it up on the weekend. Indeed, this is what most students actually do. About 10 percent of undergraduates say they sleep 8 or more hours on weekdays, but on weekends this figure rises to more than 70 percent. When recovering from final exams, the percentage of students sleeping 8 hours or more rises to an impressive but predictable 97 percent.

Keys to Smart Sleep

I now feel that one of the main keys to a sleep-smart lifestyle is to understand the implications of a small sleep debt vs. a large sleep debt. It has taken over two decades for me to learn enough to say this. Certain key research results puzzled me for years, because they seemed paradoxical. Often they were finally and very satisfying resolved when later research allowed an odd puzzle piece to fit in perfectly.

One of my favorite examples of this general process is an experiment I conducted in the late 1960s, before I had any notion there was such a thing as sleep debt, and before we had any quantitative measure of daytime sleepiness, objective or otherwise. We were commissioned by a company to evaluate their incredible high-tech bed, which cost thousands of dollars and was so huge that we couldn't fit it in the lab. (We had to do the tests in a converted loading dock.) This behemoth was essentially a huge container filled with billions of microscopic ceramic beads through which warm air was pumped. The suspension of beads in warm air felt very much like a cushion of heated mud, and everyone in our lab agreed that it was the most comfortable bed they had ever lain on. Our task was to compare how well people slept on the bead bed compared to a conventional mattress. To show how bad sleep could be and give a more dramatic comparison, we included a third condition: sleeping on a concrete floor with no padding. After the volunteer subjects had slept on all three surfaces, we were absolutely flabbergasted to find no significant differences in the amount or continuity of their sleep. I actually rescored the recordings from the concrete floor myself because I just couldn't believe it. Naturally the bead-bed company was not pleased that we found no difference between their expensive bed and a concrete floor, and summarily canceled further studies.

The lack of any measurable difference between sleep in a high-tech bed and on a concrete floor was so confusing that we set it aside; it just didn't make sense. Today these results make very good sense, as they should. The key fact was that our volunteers were mostly college students. In retrospect, we know that they had to be extremely sleep deprived because the study was carried out during spring break, right after final exams. That, in addition to their youth, led them to sleep very deeply on any surface. If we had done the test using middle-aged volunteers who had less sleep debt, I'm sure the results would have been quite different.

In addition to grasping the implications of a large sleep debt, it is also important for people to understand the implications of a small sleep debt. Last year one of the Stanford Students for Healthy Sleep, after meticulously keeping his sleep diary for several weeks, concluded that his sleep debt was approximately 35 hours. In order to lower it, he began obtaining extra sleep as often as possible. When he had reduced it to about 20 hours by his calculations, he announced that he was no longer sleepy in his 1:15 P.M. Early American History class; he could hardly believe it. However, after continuing to reduce his sleep debt the following week, he related an experience that he found somewhat unsettling. He went to bed at his regular time, but instead of falling asleep in the usual 5 to 10 minutes, it took him over an hour. He immediately decided on his own to increase his debt back to the level that would allow him to fall asleep quickly.

What delighted me was the surprise he felt when he didn't fall asleep, because it impressed upon him what I had been teaching all quarter. He realized the very important lesson that trouble falling asleep can be a predictable result of a low sleep debt, and it is totally within a person's control to reverse it. I am also quite sure that with his sleep debt as low as it was, this student would have slept much more poorly on the cold concrete floor than he would have in a regular bed or the superbed. The smaller your sleep debt, the more important will be the quality of your sleep environment and sleep surface. The corollary is that if you can sleep deeply and continuously on the floor, you've got to be very sleep deprived.

As you now know, our society has a gaping blind spot around the single most important factor in cognitive and psychological function: alertness. Being optimally wide awake enhances our productivity and enjoyment of everything, from work to recreation to family time. If adequate sleep is so important to our health and happiness, doesn't it make sense to include our sleep needs as we tailor our lifestyle?

The problem is that people don't take their sleep seriously enough to get the most out of their nights and their waking hours—in short, our society doesn't take the trouble to incorporate the principles of healthy sleep into its collective lifestyle. We can't be sleep-smart because we don't learn how much sleep we need, how to be sleep efficient, how to get into the sleep groove around bedtime. In the name of efficiency, we often end up thinking about work when we should be preparing for sleep, which makes about as much sense as trying to save time by drying off before the shower is over.

Another key to being sleep smart is understanding clock-dependent alerting and to have a feeling for when you are alert or drowsy. Many of us don't know much about what times of day we are at our best, when our peaks and valleys in alertness occur every day. Ever since I began to understand the profound balancing act that goes on between clock-dependent alerting and sleep debt, I must have asked myself at least 100,000 times, "How do I feel right now? How alert or sleepy am I, how clear-headed or foggy?" After years of practice, I think I have a very good sense of exactly how my circadian cycle plays itself out over the day, how I will likely feel at a given time, and when I will be at my best in terms of intellectual performance.

Although Stanford undergraduates have been referred to as the "cream of the crop" by some people (though not by those at Harvard), they can do things that are stunningly counterproductive. After I was satisfied that my little group of Stanford Students for

Healthy Sleep had come to know through self-evaluation their time of day for peak performance, I was talking to one of the students who had established that his peak alertness was from 7:00 P.M. to 1:00 A.M. I assumed these were the hours during which he studied, wrote papers, and the like. He said no. I was aghast to learn that he worked in a packaging business during these precious prime-time hours. The job was unskilled, repetitive, and only paid minimum wage. I could hardly believe my ears. Every day he was throwing away his peak period. It was like someone using his best shirts to scrub the floor. Since I couldn't stand to see him waste his intellectual assets this way, I offered to hire him to file reprints after lunch, during his afternoon slump, thereby freeing up his evening for study. Learning about sleep and adopting a sleep-smart lifestyle will enable each of you to put my message to use in your own life.

If you are serious about your health, nutrition, and fitness, you need to be serious about your sleep. Does this mean you have to structure your life around sleep, make huge sacrifices, give up night life, abandon your promising career for the "sleep track"? Not at all. I believe that the increase in nocturnal sleep that would be necessary to make a huge difference during the day could be very small. The key is not so much lots of extra sleep at night but rather effectively managing your sleep debt.

In fact, by definition sleep debt builds up if you are not getting enough sleep. Since sleep debt cannot build up forever, at some point it appears that most people reach a steady state of sleepiness: They appear to fulfill their daily need with deep semicomatose sleep, and their already massive sleep debt doesn't get larger or smaller. So once the sleep debt is worked down, you should be able to get by on about as much sleep as you get now, but feel much better most of the day.

A major difference is in sleep efficiency. When people have a very large sleep debt, their sleep is more efficient. They take less time to fall asleep and have fewer middle-of-the-night awakenings, so they actually get more sleep for the time they spend in bed. With a lower sleep debt, the resulting small loss in sleep efficiency means that they may need a few minutes more sleep per night.

The study by Tom Wehr described in Chapter 3 is very instructive in this regard. The subjects were in bed 8 hours and averaged slightly more than $7^1/_2$ hours of sleep per night in the seven-night baseline, which represented their normal sleep outside the experiment, and were found to be carrying a sleep debt of 25 to 35 hours. Their ultimate daily sleep requirement—the 8 hours and 15 minutes they got every night toward the end of the experiment—was only 40 minutes more than they slept normally. Many people mistakenly seem to think that I am urging them to spend 10 hours in bed every night, which probably wouldn't be practical. But this experiment suggests that people need only 40 minutes more sleep to sleep healthy.

But the amount of extra sleep people need may be even less in the real world. The subjects' daily sleep "requirement" of about 8 hours and 15 minutes in the final weeks of the study may have been the product of inefficient sleep, resulting from a very low sleep debt. We know that the subjects were often lying around in the dark for hours. It is possible that by accumulating a little more sleep debt, the subjects might have met their daily sleep requirement with slightly less sleep, say 8 hours, that was deeper and more continuous. By manipulating their sleep debt, they might have enjoyed the same improvement in mood and energy as in the final weeks of the experiment, without increasing their sleep time much at all.

Assume that your daily sleep requirement could be fulfilled, and you could maintain the right level of sleep debt, with an extra 30 minutes of sleep per night. Thirty minutes is one less sitcom, one less report read at home. It might mean deciding to skip the evening TV news and get the same information from the newspaper the next morning. Or perhaps it means skipping the newspaper. Most people have something that they can give up, if they really think about it. We can find the time to exercise or to get a balanced meal instead of eating junk food. Why not find an extra half hour for healthy sleep? If not half an hour, why not just 15 minutes more sleep per night? It may take that little. The task is to work down your sleep debt until you are alert and energetic all day and then calculate your daily sleep need at that level of sleep debt.

According to George Bernard Shaw, "A rich man is a man who makes £100 and needs £99. A poor man is a man who makes £100 and needs £101. The difference between being rich and being poor is £2." So too the difference between a rich, vital, healthy life and a diminished one may be only a few minutes of sleep. In this sense, you really don't give up any time at all: You'll work more efficiently when you are well rested, and working more efficiently will, in turn, give you more time for other activities.

When I talk to an audience I often ask, "How many of you sleep well and feel wide awake and energetic all day long?" Usually only a few hands are raised. If you are one of the majority whose daytime alertness is less than optimal because your sleep is less than optimal, here are just a few questions to determine how sleep-smart your lifestyle is:

1. Do you carefully avoid caffeinated drinks in the evening?
2. Do you typically schedule your evening meal at least three hours before you go to bed?
3. Do you have a regular bedtime, which you follow with rare exceptions?
4. Do you have a bedtime ritual, such as a hot bath and perhaps reading a few pages, relaxing, while drowsiness sneaks up on you?
5. Is your bedroom generally a quiet place all night long?
6. Is the temperature of your bedroom just right?
7. Do you think of your bed, particularly the mattress and pillows, as the most comfortable place in the world?
8. Are the bedclothes (blankets, quilts, comforters) exactly right for you?

If you answered no to any of these questions, you might look at that particular area of your life as a possible hiding place for sleep problems. Maybe caffeine in the evening doesn't affect you. Perhaps the temperature in your bedroom doesn't matter in the slightest. But if you haven't considered all the factors that might negatively affect your sleep, you aren't acting in an informed manner. It always amazes me that people may have a caffeinated cola at dinner, or even coffee, and completely fail to make the connection between consuming caffeine and their failure to fall asleep quickly.

One of the above tips is to get to bed the same time every day, but to make this idea work in your own life, you have to understand why regularity tends to make both sleep and wakefulness more robust. One of the results of such regularity is that you start falling asleep faster and waking up more easily. Psychologically and physiologically, you become conditioned for sleep. With a set presleep routine, an understanding of your natural periods of clock-dependent alerting, and a predictable bedtime, you will be relaxed and getting drowsy as you approach sleep. This psychological and physiological rhythm in turn makes it easier to fall asleep and stay asleep.

People who need an alarm clock to wake up on time are often being jolted from a deep sleep because the brain is not ready to wake up. Whoever invented the snooze button understood that it takes a barrage of wake-up calls to rouse the severely sleep deprived. On the other hand, if you're getting enough sleep the brain should usually wake up naturally at its normal time, without an alarm clock. This happens because the clock-dependent alerting rises naturally in the morning. With very low sleep debt to oppose this alerting, waking up should not be difficult. I do not mean to imply that you will wake up spontaneously at exactly the same time every morning. Relatively few individuals can claim to do this. Generally, you will awaken spontaneously at about the same time, and if it is at an hour that allows adequate time to get to work or to be somewhere, there is no problem.

Managing your sleep debt will sometimes involve sacrifice. It can be awkward, especially when you have to make excuses to friends, turn down social engagements, or leave the party early. If you're a gregarious person who thrives on social interaction, this requires self-discipline. I have been at many dinner parties (and even hosted some) where I excused myself early to make my 9:00 P.M. bedtime. I used to have to make my little "If I don't put sleep first, who will?" speech, but now my friends are so used to it that they hardly even notice. Other diners, including my wife, who sleeps in later, merely continue on without me. But I have to say it wasn't easy the first few times. You really feel like the world's champion party pooper, and especially if it is someone else's party, and you and your wife are the only guests, or half of the guests. However, it gets easier with practice.

Although regularity is a desirable part of keeping your sleep in good shape, as with any realistic lifestyle change, moderation is the key. There is room to deviate from the plan. After all, we are human. Exceptional things happen that are worth interrupting our routine for. (Just as, if you're on a strict diet it makes sense to allow yourself a treat when you're dining in a once-in-a-lifetime five-star restaurant or celebrating an annual holiday that includes special foods.) The important thing is to keep an eye on the bottom line: total sleep time. Take charge, manage your sleep, get extra sleep to make up for your short nights. Take naps either before or after the shortened sleep periods to keep your sleep time equal to your required sleep. If you stay up late or get up early, try to get back on schedule as soon as possible so your circadian rhythm doesn't shift.

We all have an innate desire to find more excitement, to feel alert and aroused. That's why we flip through the channels for a good movie or browse our bookshelves, even late at night. If we have any energy at all, we want that extra hit of excitement. That's one of the problems with working down a titanic sleep debt—people may start to feel so good, so alert, that they want to stay up and enjoy life—and sleep debt piles up again.

Evaluate Your Consumption of Caffeine, Alcohol, and Other Drugs

While most foods don't have a dramatic effect on sleep, some things we ingest do. These include coffee, alcohol, and a fair number of medications. Sleeping smart doesn't necessarily mean giving up these substances, although it can. But it absolutely does mean that you must understand how they work and how they affect you so that you can tailor their use to allow for healthy sleep.

Caffeine is a good example. I personally love coffee and always start the day with two or three cups. Coffee seems to augment my clock-dependent alerting in the morning. I am obviously not alone in this feeling. Every year, people use over 600 million kilograms of coffee beans and 2 billion kilograms of tea leaves worldwide.

To manage caffeine's effects, you should understand its behavior in the body. It takes coffee or tea about 15 to 30 minutes to start having an effect on the brain and about 1 hour to reach maximum blood levels. Thereafter, its blood concentrations decline as it is degraded by enzymes in the liver. The half-life of caffeine in the bloodstream is between three and seven hours (depending on the person's age, activity, and individual chemistry). That means that if the cup you drink has 100 milligrams of caffeine (which is pretty typical), after five hours you will have 50 milligrams floating around in the blood. Five more hours and you will have 25 milligrams. How long the effect lasts depends on other factors: the time of day, the amount of your sleep debt, your age, and your level of tolerance.

With these facts in mind, you can manage your coffee intake for maximum alertness when you want it, without interfering too much with sleep. Know that coffee will not have an immediate effect: You have to wait awhile for it to really kick in, so don't gulp it down and expect to get right behind your desk and start working. Similarly, don't think that you can drink a cup or two of coffee or tea at 6:00 P.M. and have all the caffeine out of your system by the time you go to bed at 11:00. In five hours you have rid your body of only half of its initial level of caffeine, and the remaining portion can interfere with sleep. Some people are able to have the dinnertime coffee in their 20s and 30s without noticeable effects on sleep, but in their 40s or later, as sleep becomes more fragile and sensitive to stimulants like caffeine, coffee begins to cause problems at night.

Individuals vary greatly in their reaction to caffeine. Some people can have an espresso (or several) near bedtime and have no trouble sleeping at all. This is mostly because they have built up tolerance to the stimulant. The more you drink caffeine, the more your body becomes used to it, and the less you are affected. Regular coffee drinkers may feel a stimulating effect from the caffeine for only an hour or two, because the brain doesn't react to the caffeine unless it is present at the highest levels in the blood. When you stop drinking coffee, tolerance diminishes, so that after a few weeks without exposure to caffeine you are as sensitive to it as you were when you first had some.

Years ago, my wife and I drove from Chicago to Walla Walla to visit my parents. To save money, we generally camped out when we stopped for the night. It was simply too inconvenient and time consuming to build a fire just to heat coffee, so I essentially gave it up. The first morning we returned home I had my usual three cups of coffee and I couldn't believe the effect it had on me. My heart was racing. I felt uncomfortably jittery. My thoughts were scattered. I was far too stimulated, and it took me much of the day to get back to normal.

Tolerance should be managed. If you drink more than two or three cups a day, try giving it up entirely for a week or two. You can mitigate the withdrawal symptoms somewhat by remaining very well hydrated throughout the day, drinking six to eight glasses of water. Then, when you start using caffeine again, notice how much greater the effect is. After this, drink decaffeinated coffee for the flavor and the warmth, and reserve caffeine for when you really want the pick-me-up. This might mean only one cup a day, either in the morning or during the afternoon slump in alertness. To increase the effect even more, drink caffeinated coffee or tea only once every few days.

Also take a look at your evening alcohol consumption. I do not believe that drinking a glass or two of wine, beer, or a shot of spirits will seriously disrupt sleep. In fact, a bit of alcohol can nicely uncover accumulated sleep debt and make getting to sleep easier. There is evidence, however, that three to five glasses or more of alcohol in the evening cause arousal and rebound insomnia as they wear off in the middle of the night.

Dozens of prescription drugs have some effect on sleep, and you always should ask your doctor or pharmacist about drowsiness or stimulation as a side effect. If a prescription drug makes you really drowsy when you need to perform at your peak, or hyperalert when you need to sleep, consult with your doctor about adjusting the timing of the medication; perhaps you can delay taking a particular drug until an hour or so later than usual.

Diet and Exercise

One of the favorite pitches made by me and few of my more activist colleagues is that there is a fundamental triumvirate of health: good nutrition, physical fitness, and healthy sleep. Obviously good nutrition and physical fitness are important for health. Do they also have crucial effects on sleep? Researchers have yet to find any particular food that strongly promotes sleep. If you've heard that certain foods aid sleep—such as turkey or carbohydrates—remember that any effect is minuscule compared to other factors, such as sleep load or circadian alerting. However, eating generally does cause the release of hormones from the stomach that may have a small role in revealing underlying sleep indebtedness.

Sleep problems also can exacerbate weight problems. People who have sleep disorders such as apnea or insomnia or who otherwise rack up a huge sleep debt feel terrible during the day. They barely have the energy to drag themselves around and do the things they absolutely must. They don't burn many calories. Instead, their bodies hoard calories as fat. Especially for people with apnea, fatigue and sleeplessness can lead to a horrible downward spiral: Weight gain worsens apnea at night, which increases sleepiness during the day, which leads to more weight gain.

Just as the biological clock can affect the drive to be active, exercise can affect the timing of the clock. Light is the strongest influence on circadian rhythms, but doses of exercise can shift circadian rhythms in experimental animals and in humans. In one experiment, human subjects who exercised and were exposed to light at certain times had an easier time adapting to a night shift than those who were only exposed to light.

Dale Edgar has shown that wheel running in mice is a powerful time cue, or Zeitgeber, for the biological clock. Because wheel-running activity is the most important measure used by biological rhythm researchers over the years, and laboratory rodents can be depended on to run at more or less the same time every day, an enormous amount of scientific data and conclusions are based on this approach.

This research has often been criticized on the basis that wheel-running is unnatural. An amusing story is often cited in rebuttal to this criticism: Stanford Professor of Biology Colin Pittendrihg, who was one of the world's leading circadian rhythm scientists, spent summers in a mountain cabin in Wyoming. He did some work during his time there and had discarded a number of cages and running wheels behind the cabin. At some point, a regular squeaking every night behind the cabin led him to investigate, and he found that wild rodents had discovered his running wheels and were making regular visits to run on them. I guess this shows that most mammals want to exercise, whether they have a wheel or not. Laboratory rodents will exercise at very precise points in their circadian cycle; even when they are given no outside time cues, they will start exercising at the same time every day.

About two decades ago, when jogging for fitness was becoming popular, regular joggers reported that they slept better at night. But the first studies of exercise and sleep showed the opposite: Exercise was followed by disturbed sleep. The reason illuminates nicely some of the misleading complexities of doing sleep research. The first investigators used subjects who did not work out regularly, and they didn't take into account how the soreness that follows unaccustomed exercise can disturb sleep. Later studies used trained athletes as subjects. James Horne at the University of Loughborough was the first to find that exercise in fit individuals increased stage 3 and stage 4 sleep—the deepest stages of sleep. But his further research was very interesting. He found that the increase in slow-wave sleep was due more to the increase in body temperature than to the exercise itself. Perhaps the most important effects of exercise on sleep are not the objective changes that scientists can measure, but the improvements that people feel subjectively. Recent work by Abby King at Stanford showed that in elderly volunteers, exercise can produce statistically significant improvements in the subjective quality of their sleep.

As a matter of sleep hygiene, it is not a good idea to exercise within three hours before bedtime, because the physiological arousal created by a good workout opposes the sleep process. Exercising regularly during the afternoon or early-evening hours should help entrain the brain to follow the right pattern of sleep and wakefulness. Again, a minority of the people sleep better right after exercise, so it's important to know your own proclivities.

The Sleep Environment

My experiences with Stanford students have also taught me that there are no absolutes with regard to sleep environment. I wish that I could find the words to convey a truly adequate description of Stanford students' dorm rooms. It is endlessly fascinating to walk down a dormitory hall and peer into the open doors and try to imagine how anyone could possibly sleep under such circumstances. In their rooms, students have stereos, one or two computers, phones, food— basically all their worldly goods and those of their roommate.

I recently visited a friend whose son is an authentic genius. At the age of 18 he is doing high-level computer-graphics for NASA. But the point is that his bedroom has two large computer monitors, cables running everywhere, and clutter on the bed that would hardly allow space for his dog to sleep. One of the primary "better sleep" tips I always see listed is: "The bedroom is only for sleeping." I have never seen this tip more violated, yet this young man sleeps just fine in his all-purpose bedroom.

With this major caveat in mind, I will nevertheless give you some recommendations about your sleep environment in order to get you thinking about how your bed and bedroom affect your sleep. The fundamental principle is that the bedroom should be a comfortable, secure, quiet, and dark place where all the factors that promote sleep can work best for *you individually*. That means if you feel most comfortable with a bedroom that is completely uncontaminated by work, ban the computer. If you are most comfortable with file cabinets in the room, put them there. The important principle is to be sensitive to the things in your sleep environment that put you at ease, and those that may cause tension or distraction.

One example is noise. Most sleep tips will tell you to make sure the bedroom is quiet. While this is generally good advice, I, and many others, like a little sound when falling asleep because it relaxes me and keeps my mind off obsessive thoughts. The best thing for me is falling asleep with the television quietly on in the room broadcasting routine news or the weather. I used to have the problem that when the station went off the air—the sound of static would disturb my sleep—but ever since televisions started coming with an automatic cutoff an after 30 minutes (called the "sleep" function), I don't have to worry about that.

The bedroom should generally be dark during sleep. Although people may feel more comfortable falling asleep with a little light on, too much light at night can have the effect of shifting the biological clock. For those who like a little light to fall asleep by, timers can turn lights off automatically. Today everyone can have a dark bedroom; whereas blackout curtains used to be very expensive, now you can get an inexpensive blackout liner that fits onto existing curtains. For a little more money you can buy heavy roller shades or very heavy drapes with nice patterns. Since even a short burst of bright light can reset the biological clock, use night-lights or rheostats in hallways and bathrooms so that if you need to use the bathroom in the middle of the night, you can maneuver through the house without upsetting your internal clock.

Although students with large sleep debts may be able to sleep on a cement floor, if you lower your sleep debt or are a little older you generally have to sleep on better surfaces to sleep well. Despite the negative result of the bead-bed experiment and the almost nonexistent sleep recording data that would evaluate conventional sleep surfaces, I have no doubt whatsoever that the right mattress is very important.

One of the mistakes most people make is the way they purchase a mattress. Companies must devise ways for people to adequately test mattresses before buying them. Lying on a mattress in a store in full view of everyone for maybe ten minutes doesn't even come close to a good test. I am reasonably happy with my mattress and bed, but there were two nights in the past 30 years that suggest I may have shortchanged myself. One night I slept at the Beverly Hilton, and it was like sleeping on a cloud. I have never felt more comfortable, more cozy, and more well rested. I tried to determine the brand of the mattress, but the label (against the law) had been removed. The other perfect sleeping experience was about seven years ago while campaigning for Wake Up America. I was given a free night in a bed-and-breakfast in Pasco, Washington, operated by a patient with narcolepsy. Once again I had a magical night, and again I couldn't find out what brand of mattress I had slept upon. When I retire, I am going to spend about a week, maybe a month, finding that perfect surface so I can make it my permanent bed.

I have tried to convince mattress companies for more than a decade that they should contribute support to the National Sleep Awareness Campaign because it would enhance awareness of the importance of the sleep surface. Mattress companies have not been truly enlightened members of the sleep community. They seem to have a desire, but also a fear, of understanding the role of the sleep surface. Companies would like to prove with all-night brain-wave recordings that their mattress is better than all others, but they are afraid that this type of costly scientific research might show that their mattress is no better or maybe even worse.

I may be wrong, but I do not believe a single how-to book about improving sleep recognizes or takes into account that the vast majority of adults sleep with someone: over 70 percent of Americans do not sleep alone. I have learned that the preferences and tendencies of a bedmate or roommate have a huge effect on anyone's sleep. This means that all the advice about the sleep environment and finding what really suits you must also suit your bed partner, or at least there must be a compromise. Since I am endlessly fascinated with this area, I am constantly finding that someone's wife likes a cool room, her husband likes a warm room, or the wife wants the window open and the husband wants the window closed, or the wife wants lots of covers and the husband wants few, and so on and so on.

The importance of a comfortable and pleasing bedroom brings me to my last point about good sleep hygiene: Enjoy your sleep. I think many people tend to feel guilty about sleep; staying in bed any longer than absolutely necessary feels like sheer laziness. That is wrong: Sleep quotas are biologically fixed, and there is no more shame in needing 10 hours a day of sleep than in needing a size 10 shoe.

Sleep is an essential part of life—but more important, sleep is a gift. To me, there are few things more exquisitely pleasurable than giving myself over to sleep at the end of the day or lying in bed half asleep, slowly waking to the new day. I've talked a lot in this book and in lectures about the horrors of living in the twilight zone 24 hours a day, never really awake during the day and never deeply asleep at night. But I also want to emphasize the other side of the coin: the exhilaration of being vitally awake during the day and deeply asleep at night.

That's why I chose a yin-yang as the symbol of the American Sleep Disorders Association: The dark and the light of night and day, of sleep and wakefulness, form the interlocking whole that makes up our lives. Each alternates with, reinforces, and gives substance to the other. In order to grasp the fullness of our waking life, we have to make the most of our sleeping time. We have to appreciate the many beauties of both.

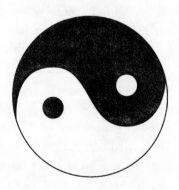

Chapter 20

Get a Good Night's Sleep
—Starting Tonight!
(A Three-Week Sleep Camp)

EVERY ONCE in a while I will bump into one of the campers or counselors who spent time at the first Stanford Sleep Camp more than two decades ago. I am delighted to find that they usually have very fond memories of that time. While the original sleep camp was intended for research rather than self-improvement, I present the following three-week sleep camp as a program for actually improving sleep and, more important, for making daytime life fuller, better, more pleasurable, and more vital.

As I have emphasized throughout this book, everyone has different sleep needs and sleep styles—there is no one magic formula for achieving healthy sleep. In this chapter I try to organize many of the ideas I have talked about in the rest of the book into a step-by-step program. The sleep camp is not the only way to accomplish the goal of healthy sleep—it is only one of many possible programs that you might follow. The important thing is to get to know your own sleep requirements and use that knowledge to acquire healthy sleep. With that in mind, I would urge you to monitor how you are responding to the sleep camp as you are doing it and to modify the regimen according to your own self-knowledge and what you have learned in the rest of this book.

People who make the commitment to work off their sleep debt and improve their sleep are often very surprised by how much better they feel during the day, both emotionally and physically. The restorative benefits of this regimen have been heartily affirmed by the members of Stanford Students for Healthy Sleep, who agreed to "go to sleep camp" this past spring and test the program. After completing camp, most were excited at how clear-minded, energetic, and alert they felt, both in and outside of class. If college students—perhaps the most sleep-deprived and stimulus-driven segment of the population—can make improving sleep their highest priority for three weeks, so can you.

I want to warn you that at first some people actually feel more tired when they start sleeping more. No one knows for sure why this is, although most likely it happens because when people finally rest they stop driving themselves so hard, stop working to stave off sleepiness, and become more sensitive to their true, underlying sleep load. These people definitely are not becoming more tired during the day because they are getting too much sleep. That is impossible. Whatever the reason for the initial increase in sleepiness, when people continue to work off sleep debt, they soon start feeling an increase in energy and vitality.

So dive right in. Start as soon as possible. But just as you would with any diet or exercise regimen, plan for success. Don't start the program right before a major work deadline or in the midst of any particularly stressful period. Picking a time when you will have a little flexibility in structuring your schedule will give you the best chance to succeed.

And even more so than with a diet, you really should try to undertake this program with your roommate or spouse. Having someone in the house staying up late and making noise or having a great time watching a movie can undermine the program. On the other hand, having someone to share the quiet domestic atmosphere the sleep camp seeks to generate can be a wonderful experience. Even if you live alone, try to find a friend to "go to camp" at the same time you do. Positive reinforcement is always a plus, and it's more interesting when you have someone to share your trials and triumphs with.

The primary goal of the sleep camp is to integrate your new knowledge about sleep and the techniques you've learned to pay off your sleep debt, and to begin building good sleep habits from scratch. Ideally, you'll build these new habits into the existing framework of your work and social life—although you may have to modify some of your behaviors to accommodate your respect for the primacy of sleep at night. Again, as long as you know the principles that drive sleep, you can be creative in how you structure your life so that you get enough quality sleep. By using your knowledge wisely, you may have to change very little to achieve success.

This is not a program for people with clinical sleep disorders. If you learned you have apnea or chronic insomnia, you should get treatment. But if you're in the habit of cannibalizing your sleep to feed the demands of work, family, and personal passions, then sleep camp is a good way to step back and reassess the imbalances in your life—to discover tangible steps you can take to realign your sleep and waking hours in a healthier fashion.

Achieving these goals will take discipline and willpower. Anyone who has been on a diet knows that good intentions alone don't lead to success. Working off sleep debt takes real sleep time, which means cutting back on some of the things you usually do at night. You may have to skip or tape favorite TV shows. You may have to turn down invitations from family or friends who are going out to a movie or a restaurant at night. But if you make the commitment and stick to it, most people find that these few weeks can set a rewarding pattern for the rest of their lives.

The sleep camp is designed as a three-week program. Week 1 is an opportunity to audit your current sleep habits and arrive at specific targets for paying off sleep debt and making your life more sleep friendly. Week 2 is when you pay off the lion's share of your sleep debt and reorient your evenings and nights toward sleep. Week 3 is for repaying any remaining debt and, most of all, finally enjoying the fruits of healthy sleep. After the three-week period is over, continue to use sleep patterns that worked for you during the sleep camp, and continue to monitor and modify your sleep to find what works best for you.

Camp Rules

The only hard-and-fast rule of my sleep camp is that for these few weeks, sleep is king (or queen, if you prefer). If you are torn between two competing activities, go with the one that favors sleep. This translates into putting sleep first and other considerations second.

One of the great lessons of sleep camp is that the planet will continue to spin on its axis, even if you take an extra hour a day to catch up on sleep.

Week 1

Goals:

Familiarize yourself with your current sleep habits. Figure out how much sleep you need and how much you're getting. Meanwhile, audit your lifestyle to see where it's most sleep unfriendly. Turn your bedroom into a sleep room and begin to ease into the sleep regimen of week 2.

The Program

1. *Start a sleep diary.* You will use a sleep diary throughout the three weeks of sleep camp, but this week you should record your normal patterns as a baseline of comparison. Choose the type of sleep diary you want (fill-in-the-blanks or a chart) and carry it with you through the day.

2. *Calculate your total sleep time.* Record what time you go to bed, go to sleep, and wake up. Note down any naps you take during the day and any nighttime awakenings that you can remember (or vice versa, if you work at night). Calculate your total sleep time for each day and about how long it took to go to sleep at night. (But don't keep yourself awake trying to figure out when you are going to sleep.)

3. *Record your alertness during the day* using the Stanford Sleepiness Scale. Measure your sleepiness as many times as possible, but definitely measure it one hour after you wake up, and during the midday dip in alertness. If you decide to take a home Multiple Sleep Latency Test, do it during these times too. If you can't take the MSLT, the Stanford Sleepiness Scale rating will suffice.

4. *Keep track of what you're drinking,* particularly coffee, tea, caffeinated sodas, and alcoholic drinks (beer, wine, distilled liquor). Many drinks list caffeine content on the label. Write down or mark on the graph a "C" for each caffeinated drink and an "A" for each alcoholic drink.

5. *Note any exercise you get each day* and how much time you spend outdoors in the sunlight.

6. *Record your normal going-to-bed routine.* Pay attention to whether nighttime television makes you more or less tired. Do you read before bed? Does reading make you sleepy or wake you up? Do you work in bed? Talk on the phone? Do you check your e-mail before going to bed? Your office voice mail? Once you climb into bed, what kinds of things do you normally think about? Do you worry about the next day's work? Do you have a set routine in the half hour before you go to bed, or does it change?

7. *Note which drugs you are taking,* including over-the-counter medications, prescription drugs, and recreational drugs.

8. *Review your diary at the end of each day* and write a short note summing up how stressful, relaxed, alert, or sleepy a day you had.

Days and Nights

Here are some suggested sleep-friendly activities for the first week. Remember, though, that you can discard ideas that you know absolutely would not work for you and add ideas that you think will work.

Sunday: Buy something indulgent for your bedroom: a comfortable pillow or new sheets.

Monday: If light bothers you, figure out a way to black out your room at night. Heavy blankets or curtains help keep out light as well as sound.

Tuesday: Make a note of how sleepy or alert you feel every two hours on this day, in order to get a complete picture of your peaks and troughs during the day.

Wednesday: If you consume lots of coffee or tea, start cutting back now so you can try to cut out caffeine completely next week.

Thursday: Get a few night-lights to use instead of overhead lights at night, particularly for the bathroom.

Friday: Based on your diary count of how much alcohol you drink, try to cut that amount in half, starting tonight.

Saturday: Take a hot bath and prepare for your upcoming sleep week.

Week 2

Goals

Now that you have a good handle on your current sleep life, it's time to put your house in order and pay off the mortgage. This week you start working off your sleep debt and building sleep-friendly activities into your days and nights.

Based on your diary from week 1, you should have a good sense of how much sleep debt you're carrying around. (Don't try to get an exact number—get an estimate using methods from Chapter 15.) My own feeling is that you should work at paying off your sleep debt as fast as possible. That means getting as much extra sleep as you can. Remember that the volunteers in previous sleep camps slept for over 9 to 10 hours on the first nights. These were average people, not subjects who were picked because they had large sleep debts. Those subjects who slept for 9 to 10 hours per night hadn't even paid off all their sleep debt over the course of two weeks. So if you are just average, you have a large sleep debt to work off.

The Program

1. *Go to bed as early as you can at night*—at least an hour earlier than normal. Since it's hard for many people to sleep in past your normal wake-up time—because of work or personal commitments or force of circadian habit—going to bed early is the best way to pay off debt.

2. *Watch no television after 9:00 P.M.* If TV helps you feel drowsy, watch a little (15 to 20 minutes of news or a talk show) before you go to sleep. If television stimulates you, move it out of the bedroom entirely.

3. *Completely cut out coffee, tea, or anything else that contains caffeine.* For the next 10 days you should try to abstain from caffeine. If caffeine withdrawal is too much to handle, you should just cut down to a minimal dose—one or two cups of caffeinated coffee, tea, or soda per day. (People who are physiologically dependent on caffeine can get headaches when they stop taking this stimulant. Aspirin can help alleviate the headache, but be careful not to

use aspirin compounds that contain caffeine. Drinking decaffeinated coffee, tea, or cola can help fulfill your habitual desire to sip something.) Cutting out caffeine will help make your sleep debt obvious to you as well as highlight the effects of caffeine. And a break from caffeine will decrease the tolerance you have built up over time. When it is time to start drinking coffee again, it will carry a much more powerful punch, and you can use it strategically, drinking only when you really need it, such as at the lowest points of the day.

4. *In addition to keeping your normal sleep diary, you might want to begin a dream log.* Don't work hard at it. Just remain receptive to your dreams and write them down when you remember them.

5. *Try to sleep a little longer each night.* Add a few minutes of sleep time in the morning or night, whichever is easier, every day.

If you are a night owl and have to get up early, you will have to be creative about getting more sleep. Expose yourself to bright lights in the morning to try to shift your clock. Take a walk in the morning sun. In the evening, wear dark glasses, turn the lights in your house very low, and don't sit in front of a computer screen. If you are a lark, you will have trouble staying asleep in the morning no matter what time you go to bed. To get extra sleep, you will have to get to bed earlier. Usually larks will not have a problem doing so, but if you do, some of the techniques I have mentioned previously might help.

6. *Be businesslike about your sleep.* Look at what helped you sleep better last week, and do those things regularly. Don't let yourself get distracted with "more important" things. Work at helping yourself get sleepy.

7. *Cut out any over-the-counter or recreational drugs you may be taking, including alcohol.* Don't go off any prescription drugs without consulting your doctor. And if cutting out alcohol completely strikes you as too Spartan, cut back to one glass of beer or wine with your evening meal.

8. *Don't check your e-mail or office voice mail after 7:00 P.M.* Don't use the time before bed to worry about what you are going to do tomorrow. Don't try to fight tomorrow's battles the evening before.

9. *Be active during the day.* Try to take walks in sunlight every day.

Being physically active and mentally excited during the day also helps you sleep better at night.

10. *Take naps during the afternoon dip in alerting.* Again, the main goal this week is paying off sleep debt. Grab sleep where you can.

11. Tell yourself and others, "I'm putting sleep first."

Days and Nights

Sunday: Turn off the phone after dinner and turn the sound down on the answering machine.

Monday: Use dim lights or night-lights instead of overhead lights for an hour before going to bed.

Tuesday: If you do not already do so, take a leisurely bath as a way to crank down before bedtime. If this agrees with you, replace your morning shower with a nightly bath.

Wednesday: Take a walk at lunch. Do stretching exercises after dinner.

Thursday: If you're a news junkie, cut out one of your media hits and keep it out of your daily routine for the next 10 days.

Friday: Have your spouse or partner give you a gentle massage in the evening. (Or hire a masseur/masseuse.)

Saturday: Get into the outdoors. Have a picnic, or better yet, go for a long hike. If you are working on getting to bed earlier, take your walk in the early-morning sun.

Week 3

Goals:

Keep working off sleep debt and begin enjoying the fruits of a healthy sleep routine. This is the week to stabilize your sleep rhythms and find the routine that's right for you. As you pay back your remaining sleep debt, look for the optimal point short of total repayment. A little bit of sleep debt is good for consolidating nighttime sleep in order to achieve an ideal state of alertness through the day.

The Program

1. *Stabilize your sleep routine.* By now you should be feeling the effects of last week's extra sleep. You will also have a better feeling for what kind of schedule works well for your circadian rhythm and for your schedule. Set your routine—your bedtime and rising time—and stick with it all week.

2. *Restrict naps to your afternoon dip.* You still may need daytime naps to pay off residual sleep debt, but try to keep them to your midafternoon dip. Otherwise, naps could begin interfering with your nighttime sleep.

3. *Keep up your sleep diary.* Start to graph your sleep patterns, now that their natural contours are taking shape. Keep track of your moods and alertness and compare them to those of week 1.

4. *Make strategic use of caffeine.* Now that you've flushed out your system, you can start drinking moderate amounts of caffeinated beverages again—but start using the stimulant strategically. Have caffeine only at your lowest energy points of the day, and keep consumption down. Have a maximum of two cups a day of coffee, tea, or soda. One cup would be even better. (If you like the feeling of being off caffeine altogether, by all means maintain your abstinence.)

5. *Get in touch with your dreams.* Lie in bed in the morning and think about the dreams you have just had. Writing down complete narratives of dreams is difficult for most people, so for starters, write or tape record just enough details to remember the dream by. One of the biggest obstacles to dream recall is a large sleep debt. Now that you've cut out some of the competing media in your nights, this is a golden opportunity to enter your dream world in earnest.

6. *Try to build physical and mental activity into every day.* Keep exercising and stretching. Do something—any little thing—exciting or fun each day this week. The higher your activity during the day, the deeper your sleep at night.

7. *Expose yourself to sunlight every day.* Keep track of what time the sun rises and sets. Try to find the moon in the night or morning

sky. Note any sunrises, sunsets, moon rises, and moon sets in your diary.

Days and Nights

Sunday: Go out to dinner. Beat the rush and get back in time for an early bedtime.

Monday: Have a strategic cup of coffee and tear into work you've been dreading doing, like doing taxes or cleaning the garage.

Tuesday: Try setting your alarm clock for 15 minutes later than you usually would—see if you can wake up naturally and easily before it goes off.

Wednesday: Record your dreams.

Thursday: Get another massage. (Life is short.)

Friday: Stay out later tonight. Every program should have a break. Take a nap in the afternoon, then stay out a little later than you have been doing. Get up the next morning at the usual time. Make sure that tomorrow's nap is long enough to make up for any sleep lost.

Saturday: Take stock of how far you've come in these three weeks. Set sleep goals for the next three months. Write them down and revisit them weekly.

Congratulations! You're a sleep camp graduate. Welcome to the world of the fully living. Now that you've experienced life without punishing sleep debt, consider the possibility of adopting a maintenance sleep diet for life. You don't have to cut out the things you love—you just have to make room for the things you need: sleep, health, and vitality.

Afterword

FOR A NUMBER of years, my lectures about sleep to students were limited to an hour here or there as part of someone else's course. Nonetheless, I was always interested in what students remembered beyond the exam. If I ran into students after the quarter ended, I would ask if they recalled some specific thing I had covered in the lecture. They never did. About this time, I came across a very slim, funny book entitled *1066 and All That,* written in 1931 by two English historians. In this book, the authors firmly state that "History is what you can remember." They claim that the average Englishman can remember only one event in history, the Battle of Hastings in 1066.

By the time I offered my course "Sleep and Dreams" for the first time in the Winter Quarter 1971, there were definitely a few facts about sleep that I thought the students should remember vividly for the rest of their lives. So, in my very first lecture I described the thesis that history is what you can remember and reported to the students that the average Englishman could remember only one date, 1066. With this idea in mind, I declared I would not burden them with volumes of detail about the world of sleep but would instead emphasize "a few very important facts and principles" that I would expect them to remember for the remainder of their days. In every lecture throughout the quarter, I repeatedly underscored the few facts and principles that the students should always remember. I told them that if I ever ran into any of them, I would be very likely to give them an oral quiz, and they should get a perfect score.

At the end of the quarter, as the very last question of the final exam, I asked students to "write one thing from the course that you promise you will remember for the rest of your life." When I corrected the exams, the answer to this question was an incredible surprise. Nearly all of the several hundred students had answered "1066." To this day, I am not sure whether they were telling me something very profound about the educational process or whether this amazing result was just an extremely well-executed practical joke.

But what a great story! More than 10 years' worth of undergraduate "Sleep and Dreams" students heard me tell this story in the course's opening lecture, and soon a sort of cult phenomenon began. If I was recognized by students on a walk across the campus, the students would not say "Hello, Professor Dement," but simply "1066." When I mentioned these encounters in my first lecture each year, the phenomenon rose to a new level. I was on a ferry in Vienna going under a bridge, and I heard the words "1066" shouted from above me by a young person waving on the bridge. Someone shouted "1066" to me in Tokyo on the Ginza. I began to get phone messages that were just "1066." Once when I arrived at a hotel in Mexico City, the message light was blinking, and sure enough: "1066."

The occasion I remember best was at the Oakland Coliseum. The place was packed for a Bob Dylan concert. During intermission, I noticed that a piece of paper was being passed from hand to hand toward me. I thought it might be from Mr. Dylan himself, but when I opened it: "1066."

My hope is that in addition to indelibly imprinting the date 1066 on the minds of my students, I also imparted a lifelong knowledge of the fundamental truths about healthy and unhealthy sleep. Only when people are armed with fundamental knowledge about sleep can they understand what it takes to make their sleep healthy and actively manage their lives to achieve that goal. I've spent the better part of four decades constantly creating and revising my list of what everyone must know at the very minimum about sleep, sleep deprivation, biological rhythms, and sleep disorders. Despite the fact that we have learned more about sleep in the last four decades than we have in the last four millennia, almost nobody among the public at-large even knows these fundamentals exist let alone what they are.

I'm not saying we should stop research and turn our attention to education. There's a tremendous amount of exciting clinical research currently under way that is elegant, complex, and at the very cutting edge of medical technology. At the basic science level, my sleep colleagues are utilizing the vast weaponry of modern molecular neurobiology and genetics. Hugely important research projects remain to be done. We have yet to find out what sleep is for, how sleep works, and how it affects us on a cellular level.

For my part, I would like to know what happens to sleep debt in the long term—not just the two-week period that we currently know about. For instance, parents claim that they accumulate about 300 hours of sleep debt over the months after a child is born. What happens to this sleep debt? We also need to know how the brain keeps track of long-term sleep indebtedness.

I believe we desperately need a National Sleep Laboratory to answer these latter types of questions—a place where there can be many bedrooms, a permanent technical and scientific staff, an adequate budget, access to computerized data-gathering technology, and comfortable work space for maintaining large numbers of volunteers for long periods of time. Such a laboratory could be an international effort.

The technology required to perform such sleep studies is not terribly expensive. The major costs are housing and feeding subjects during the experiments and paying for technicians. That means it may be best to place such a laboratory in China, India, or anywhere there is a base of educated technicians available but where the cost of living is relatively low. Another extremely intriguing possibility was brought to my attention by the headline "Shelter Secret Exposed!" It turns out that the Cold War gave rise to the creation of a secret government-controlled underground bunker, 64 feet beneath the ritzy Greenbrier Resort in White Sulphur Springs, West Virginia. The bunker was designed to protect members of the Congress and their staff from nuclear fallout, although not from a direct nuclear strike. The report stated that the bunker could house 1,152 people. It has dormitories, bathrooms, communal showers, lounges, and so on. I don't know what anyone is doing with this facility now, but it would be the perfect site for a national or international laboratory. It would be extremely easy to develop time isolation facilities, to shield individuals from outside clues as to the true time of day, and there is easy access to catering at the Greenbrier Resort (which has one of the world's better golf courses, in addition to everything else).

I sincerely hope that people will learn enough about sleep to live their lives more fully, with a greater sense of joy. Too many people think that it is normal to feel sleepy during the day, and they move through their lives wrapped in the gauze of drowsiness. At the very least, it is essential that people learn enough to avoid accidents. I was recently talking about sleep with an administrative assistant at Stanford, and she remarked, "I wish my son had heard your lecture—he fell asleep while driving and was killed at the age of 19." Too many lives have been lost already.

But my greatest hope for the future is that the Walla Walla project may be repeated in one form or another in every small and large town in America and around the world. Our studies have established beyond the shadow of a doubt that serious sleep disorders permeate primary care patient populations. As the gatekeepers of managed care and medical practice in general, primary care physicians can and must include sleep disorders in their domain. I have no doubt that data demonstrating lower total health care costs by treating sleep disorders will continue to pour in, and that the mountain of evidence will eventually be so huge that the necessary wise public policy decisions will come to pass. Sleep will finally and truly be included in the mainstream of the health care system, the educational system, and throughout society.

Everything I am working for, and everything I believe can be done for my fellow human beings, is being done in Walla Walla. Since Walla Walla is typical of most small towns, *if it can happen there, it can happen anywhere.* Hundreds of people have literally been rescued from premature death in this sleepy little town, and the lives of many more have been greatly enhanced by restored health and energy. In 1998 the National Sleep Foundation sponsored the first annual National Sleep Awareness Week, during which I was interviewed a number of times by various media representatives. It occurred to me that Walla Walla had become the model of what we want to happen in every community in America and eventually throughout the world. I told reporters that my hometown was now the "healthy sleep capital of the world," and it is.

I'm sure it's probably my imagination, but I swear that when I walk through Walla Walla's one large shopping mall, people seem more energetic, more friendly, happier than they were several years ago. On every visit, I try to guess which of the people I encounter on the street or in stores would not be there if my own life and career had not come full circle. Is it possible that this was my true destiny—to search for the gift of life and when found, to bring it back to the place of my origins? These musings are great fun!

We still have miles to go before we sleep. In other communities, the rivers of sleep disorders continue to flow past the unseeing eyes of primary care physicians. In Walla Walla, we have clearly shown that these patients can be easily identified and managed largely within the constraints of office-based medical practice. The loudest and clearest message from Walla Walla is that doctors who truly care about their patients must ask about their sleep. "How are you sleeping?" must be as routine as "How are you feeling?" What's more, doctors must know how to respond to the answers they hear.

Primary care physicians are in an ideal position to diagnose sleep disorders early. Our Walla Walla experience suggests an even more exciting possibility: that primary care physicians are also in an ideal position to educate the entire community about sleep as a component of good health and quality of life. People everywhere do not know how sleep debt works, or the consequences of inadequate sleep. Imagine if physicians everywhere would spread this life-saving information among their patients.

One of my favorite letters arrived a few years ago from someone who wanted to tell me that the minister at her church taught from both the Bible and a book called *The Sleepwatchers,* a small book I wrote for the Stanford Alumni Association. The writer of the letter thought I would appreciate knowing that her minister at one time had my book in one hand and the Bible in the other as he preached from the pulpit. What we need in every neighborhood community is one person—a physician, a patient, a parent—who will preach the gospel of sleep. Our quality of life, and often life itself, hangs in the balance. But armed with some simple knowledge, all of us can fulfill sleep's abundant promise and reclaim our birthright of healthy sleep.

Appendix A

Sleep Centers

American Sleep Disorders Association–accredited member centers and laboratories.

ALABAMA

Athens

Sleep-Related Breathing
  Disorders Lab
Athens-Limestone Hospital
700 West Market Street
P.O. Box 999
Athens, AL 35612
Andy Jackson
Cherri Walker
256-771-REST (7378)
256-233-9575

Birmingham

Brookwood Sleep Disorders
  Center
Brookwood Medical Center
2010 Brookwood Medical
  Center Drive
Birmingham, AL 35209
Attn: Robert C. Doekel, M.D.

205-877-2486
FAX: 205-877-1663

Sleep Disorders Center of
  Alabama, Inc.
790 Montclair Road, Suite 200
Birmingham, AL 35213
Attn: Vernon Pegram, Ph.D.
Robert C. Doekel, M.D.
205-599-1020
FAX: 205-599-1029

Sleep-Wake Disorders Center
University of Alabama at
  Birmingham
1713 6th Avenue South
CPM Building, Room 270
Birmingham, AL 35233-0018
Attn: Susan Harding, M.D.
Vernon Pegram, Ph.D.
205-934-7110

Sleep Disorders Lab
Carraway Methodist Medical
  Center
1600 Carraway Boulevard
Birmingham, AL 35234
Attn: Kurvilla George
Aneshia Williams
205-502-6164
205-502-5210

Boaz

Breathing Related Sleep
  Disorders Center
Marshall Medical Center South
P.O. Box 758
601A Corley Avenue
Boaz, AL 35957
Attn: Tony Rollins, RRT
Robert Doekel, Jr., M.D.
205-593-1226
FAX: 205-593-9945
E-MAIL: tony.rollins@
  mmcs.org

Decatur

Sleep Disorders Center
Decatur General
1201 7th Street SE
Decatur, AL 35605
Attn: Edward M. Turpin, M.D.
Marc A. Hays, RRT
256-340-2558
FAX: 256-340-2566.

Dothan

Sleep-Wake Disorders Center
Flowers Hospital
4370 West Main Street
P.O. Box 6907
Dothan, AL 36302
Attn: Ronald C. Kornegay,
  RPSGT
Ann B. McDowell, M.D.
Alan Purvis, M.D.
David Davis, M.D.
334-793-5000 ext. 1685

Florence

ECM Sleep Disorders Lab
Eliza Coffee Memorial Hospital
205 Marengo Street
P.O. Box 818
Florence, AL 35631
Attn: Felix Morris, M.D.
Byron Jamerson, RPSGT
256-768-9153
FAX: 256-740-8524.

Gadsden

GRMC Sleep Lab
Gadsden Regional Medical
  Center
1007 Goodyear Avenue
Gadsden, AL 35999
Attn: Regina McClain, RPSGT
205-494-4551
FAX: 205-494-4602

Huntsville

The Columbia Center for Sleep
  Disorders
250 Chateau Drive, Suite 235
Huntsville, AL 35801
Attn: Alan H. Arrington, M.D.
Thomas H. Arrington, RPSGT
205-880-4710
FAX: 205-880-4708
Web site: www.columbia.net

The Sleep Center at Huntsville
  Hospital
911 Big Cove
Huntsville, AL 35801
Attn: Paul LeGrand, M.D.
Debra J. Vaughn, MBA, RRT,
  RPSGT
256-517-8553
FAX: 256-533-8388
E-MAIL: paull@md.hhsys.org

Mobile

Sleep Disorders Center
Mobile Infirmary Medical
  Center
P.O. Box 2144
Mobile, AL 36652
Attn: Robert Dawkins, Ph.D.,
  M.P.H.
334-431-5559
FAX: 334-431-5222

Southeast Regional Center for
  Sleep/Wake Disorders

Springhill Memorial Hospital
3719 Dauphin Street
Mobile, AL 36608
Attn: Lawrence S. Schoen,
  Ph.D.
334-460-5319
FAX: 334-460-5464

USA Knollwood Sleep
  Disorders Center
University of South Alabama
  Knollwood Park Hospital
5644 Girby Road
Mobile, AL 36693-3398
Attn: William A. Broughton,
  M.D.
Michael P. Houston, M.D.
334-660-5757
FAX: 334-660-5254
E-MAIL: memnoch1@
  concentric.net

Montgomery

Sleep Disorders Center
Baptist Medical Center
2105 East South Boulevard
Montgomery, AL 36116-2498
Attn: David P. Franco, M.D.
Tammy Taylor, RPSGT
334-286-3252
FAX: 334-286-3108

Opelika

Sleep Disorders Lab
East Alabama Medical Center
2000 Pepperell Parkway
Opelika, AL 36801-5452
Attn: Nancy Strickland, RRT
Steven E. Dekich, M.D.
334-705-2404
334-705-2409
E-MAIL: NancyStrickland@
  EAMC.org

Tuscaloosa

Tuscaloosa Clinic Sleep Center
701 University Boulevard East
Tuscaloosa, AL 35401
Attn: Richard M. Snow, M.D.,
  FCCP
205-349-4043

ALASKA

Anchorage

Sleep Disorders Center
Providence Alaska Medical
  Center
3200 Providence Drive
P.O. Box 196604
Anchorage, AK 99519-6604

Attn: Anne H. Morris, M.D.,
  Medical Director
Katie Boyle Colborn, RPSGT,
  Clinical Manager
907-261-3650
FAX: 907-261-4810
E-MAIL: anne morris@sppha-
  03.ccmail.compuserve.com

ARIZONA

Mesa

Samaritan Regional Sleep
  Disorders Program
Desert Samaritan Medical
  Center
1400 South Dobson Road
Mesa, AZ 85202
Attn: Paul Barnard, M.D.
Tom Munzlinger, BS, RPSGT
602-835-3684
FAX: 602-835-8788

Glendale

The Sleep Center at
  Thunderbird Samaritan
  Medical Center
5555 West Thunderbird Road
Glendale, AZ 85306-4622
Attn: Paul Barnard, M.D.
Tom Munzlinger, BS, RPSGT
602-588-4800

Phoenix

Samaritan Regional Sleep
  Disorders Program
Good Samaritan Regional
  Medical Center
1111 East McDowell Road
Phoenix, AZ 85006
Attn: Bernard Levine, M.D.
Connie Boker, RPSGT
602-239-5815
FAX: 602-239-2129

Scottsdale

Sleep Disorders Center at
  Scottsdale Healthcare
Scottsdale Healthcare Shea
9003 East Shea Boulevard

Scottsdale, AZ 85260
Attn: Jeffrey S. Gitt, D.O.
Sharon E. Cichocki, RPSGT
602-860-3200
FAX: 602-860-3251

Tucson

Sleep Disorders Center
University of Arizona
1501 North Campbell Avenue
Tucson, AZ 85724
Attn: Stuart F. Quan, M.D.
520-694-6112 or 520-626-6115
FAX: 520-694-2515
E-MAIL: squan@sneeze.resp-
  sci.arizona.edu

ARKANSAS

Fayetteville

Sleep Disorders Center
Washington Regional Medical
  Center
1125 North College Avenue
Fayetteville, AR 72703
Attn: David L. Brown, M.D.,
  Director
William A. Rivers, RPSGT,
  Coordinator
501-442-1272

Little Rock

Pediatric Sleep Disorders
Arkansas Children's Hospital
800 Marshall Street

Little Rock, AR 72202-3591
Attn: May Griebel, M.D.
Linda Rhodes, EMT, RPSGT
501-320-1893
FAX: 501-320-6878

Sleep Disorders Center
Baptist Medical Center
9601 I-630, Exit 7
Little Rock, AR 72205-7299
Attn: David Davila, M.D.
Buddy Marshall, CRTT,
  RPSGT
501-202-1902
FAX: 501-202-1874
E-MAIL: dgdavila@baptist-
  health.org

CALIFORNIA

Anaheim

Western Medical Centers' Sleep
  Disorders Center
1101 South Anaheim Boulevard
Anaheim, CA 92805
Attn: Clyde Dos Santos, M.D.,
  Medical Director
Deborah Strangio, Director
714-491-1159
FAX: 714-563-2865

Carmichael

Mercy Sleep Laboratory
Mercy San Juan Hospital
6401 Coyle Avenue, Suite 109
Carmichael, CA 95608
Attn: Janice K. Herrmann,
  RPSGT, MA
Richard Stack, M.D.
916-864-5874
FAX: 916-864-5870

Fullerton

Sleep Disorders Institute
St. Jude Medical Center
1915 Sunny Crest Drive
Fullerton, CA 92835
Attn: Louis J. McNabb, M.D.
Justine Petrie, M.D.
Robert Roethe, M.D.
714-446-7240
FAX: 714-446-7245

Glendale

Glendale Adventist Medical
  Center Sleep Disorders Center
Glendale Adventist Medical
  Center
1509 Wilson Terrace
Glendale, CA 91206
Attn: David A. Thompson, M.D.
Kathy Cavander
818-409-8323
FAX: 818-546-5625

La Jolla

Pacific Sleep Medicine Services
La Jolla Center
9834 Genesee Avenue, Suite 328
La Jolla, CA 92037-1223
Attn: Milton Erman, M.D.
Stuart Menn, M.D.
619-657-0550
FAX: 619-657-0559
E-MAIL: merman@scripps.
Eedu and 75620.37@
compuserve.com
Web site: www.sleepmed
  services.com

La Mesa

Sleep Disorders Center
Grossmont Hospital
P.O. Box 158
La Mesa, CA 91944-0158
Attn: Ellie Hoey, RPSGT
619-644-4488
FAX: 619-644-4021

Loma Linda

Loma Linda Sleep Disorders
Center
Loma Linda University
Community Medical Center
25333 Barton Road
Loma Linda, CA 92354
Attn: Ralph Downey, III,
Ph.D.
Joanne MacQuarrie, RRT,
RPSGT
909-478-6344

Long Beach

Sleep Disorders Center
Long Beach Memorial Medical
Center
2801 Atlantic Avenue
P.O. Box 1428
Long Beach, CA 90801-1428
Attn: Stephen E. Brown, M.D.
Monir Kashani, RRT, RPSGT,
Technical Coordinator
562-933-0208
FAX: 562-933-0201

Los Angeles

UCLA Sleep Disorders Center
24-221 CHS, Box 957069
Los Angeles, CA 90095-7069
Attn: Frisca Yan-Go, M.D.
Jerald Simmons, M.D.

310-206-8005
FAX: 310-825-3167

Los Gatos

Clinical Monitoring Center,
Inc.
Sleep Disorders Center
555 Knowles Drive, Suite 218
Los Gatos, CA 95032
Attn: Tom Pace, RPSGT,
Clinical Coordinator
Laughton Miles, M.D., Ph.D.
Augustin de la Pena, Ph.D.
Roger Smith, D.O.
408-341-2080
FAX: 408-341-2088
E-MAIL: cmc@sleep
scape.com

Newport Beach

Sleep Disorders Center
Hoag Memorial Hospital
Presbyterian
One Hoag Drive
P.O. Box 6100
Newport Beach, CA 92658-
6100
Attn: Paul A. Selecky, M.D.
949-760-2070
FAX: 949-574-6297
Web site: www.hoag.org

Northridge

Sleep Evaluation Center
Northridge Hospital Medical
 Center
18300 Roscoe Boulevard
Northridge, CA 91328
Attn: Jeremy Cole, M.D.
David Brandes, M.D.
Dennis McGinty, Ph.D.
Ron Szymusiak, Ph.D.
818-885-5344

Oakland

California Center for Sleep
 Disorders
3012 Summit Street
5th Floor, South Building
P.O. Box 23544
Oakland, CA 94623-0544
Attn: Jerrold Kram, M.D.
Glenn Roldan, BS, RPSGT
510-834-8333
FAX: 510-834-4728

Orange

Sleep Disorders Center
University of California, Irvine
101 City Drive, Route 23
Orange, CA 92668
Attn: Peter A. Fotinakes, M.D.
714-456-5105
FAX: 714-456-7822

St. Joseph Hospital Sleep
 Disorders Center
1310 West Stewart Drive, Suite
 403
Orange, CA 92868

Attn: Sarah Mosko, Ph.D.
714-771-8950
FAX: 714-744-8541

Oxnard

Premier Diagnostics, Inc.
1851 Holser Walk, Suite 210
Oxnard, CA 93030
Attn: Jerry Harris, RPCP, RRT
Rebecca Palmieri, RCP, RRT,
 RN, BS
George Yu, M.D.
805-485-2633
805-485-6650

Pasadena

Sleep Disorders Center
Huntington Memorial Hospital
100 West California Boulevard
P.O. Box 7013
Pasadena, CA 91109-7013
Attn: Charles A. Anderson, M.D.
Richard A. Shubin, M.D.
626-397-3061
FAX: 626-397-3211
E-MAIL: sleeplab@ix.
 netcom.com

Pinole

Sleep Disorders Center
Doctors Medical Center—Pinole
2151 Appian Way
Pinole, CA 94564-2578
Attn: Darlene Connolly, R.N.
Frederick Nachtwey, M.D.
Richard Sankary, M.D.
510-741-2525 or 800-640-9440
FAX: 510-724-2189

Pomona

Sleep Disorders Center
Pomona Valley Hospital Medical
  Center
1798 North Garey Avenue
Pomona, CA 91767
Attn: Dennis Nicholson, M.D.
Fares Elghazi, M.D.
Robert Jones, M.D., FCCP
909-865-9587
FAX: 909-865-9969

Redding

The Center for Sleep Apnea
Redding Medical Center
2801 Eureka Way
Redding, CA 96001
Attn: Everett Trevor, M.D.
Jean Amari-Melancon, RPSGT
916-245-4187
FAX: 916-245-4116

Redwood City

Sequoia Sleep Disorders Center
Sequoia Hospital
170 Alameda de las Pulgas
Redwood City, CA 94062-
  2799
Attn: J. Al Reichert, RPSGT
Bernhard Votteri, M.D.,
  Medical Director
650-367-5137
FAX: 650-363-5304
E-MAIL: sleep@sleepscene.com
Web site: www.sleepscene.com

Sacramento

Sutter Sleep Disorders Center
650 Howe Avenue, Suite 910
Sacramento, CA 95825
Attn: Sue Van Duyn, RPSGT,
  RCP, BA
Lydia Wytrzes, M.D.
916-646-3300

UCDMC Sleep Disorders Center
University of California Davis
  Medical Center, Room 5305
2315 Stockton Boulevard
Sacramento, CA 95817
Attn: Masud Seyal, M.D.
William Bonekat, D.O.
916-734-0256
FAX: 916-452-2739

San Bernardino

Inland Sleep Center
401 East Highland Avenue,
  Suite 552
San Bernardino, CA 92404
Attn: Sunil Arora, M.D.
909-883-8058
FAX: 909-881-4607

San Diego

Mercy Sleep Disorders Center
Mercy-Scripps Health
4077 Fifth Avenue
San Diego, CA 92103-2180
Attn: Alex Mercandetti, M.D.,
  FCCP, Medical Director
Cheryl L. Spinweber, Ph.D.,
  Clinical Director
619-260-7378
FAX: 619-686-3990

San Francisco

Stanford Health Services
Sleep Clinic in San Francisco
2340 Clay Street, Suite 237
San Francisco, CA 94115-1932
Attn: Bruce T. Adornato, M.D.
Christopher R. Brown, M.D.
Rowena Korobkin, M.D.
Clete Kushida, M.D., Ph.D.
415-923-3336
FAX: 415-923-3584

UCSF/Stanford Sleep Disorders
  Center
University of California, San
  Francisco
1600 Divisadero Street
San Francisco, CA 94115
Attn: David Claman, M.D.
Kimberly A. Trotter, MA,
  RPSGT
415-885-7886
FAX: 415-885-3650

Santa Barbara

The Sleep Disorders Center of
  Santa Barbara
2410 Fletcher Avenue, Suite
  201
Santa Barbara, CA 93105
Attn: Andrew S. Binder, M.D.
Laurie Laatsch, RPSGT
805-898-8845
FAX: 805-898-8848

Stanford

Sleep Disorders Clinic
Stanford University Medical
  Center
401 Quarry Road
Stanford, CA 94305
Attn: Alex Adu Clerk, M.D.
650-723-6601
FAX: 650-725-8910

Thousand Oaks

Southern California Sleep
  Apnea Center
Lombard Medical Group
2230 Lynn Road
Thousand Oaks, CA 91360
Attn: Ronald A. Popper, M.D.
805-449-1096
FAX: 805-497-1782

Torrance

Torrance Memorial Medical
  Center
Sleep Disorders Center
3330 West Lomita Boulevard
Torrance, CA 90505
Attn: Lawrence W. Kneisley,
  M.D.
310-517-4617
FAX: 310-784-4869

Visalia

Sleep Disorders Laboratory
Kaweah Delta District Hospital
400 West Mineral King Avenue
Visalia, CA 93291
Attn: William R. Winn, M.D.
Gregory C. Warner, M.D.
Larry Kellett, BS, RCPT,
  Clinical Coordinator
209-625-7338
FAX: 209-635-4059
E-MAIL: lkellsleep@
  aol.com
Web site: www.KDHCD.org

West Hills

West Valley Sleep Disorders
  Center
7320 Woodlake Avenue, Suite
  140
West Hills, CA 91307
Attn: Gordon Dowds, M.D.
Pamela Pierce
818-715-0096
FAX: 818-716-1875
E-MAIL: gordon@dowds.com

Woodland

Sleep Disorders Center
Woodland Memorial Hospital
1325 Cottonwood Street
Woodland, CA 95695
Attn: Richard A. Beyer, M.D.
Marie Kearney, Manager
916-668-2695
FAX: 916-668-5787

COLORADO

Denver

National Jewish/University of
  Colorado
Sleep Center
1400 Jackson Street, A200
Denver, CO 80206
Attn: Robert D. Ballard, M.D.
303-398-1523

Sleep Disorders Center
Columbia Presbyterian St.
  Luke's Medical Center
1719 East 19th Avenue
Denver, CO 80218

Attn: Thomas Cordas, RPGST
303-839-6049

Pueblo

Sleep Center of Southern
  Colorado
Parkview Medical Center
400 West Sixteenth Street
Pueblo, CO 81003
Attn: James Pagel, M.D.
Ron Fossceco, RRT, RPSGT
719-584-4659
FAX: 719-584-4929
E-MAIL: slabsoco@usa.net

CONNECTICUT

Danbury

Danbury Hospital Sleep
  Disorders Center
Danbury Hospital
24 Hospital Avenue
Danbury, CT 06810
Attn: Arthur Kotch, M.D.
Arthur Spielman, Ph.D.
203-731-8033
FAX: 203-731-8628
E-MAIL: kotcha@danhosp.
  chime.org

Wallingford

Gaylord-Yale Sleep Disorders
  Laboratory
Gaylord Hospital
Gaylord Farms Road
Wallingford, CT 06492
Attn: Thomas Whelan, RPSGT
Vahid Mohsenin, M.D.
203-284-2853

DELAWARE

Newark

Sleep Disorders Center
Christiana Hospital
4755 Olgetown-Stanton Road
P.O. Box 6001
Newark, DE 19718
Attn: John B. Townsend, III,
  M.D.
Thomas C. Mueller, M.D.
Mary Rose Hancock
302-478-4600
FAX: 302-733-2533
E-MAIL: hancock.m@christian
  acare.org

Wilmington

Sleep Disorders Center
Christiana Care Health Services
Wilmington Hospital
501 West 14th Street
Wilmington, DE 19899
Attn: John B. Townsend, III,
  M.D.
Thomas C. Mueller, M.D.
Mary Rose Hancock
302-478-4600
FAX: 302-733-2533
E-MAIL: hancock.m@christian
  acare.org

DISTRICT OF COLUMBIA

Washington

Sibley Memorial Hospital Sleep
  Disorders Center
5255 Loughboro Road
Northwest Washington, DC
  20016
Attn: Estela Prieto
David N.F. Fairbanks, M.D.
Samuel J. Potolicchio, M.D.
202-364-7676
FAX: 202-362-9378

Sleep Disorders Center, 5 Main
  Hospital
Georgetown University Hospital
3800 Reservoir Road
Northwest Washington, DC
  20007-2197
Attn: Marilyn L. Faucette,
  RPSGT
Anne O'Donnell, M.D.
Kenneth Plotkin, M.D.
Richard E. Waldhorn, M.D.,
  Medical Director
202-784-3610
FAX: 202-784-2920

FLORIDA

Boca Raton

Boca Raton Sleep Disorders
  Center
899 Meadows Road, Suite 101
Boca Raton, FL 33486
Attn: Natalio J. Chediak, M.D.
Sheila R. Shafer, CMA
561-750-9881
FAX: 561-750-9644

Fort Lauderdale

Sleep Disorder Laboratory
Broward General Medical
  Center
1600 South Andrews Avenue
Fort Lauderdale, FL 33316
Attn: Glenn R. Singer, M.D.
954-355-5534
Web site: www.nbhd.org

Jacksonville

Mayo Sleep Disorders Center
Mayo Clinic Jacksonville
4500 San Pablo Road
Jacksonville, FL 32224
Attn: Paul Fredrickson, M.D.
Joseph Kaplan, M.D.
904-953-7287
FAX: 904-953-7388

Lakeland

Watson Clinic Sleep Disorders
  Center
The Watson Clinic, LLP
1600 Lakeland Hills Boulevard
P.O. Box 95000
Lakeland, FL 33804-5000
Attn: Eberto Pineiro, M.D.
941-680-7627
FAX: 941-680-7430

Melbourne

Atlantic Sleep Disorders Center
1401 South Apollo Boulevard,
  Suite A
Melbourne, FL 32901
Attn: Dennis K. King, M.D.
407-952-5191

Miami

Sleep Disorders Center
Miami Children's Hospital
6125 Southwest 31st Street
Miami, FL 33155
Attn: Marcel J. Deray, M.D.
305-662-8330

Miami Beach

Sleep Disorders Center
Mt. Sinai Medical Center
4300 Alton Road
Miami Beach, FL 33140
Attn: Alejandro D. Chediak, M.D.
305-674-2613

University of Miami School of
  Medicine
JMH and VA Medical Center
  Sleep Disorders Center
Department of Neurology (D4-5)
P.O. Box 016960
Miami, FL 33101
Attn: Bruce Nolan, M.D.
305-324-3371

Ocala

Munroe Regional Medical Center
  Sleep Laboratory
Munroe Regional Medical Center
131 Southwest 15th Street
Ocala, FL 34473
Attn: Keith Tighe, Director
Joy Nunez, Assistant Director
352-351-7385
FAX: 352-351-7280

Orlando

Florida Hospital Sleep Disorders
  Center
601 East Rollins Avenue
Orlando, FL 32803
Attn: Morris T. Bird, M.D.
Robert S. Thornton, M.D.
407-897-1558
FAX: 407-897-1775

Palm Bay

Health First Sleep Disorders
  Center
Palm Bay Community Hospital
1425 Malabar Road Northeast,
  Suite 255

Palm Bay, FL 32907
Attn: Michael Miller, M.D.
Anna Barker, BA, RPSGT
407-434-8087
FAX: 407-434-8496

Pensacola

Sleep Disorders Center
West Florida Regional Medical
  Center
8383 North Davis Highway
Pensacola, FL 32514
Attn: Jane Wilkinson, Director
David Shaw, M.D., Medical
  Director
850-494-4850
FAX: 850-494-4809

St. Petersburg

St. Petersburg Sleep Disorders
  Center
2525 Pasadena Avenue South,
  Suite S
St. Petersburg, FL 33707
Attn: Neil T. Feldman, M.D.
813-360-0853 or 800-242-3244
  (in Florida)

Sarasota

Sleep Disorders Center
Sarasota Memorial Hospital
1700 South Tamiami Trail
Sarasota, FL 34239
Attn: Glenn D. Adams, M.D.,
  Medical Director
941-917-2525
FAX: 941-917-6187

Tallahassee

Tallahassee Sleep Disorders
  Center
1304 Hodges Drive, Suite B
Tallahassee, FL 32308-4613
Attn: George F. Slade, M.D.
800-662-4278 ext. 4 or 850-
  878-7271
FAX: 850-878-15093

Tampa

Laboratory for Sleep Related
  Breathing Disorders
University Community Hospital
3100 East Fletcher Avenue
Tampa, FL 33613
Attn: Daniel J. Schwartz, M.D.
Mike Longman, RPSGT, RRT
813-979-7410
FAX: 813-632-7517

GEORGIA

Atlanta

Atlanta Center for Sleep
  Disorders
303 Parkway Drive
Box 44
Atlanta, GA 30312
Attn: Patrick Merrill, RPSGT
Francis Buda, M.D.
Jonne Walter, M.D.
Robert Schnapper, M.D.
404-265-3722
FAX: 404-265-3833

Sleep Disorders Center
Northside Hospital
5780 Peachtree Dunwoody
  Road
Suite 150
Atlanta, GA 30342
Attn: Russell Rosenberg, Ph.D.
404-851-8135
FAX: 404-252-9946
E-MAIL: nshsleep@-
  mindspring.com

Sleep Disorders Center of
  Georgia
5505 Peachtree Dunwoody
  Road
Suite 370
Atlanta, GA 30342
Attn: D. Alan Lankford, Ph.D.
James J. Wellman, M.D.
404-257-0080
FAX: 404-257-0592

Macon

Central Georgia Sleep Disorders
  Center
777 Hemlock Street, Second
  Floor
P.O. Box 1035
Macon, GA 31202
Attn: Charles C. Wells, M.D.,
  Medical Director
J. Mark Parrish, CRTT,
  RPSGT, Technical Director
912-633-7222
FAX: 912-745-5125

Marietta

Sleep Disorders Center
Promina Kennestone Hospital
677 Church Street
Marietta, GA 30060
Attn: William Dowdell, M.D.
David Lesch, M.D.
Susan K. Thomlinson, RPSGT
770-793-5353
FAX: 770-793-5357

Savannah

Department of Sleep Disorders
  Medicine
Candler Hospital
5353 Reynolds Street
Savannah, GA 31405
Attn: James A. Daly III, M.D.
Pamela Rockett, RPSGT, RRT
912-692-6673
FAX: 912-692-6931

Savannah Sleep Disorders
  Center
Saint Joseph's Hospital
#6 St. Joseph's Professional
  Plaza
11706 Mercy Boulevard
Savannah, GA 31419
Attn: Anthony M. Costrini,
  M.D.
Paul Donnellan, RPSGT
Steven Lurtz, RPSGT
912-927-5141
FAX: 912-921-3380

Sleep Disorders Center
Memorial Medical Center, Inc.
4700 Waters Avenue
Savannah, GA 31403
Attn: Herbert F. Sanders, M.D.
Stephen L. Morris, M.D.
912-350-8327

HAWAII

Hilo

Orchid Isle Sleep Disorders
  Laboratory
1404 Kilauea Avenue
Hilo, HI 96743
Attn: Gilbert J. Ransley, RRT,
  Technical Director
John P. Dawson, M.D., MPH,
  Medical Director
808-935-6105
FAX: 808-935-0016

Honolulu

Pulmonary Sleep Disorders
  Center
Kuakini Medical Center
347 North Kuakini Street
Honolulu, HI 96817
Attn: Edward J. Morgan, M.D.
Sonia Lee-Gushi, RPSGT,
  CRTT
808-547-9119
FAX: 808-547-9225
E-MAIL: 110047.504@-
  compuserve.com

Sleep Disorders Center of the
Pacific
Straub Clinic & Hospital
888 South King Street
Honolulu, HI 96813
Attn: James W. Pearce, M.D.
Linda Kapuniai, Dr. Public
Health
808-522-4448
FAX: 808-522-3048
E-MAIL: sdcop@aloha.net

Queen's Medical Center Sleep
Laboratory
The Queen's Medical Center
1301 Punchbowl Street
Honolulu, HI 96813
Attn: Bruce A.G. Soll, M.D.
Jamil Sulieman, M.D.
808-547-4396
FAX: 808-537-7830

Kamuela

Orchid Isles Respiratory
Services
Waimea Town Plaza
64-1063 Mamalahoa Highway
105
Kamuela, HI 96743
Attn: Jon P. Dawson, M.D.,
MPH, Medical Director
Gilbert J. Ransley, RRT,
Technical Director
808-885-7351
FAX: 808-935-0016

IDAHO

Boise

Idaho Sleep Disorders
Laboratory
St. Luke's Regional Medical
Center
190 East Bannock Street
Boise, ID 83712
Attn: Brett Troyer, M.D.
David K. Merrick, M.D.
Stephen W. Asher, M.D.
Mary R. Gable, RPSGT
208-381-2440

Twin Falls

Idaho Diagnostic Sleep Lab
526-C Shoup Avenue West
Twin Falls, ID 83301
Attn: Diana Lincoln-Haye
Robin Baggett
208-736-7646
FAX: 208-736-1569

ILLINOIS

Chicago

Center for Sleep and
  Ventilatory Disorders
University of Illinois at Chicago
1740 West Taylor Street
M/C 787
Chicago, IL 60612
Attn: Robert C. Basner, M.D.
Edward J. Stepanski, Ph.D.
312-996-7708

Sleep Disorders Center
Northwestern Memorial
  Hospital
303 East Superior
Passavant 1044
Chicago, IL 60611
Attn: Phyllis C. Zee, M.D.,
  Ph.D., Director
James Stockard, M.D., Ph.D.,
  Co-director
312-908-8120 or 312-908-8508
FAX: 312-908-6637
E-MAIL: pczee@merle.
acns.nw.edu

Sleep Disorder Service and
  Research Center
Rush-Presbyterian-St. Luke's
  Medical Center
1653 West Congress Parkway
Chicago, IL 60612
Attn: Rosalind Cartwright,
  Ph.D.
312-942-5440
FAX: 312-942-4990
E-MAIL: rcartwri@rpslmc.edu

Sleep Disorders Center
The University of Chicago
  Hospitals
5841 South Maryland
MC2091
Chicago, IL 60637
Attn: Jean-Paul Spire, M.D.
Wallace B. Mendelson, M.D.,
  Co-director
773-702-1782
FAX: 773-702-7998
E-MAIL: eegs@midway.
uchicago.edu

Evanston

Sleep Disorders Center
Evanston Hospital
2650 Ridge Avenue
Evanston, IL 60201
Attn: Richard S. Rosenberg,
  Ph.D.
847-570-2567
FAX: 847-570-2984
E-MAIL: r-rosenberg@nwu.edu

Park Ridge

Sleep Disorders Center
Lutheran General Hospital
1775 Dempster Street
Parkside Center, Suite B06
Park Ridge, IL 60068
Attn: Barry Weber, M.D.
Wayne Rubinstein, M.D.
Lauren Witcoff, M.D.
847-723-7024
FAX: 847-723-7369

Peoria

C. Duane Morgan Sleep
Disorders Center
Methodist Medical Center of
Illinois
221 Northeast Glen Oak
Avenue
Peoria, IL 61636
309-672-4966 or 309-671-5136
FAX: 309-672-4117

Rockford

Sleep Disorders Laboratory
Rockford Health System
2400 North Rockton Avenue
Rockford, IL 61103
Attn: Theodore S. Ingrassia III,
M.D.
815-971-5595
FAX: 815-971-9894

Springfield

SIU School of Medicine/
Memorial Medical Center
Sleep Disorders Center
Memorial Medical Center
800 North Rutledge
Springfield, IL 62781

Attn: Joseph Henkle, M.D.
Steven Todd, RRT, RPSGT
217-788-4269

Urbana

Carle Regional Sleep Disorders
Center
Carle Foundation Hospital
611 West Park Street
Urbana, IL 61801-2595
Attn: Daniel Picchietti, M.D.
Donald A. Greeley, M.D.
217-383-3364

Winfield

Sleep Disorders Center
Central Du Page Hospital
25 North Winfield Road
Winfield, IL 60190
Attn: Michael McCormick
630-682-1600, ext. 6982
FAX: 630-260-2629
E-MAIL: mike_mccormick@-
cdh.org

INDIANA

Beech Grove

Sleep Disorders Center
St. Francis Hospital and Health
Centers
1500 Albany Street, Suite 1110
Beech Grove, IN 46107

Attn: Dianna L. Fields, RPSGT
Manfred P. Mueller, M.D.,
FCCP
317-783-8144
FAX: 317-781-1402
Web site: www.stfrancis-
indy.org

Evansville

St. Mary's Sleep Disorders
Center
St. Mary's Medical Center
3700 Washington Avenue
Evansville, IN 47750
Attn: David Cocanower, M.D.
Rebecca N. Dicus
812-485-4960
FAX: 812-485-7953

Fort Wayne

St. Joseph Sleep Disorders
Center
St. Joseph Medical Center
700 Broadway
Fort Wayne, IN 46802
Attn: James C. Stevens, M.D.
Thomandram Sekar, M.D.
219-425-3552
FAX: 219-425-3553

Indianapolis

Sleep Disorders Center
St. Vincent Hospital and Health
Services
8401 Harcourt Road
Indianapolis, IN 46260-0160
Attn: Rex McKinney

Thomas Cartwright, M.D.
317-338-2152
FAX: 317-338-4917

Sleep/Wake Disorders Center
Community Hospitals of
Indianapolis
1500 North Ritter Avenue
Indianapolis, IN 46219
Attn: Marvin E. Vollmer, M.D.
317-355-4275
FAX: 317-351-2785

Sleep/Wake Disorders Center
Winona Memorial Hospital
3232 North Meridian Street
Indianapolis, IN 46208
Attn: Kenneth N. Wiesert,
M.D.
317-927-2100

Lafayette

Sleep Alertness Center
Lafayette Home Hospital
2400 South Street
Lafayette, IN 47904
Attn: Frederick Robinson,
M.D.
317-447-6811 ext. 2840

IOWA

Ames

Sleep Disorders Center
Mary Greeley Medical Center
1111 Duff Avenue
Ames, IA 50010
Attn: Selden Spencer, M.D.,
  Director
Mark Hislop, RRT
515-239-2353

Iowa City

Sleep Disorders Center
The Department of Neurology
The University of Iowa
  Hospitals and Clinics
Iowa City, IA 52242
Attn: Mark Eric Dyken, M.D.
319-356-3813
FAX: 319-356-4505
E-MAIL: mark-dyken@
  uiowa.edu

KANSAS

Topeka

Sleep Disorders Center
St. Francis Hospital and Medical
  Center
1700 Southwest 7th Street
Topeka, KS 66606-1690
Attn: Ted W. Daughety, M.D.
David D. Miller, RPSGT
785-295-7900

Wichita

Sleep Disorders Center
Wesley Medical Center
550 North Hillside
Wichita, KS 67214-4976
Attn: Jeff D. Newby, RPSGT
Emilio D. Soria, M.D.
316-688-2663
FAX: 316-688-3256
Web site: http://
  www.columbia-Wesley.com/
  wessleep.html#

KENTUCKY

Bowling Green

Physicians' Center for Sleep
  Disorders
Graves-Gilbert Clinic
201 Park Street
P.O. Box 90007

Bowling Green, KY 42102-
  9007
Attn: Craig D. Heckman
502-781-5111
FAX: 502-782-4263
E-MAIL: heckmanc@graves-
  gilbertclinic.com

Sleep Diagnostics Lab
Columbia/Greenview Regional
  Hospital
1801 Ashley Circle
Bowling Green, KY 42101
Attn: Steven Zeller, RPSGT
Gul K. Sahetya, M.D. E.
Chandler Deal, M.D.
502-793-2175
FAX: 502-793-2177

Sleep Lab
The Medical Center at Bowling
  Green
250 Park Street
P.O. Box 90010
Bowling Green, KY 42101-9010
Attn: Chris A. Barnett, RRT
Rosanne M. Boyer, RPSGT
502-745-1024

Florence

Sleep Disorders Center
St. Luke Hospital West
7380 Turfway Road
Florence, KY 41042
Attn: Bruce Corser, M.D.
606-525-5347
FAX: 606-572-3375
E-MAIL: fletcher@healthall.com

Fort Thomas

The Sleep Disorder Center of
  St. Luke Hospital
St. Luke Hospital, Inc.
85 North Grand Avenue
Fort Thomas, KY 41075
Attn: Bruce Corser, M.D.
Michael Fletcher, RPSGT
606-572-3535

Hopkinsville

Sleep Apnea Center
Jennie Stuart Medical Center
320 West 18th Street
Hopkinsville, KY 42240
Manoj H. Majmudar, M.D.
Mark L Pierce, RRT, RPSGT
502-887-0410
FAX: 502-887-0412

Lexington

Sleep Apnea Center
Samaritan Hospital
310 South Limestone
Lexington, KY 40508
Attn: Barbara Phillips, M.D.,
  MSPH, FCCP
Gary King, RRT, Director
606-252-6612 ext. 7331
FAX: 606-252-6612 ext. 7292
E-MAIL: bphil95@aol.com

Sleep Disorders Center
St. Joseph's Hospital
One St. Joseph Drive
Lexington, KY 40504
Attn: Kathryn Hansen
606-278-0444

Louisville

Caritas Sleep Apnea Center
Caritas Medical Center
1850 Bluegrass Avenue
Louisville, KY 40215
Attn: Peter Moore, M.D.
William Lacy, M.D.
Richard Baker, M.D.
502-361-6555

Sleep Disorders Center
Columbia Audubon Hospital
One Audubon Plaza Drive
Louisville, KY 40217
Attn: Pamela McCullough
David Winslow, M.D.
502-636-7459

Sleep Disorders Center
University of Louisville Hospital
530 South Jackson Street
Louisville, KY 40202
Attn: Barbara J. Rigdon,
  RPSGT, R.EEG.T.
Vasudeva G. Iyer, M.D.
Eugene C. Fletcher, M.D.
502-562-3792
FAX: 502-562-4632

Sleep Medicine Specialists
1169 Eastern Parkway, Suite
  3357
Louisville, KY 40217
Attn: David H. Winslow, M.D.,
  Director
Darlene R. Herps, RPSGT,
  Clinical Manager
502-454-0755
FAX: 502-454-3497

Madisonville

Regional Medical Center Lab
  for Sleep-Related Breathing
  Disorders
900 Hospital Drive
Madisonville, KY 42431
Attn: Thomas Gallo, M.D.
Frank Taylor, M.D.
502-825-5918
FAX: 502-825-5159

Paducah

Diller Regional Sleep Disorders
  Center
Lourdes Hospital
1530 Lone Oak Road
Paducah, KY 42001
Attn: James Metcalf, M.D.
Rick Irvan, R.EEG.T.,
  Coordinator
502-444-2660
FAX: 502-444-2661

Pikeville

Breathing Disorders Sleep Lab
Pikeville Methodist Hospital
911 South Bypass Road
Pikeville, KY 41501
Attn: Ramanarao V. Mettu,
  M.D., FACP, FCCP, Medical
  Director
Sally Stamper Compton, RRT,
  Director
Linda Greer, CRTT, Manager
Jerry Miller, Vice-President
606-437-3989
FAX: 606-437-9649

Richmond

P.A.C. Sleep Disorders Lab
Pattie A. Clay Hospital
P.O. Box 1600
801 Eastern Bypass
Richmond, KY 40475
Attn: Tom Grant
David Broughton
606-625-3334
FAX: 606-625-3104

LOUISIANA

New Orleans

Memorial Medical Center Sleep
  Disorders Center
2700 Napoleon Avenue
New Orleans, LA 70115
Attn: Gregory S. Ferriss, M.D.
Lynn Causey, R.EEG.T.
504-896-5439
FAX: 504-897-4403

Tulane Sleep Disorders Center
1415 Tulane Avenue
New Orleans, LA 70112
Attn: Mark A. McCarthy, M.D.
504-588-5231
FAX: 504-584-1727

Shreveport

LSU Sleep Disorders Center
Louisiana State University
  Medical Center
P.O. Box 33932
Shreveport, LA 71130-3932
Attn: Andrew L. Chesson, Jr.,
  M.D.
318-675-5365
FAX: 318-675-4440

E-MAIL: achess@
  lsumc.edu

The Neurology and Sleep
  Clinic
2205 East 70th Street
Shreveport, LA 71105
Attn: Nabil A. Moufarrej, M.D.
Annette Berry, RPFT, RPSGT
318-797-1585
FAX: 318-797-6077
E-MAIL: namouf@
  msn.com

Slidel

NSRMC Sleep Disorders
  Center
North Shore Regional Medical
  Center
100 Medical Center Drive
Slidell, LA 70461
Attn: Anwant Chawla, M.D.
Mary B. Jones, BS, MT,
  RPSGT
504-646-5711
FAX: 504-646-5013

MAINE

Lewiston

St. Mary's Sleep Disorders
  Laboratory
St. Mary's Regional Medical
  Center
97 Campus Avenue
Lewiston, ME 04240
Attn: Ralph V. Harder, M.D.
Peter J. Leavitt, RRT
207-777-8959

Portland

Maine Institute for Sleep
  Breathing Disorders
930 Congress Street
Portland, ME 04102
Attn: George E. Bokinsky, Jr.,
  M.D.
207-871-4535

MARYLAND

Baltimore

Maryland Sleep Disorders Center
Greater Baltimore Medical
  Center
6701 North Charles Street,
  Suite 4140
Baltimore, MD 21204-6808
Attn: Thomas E. Hobbins, M.D.
410-494-9773
FAX: 410-823-6635
E-MAIL: psrmdteh@igc.apc.org

The Johns Hopkins Sleep
  Disorders Center
Asthma and Allergy Building,
  Room 4B50
Johns Hopkins Bayview
  Medical Center
5501 Hopkins Bayview Circle
Baltimore, MD 21224
Attn: Philip L. Smith, M.D.
Alan Schwartz, M.D.
410-550-0571
FAX: 410-550-3374

Frederick

Frederick Sleep Disorders Center
Frederick Memorial Hospital
400 West Seventh Street
Frederick, MD 21701
Attn: Marc Raphaelson, M.D.
Konrad W. Bakker, M.D.
301-698-3802

Hagerstown

The Sleep-Breathing Disorders
  Center of Hagerstown
12821 Oak Hill Avenue
Hagerstown, MD 21742
Attn: Abdul Waheed, M.D.
Shaheen Iqbal, M.D.
Johnny Alencherry, M.D.
301-733-5971

Rockville

Shady Grove Sleep Disorders
  Center
14915 Broschart Road, Suite 102
Rockville, MD 20850
Attn: Jean Neuenkirch, RPSGT
301-251-5905
FAX: 301-251-6189

Takoma Park

Washington Adventist Sleep
  Disorders Center
7525 Carroll Avenue
Takoma Park, MD 20912
Attn: Marc Raphaelson, M.D.
Konrad W. Bakker, M.D.
301-891-2594

MASSACHUSETTS

Boston

Sleep Disorders Center
Beth Israel Deaconess Medical
  Center
330 Brookline Avenue KS430
Boston, MA 02215
Attn: Jean K. Matheson, M.D.
Janet Mullington, Ph.D.
617-667-3237
FAX: 617-667-5216

Burlington

Sleep Disorders Center
Lahey-Hitchcock Clinic
41 Mall Road
Burlington, MA 01805
Attn: Paul T. Gross, M.D.
Susan M. Dignan, RPSGT
781-744-8251 FAX:
781-744-5243

Worcester

Sleep Disorders Institute of
  Central New England
St. Vincent Hospital
25 Winthrop Street
Worcester, MA 01604
Attn: Jayant G. Phadke, M.D.
508-798-6212
FAX: 508-798-6373

MICHIGAN

Ann Arbor

Sleep Disorders Center
St. Joseph Mercy Hospital
P.O. Box 995 Ann Arbor, MI
  48106
Attn: James R. Weintraub,
  D.O.
Sharon S. Potoczak, RPSGT
  734-712-4651

Sleep Disorders Center
University of Michigan
  Hospitals
1500 East Medical Center
  Drive UH8D 8702, Box 0117
Ann Arbor, MI 48109-0115
Attn: Brenda Livingston,
  Coordinator
Michael S. Aldrich, M.D.
Ronald Chervin, M.D.
Beth Malow, M.D.
734-936-9068
FAX: 734-936-5377

Bay City

Sleep Disorders Clinic
Bay Medical Center
1900 Columbus Avenue
Bay City, MI 48708
Attn: John M. Buday, M.D.
Mary K. Taylor, RPSGT, RRT
517-894-3332
FAX: 517-894-6114

Detroit

Harper Hospital Sleep Disorders
  Center
Hutzel Hospital Center
4707 St. Antoine
Detroit, MI 48201
Attn: James A. Rowley, M.D.
Larry Thomas, RPSGT
313-745-9009
FAX: 313-745-8725

Sleep/Wake Disorders
  Laboratory (127B)
VA Medical Center
4646 John R. Street
Detroit, MI 48201-1916
Attn: Sheldon Kapen, M.D.
M. Safwan Badr, M.D.
Greg Kashorek
313-576-1000 ext. 3663

Sinai Sleep Center
DMC Sinai Hospital
6767 West Outer Drive
Detroit, MI 48235-2899
Attn: Bradley Rowens, M.D.
Keith Williams
313-493-5148
313-493-5036

Grand Rapids

West Michigan Sleep Disorders
Center
Butterworth Hospital
100 Michigan Street Northeast
Grand Rapids, MI 49503
Attn: Lee Marmion, M.D.
Ronald Van Drunen, RPSGT
616-391-3759
FAX: 616-391-3052

Kalamazoo

Sleep Disorders Center
Borgess Medical Center
1521 Gull Road
Kalamazoo, MI 49001
Attn: Sue Cammarata, M.D.
Thomas Wittenberg, RRT
Sheri Dillon, RRT
616-226-7081
FAX: 616-226-6909

Lansing

Ingham Regional Medical
Center
Sleep/Wake Center
2025 South Washington
Avenue, Suite 300
Lansing, MI 48910-0817
Attn: Pamela Minkley, RRT,
RPSGT
Gauresh Kashyap, M.D., FACP,
FCCP
517-372-6444
FAX: 517-372-6440
E-MAIL: pminkley@juno.com

Sparrow Sleep Center
Sparrow Hospital
1215 East Michigan Avenue
P.O. Box 30480
Lansing, MI 48909-7980
Attn: Alan M. Atkinson, D.O.
David K. Young, D.O.
517-364-5370
FAX: 517-364-5373

Southfield

Sleep & Respiratory Associates
of Michigan
28200 Franklin Road
Southfield, MI 48034
Attn: Harvey W. Organek,
M.D.
248-350-2722
FAX: 248-350-0154

Traverse City

Munson Sleep Disorders Center
Munson Medical Center
1105 6th Street MPB, Suite 307
Traverse City, MI 49684-2386
Attn: David A. Walker, D.O.,
FCCP,
Medical Director Leon R.
Olewinski, RRT
Director Marcia Rinal, CRTT,
RPSGT, Manager
800-358-9641 or 616-935-6600
FAX: 616-935-6610

Troy

Sleep Disorders Institute
44199 Dequindre, Suite 311
Troy, MI 48098

Attn: R. Bart Sangal, M.D.
248-879-0707
FAX: 248-879-2704

MINNESOTA

Duluth

Duluth Regional Sleep
  Disorders Center
St. Mary's Duluth Clinic Health
  System
407 East Third Street
Duluth, MN 55805
Attn: Peter K. Franklin, M.D.
Paul J. Windberg, M.D.
Mary Carlson, RPSGT
218-726-4692
FAX: 218-726-4083

Edina

Fairview Sleep Center
Fairview Southdale Hospital
6401 France Avenue S.
Edina, MN 55435
612-924-5053,
E-MAIL: epeters1@fairview.org

Minneapolis

Minnesota Regional Sleep
  Disorders Center
#867B Hennepin County
  Medical Center
701 Park Avenue South
Minneapolis, MN 55415
Attn: Mark Mahowald, M.D.
612-347-6288
FAX: 612-904-4207
E-MAIL:mahowoo2@
  maroon.tc.umn.edu

Sleep Disorders Center
Abbott Northwestern Hospital
800 East 28th Street at Chicago
  Avenue
Minneapolis, MN 55407
Attn: Wilfred A. Corson, M.D.
612-863-4516
FAX: 612-863-2837

Rochester

Mayo Sleep Disorders Center
Mayo Clinic
200 First Street Southwest
Rochester, MN 55905
Attn: Peter Hauri, Ph.D.
John W. Shepard, Jr., M.D.
507-266-8900
FAX: 507-266-7772

St. Louis Park

Sleep Disorders Center
Methodist Hospital
6500 Excelsior Boulevard
St. Louis Park, MN 55426
Attn: Barb Feider, RPSGT
Salim Kathawalla, M.D.
612-993-6083
FAX: 612-993-7026

St. Paul

St. Joseph's Sleep Diagnostic
  Center
St. Joseph's Hospital
69 West Exchange Street
St. Paul, MN 55102
Attn: Thomas Mulrooney,
  M.D.
612-232-3682 FAX:
612-232-4111

MISSISSIPPI

Gulfport

Sleep Disorders Center
Memorial Hospital at Gulfport
P.O. Box 1810
Gulfport, MS 39501
Attn: Sydney Smith, M.D.
601-865-3152
FAX: 601-865-3259

Hattiesburg

Sleep Disorders Center
Forrest General Hospital
6051 Highway 49
P.O. Box 16389
Hattiesburg, MS 39404-6389
Attn: Geoffrey B. Hartwig,
  M.D.
John R. Harsh, Ph.D.
Dennis Kramer
601-288-4790 or 800-280-8520
FAX: 601-288-4791
E-MAIL: fghsdc@netdoor.com.
Web site: www.forrest
  general.com

Jackson

Sleep Disorders Center
University of Mississippi
  Medical Center
2500 North State Street
Jackson, MS 39216-4505
Attn: Howard Roffwarg, M.D.,
  Director
Alp Sinan Baran, M.D.,
  Medical Director
601-984-4820
FAX: 601-984-5885
E-MAIL: asbaran@pol.net

MISSOURI

Chesterfield

Unity Sleep Medicine and
  Research Center
St. Luke's Hospital
232 South Woods Mill Road
Chesterfield, MO 63017
Attn: James K. Walsh, Ph.D.
Gihan Kader, M.D.
314-205-6030
FAX: 314-205-6025
E-MAIL: jkw@stlo.smhs.com
  and gak@stlo.smhs.com

Columbia

University of Missouri Sleep
  Disorders Center
M-741 Neurology University
  Hospital and Clinics
One Hospital Drive
Columbia, MO 65212
Attn: Pradeep Sahota, M.D.
573-884-SLEEP or 800-ADD-
  SLEEP
FAX: 573-884-4785
E-MAIL: sahotp@brain.
  missouri.edu

Kansas City

Sleep Disorders Center
Research Medical Center
2316 East Meyer Boulevard
Kansas City, MO 64132-1199

Attn: Jon D. Magee, Ph.D.
816-276-4334
FAX: 816-276-3488

Sleep Disorders Center
St. Luke's Hospital
4400 Wornall Road
Kansas City, MO 64111
Attn: Ann Romaker, M.D.
Wendy L. Fluegel, M.D.
816-932-3207

St. Louis

Sleep Disorders & Research
  Center
Deaconess Medical Center
6150 Oakland Avenue
St. Louis, MO 63139
Attn: Sidney D. Nau, Ph.D.
Korgi V. Hegde, M.D.
314-768-3100
FAX: 314-768-3594

Sleep/Wake Disorders Center
SLU Care,
The Health Services Division of
  Saint Louis University
1221 South Grand Boulevard
St. Louis, MO 63104
Attn: Shashidhar M. Shettar,
  M.D.
314-577-8705
FAX: 314-664-7248

Springfield

Cox Regional Sleep Disorders
  Center
3800 South National Avenue,
  Suite LL 150
Springfield, MO 65807
Attn: Edward Gwin, M.D.
417-269-5575
FAX: 417-269-5578

St. John's Sleep Disorders
  Center
St. John's Regional Health
  Center
1235 East Cherokee
Springfield, MO 65804
Attn: John Brabson, M.D.,
  Medical Director
Terry M. Yarnell, REEGT,
  RCPT, Administrative
  Director
417-885-5464
FAX: 417-885-5465

MONTANA

Billings

Sleep Disorders Center
Deaconess Billings Clinic
2800 10th Avenue North
P.O. Box 37000
Billings, MT 59107
Attn: Rich Lundy, RRT
Robert K. Merchant, M.D.
406-657-4075
FAX: 406-657-4717
E-MAIL: rlundy@billings
  clinic.org

The Sleep Center at St. Vincent
  Hospital

Saint Vincent Hospital and
  Health Center
1233 North 30th Street
Billings, MT 59101
Attn: William C. Kohler,
M.D. Karen Y. Allen, CRTT,
  RPSGT
406-238-6815
FAX: 406-238-6262
E-MAIL: karenya@aol.com or
  kallen@svhhc.org

NEBRASKA

Lincoln

Adult and Pediatric Sleep
  Related Breathing Disorders
  Laboratory
Bryan Memorial Hospital
1600 South 48th Street
Lincoln, NE 68506
Attn: Debra Bailey, R.N.,
  Clinical Manager
Jack Mathews, M.D., Medical
  Director
402-483-3950
FAX: 402-483-8374

Great Plains Regional Sleep
  Physiology Center
Lincoln General Hospital 2300
  South 16th Street
Lincoln, NE 68502
Attn: Timothy R. Lieske, M.D.
Leigh Heithoff, RPSGT,
  R.EEG.T.
402-473-5338
FAX: 402-473-5380

Omaha

Sleep Disorders Center
Methodist/Richard Young
  Hospital
2566 St. Mary's Avenue
Omaha, NE 68105
Attn: Robert J. Ellingson,
  Ph.D., M.D.
John D. Roehrs, M.D.
402-354-6305 or 402-354-6309
FAX: 402-354-6334

Sleep Disorders Center
Nebraska Health System
4350 Dewey Avenue Omaha,
  NE 68105-1018
Attn: Carie L. Smith, RRT,
  RPSGT
Stephen B. Smith, M.D.
402-552-2286
FAX: 402-552-2057

NEVADA

Las Vegas

The Sleep Clinic of Nevada
1012 East Sahara Avenue
Las Vegas, NV 89104 Attn:
  Darlene Steljes, CEO
702-893-0020
FAX: 702-893-0025
E-MAIL: yingyang@ix.
  netcom.com

Reno

Washoe Sleep Disorders Center
  and Sleep Laboratory
Washoe Professional Building
  and Washoe Medical Center
  Sleep Management, Inc.
75 Pringle Way, Suite 701
Reno, NV 89502
Attn: William C. Torch, M.D.
John T. Zimmerman, Ph.D.
Kathleen Auld, D.O.
702-328-4700 or 800-
  JETLAGG
FAX: 702-329-2715

NEW HAMPSHIRE

Lebanon

Sleep Disorders Center
Dartmouth-Hitchcock Medical
  Center
One Medical Center Drive
Lebanon, NH 03756
Attn: Michael Sateia, M.D.
603-650-7534 FAX:
603-650-7820
E-MAIL: sleep@dartmouth.edu

Manchester

Center for Sleep Evaluation
Catholic Medical Center
100 McGregor Street
Manchester, NH 03102
Attn: Peter E. Corrigan, M.D.,
  Medical Director
Jeanetta C. Rains, Ph.D.,
  Clinical Director
603-663-6680
FAX: 603-663-6699

NEW JERSEY

Cherry Hill

SleepCare Center of Cherry Hill
457 Haddonfield Road, Suite
  520
Cherry Hill, NJ 08002
Attn: James LaRusso, Chief
  Executive Officer
John D. Miladin, President/
  Chief Operating Officer
Kathleen L. Ryan, M.D.,
  FCCP, FACP
800-753-3770
FAX: 609-662-5187

Hackensack

Institute for Sleep/Wake
  Disorders
Hackensack University Medical
  Center
30 Prospect Avenue
Hackensack, NJ 07601
Attn: Hormoz Ashtyani, M.D.
Sue Zafarlotfi, Ph.D.
201-996-2992

Morristown

Sleep Disorder Center
Morristown Memorial Hospital
95 Mount Kemble Avenue
Morristown, NJ 07962
Attn: Robert A. Capone, M.D.,
  FCCP
Pamela Wolfsie, RPSGT
973-971-4567
FAX: 973-290-7620

New Brunswick

Comprehensive Sleep Disorders
  Center
Robert Wood Johnson
  University Hospital/
UMDNJ - Robert Wood
  Johnson Medical School
One Robert Wood Johnson
  Place
P.O. Box 2601
New Brunswick, NJ 08903-
  2601
Attn: Richard A. Parisi, M.D.
Raymond Rosen, Ph.D.
732-937-8683
FAX: 732-418-8448

Newark

Sleep Disorders Center
Newark Beth Israel Medical
  Center
201 Lyons Avenue
Newark, NJ 07112
Attn: Monroe Karetzky, M.D.
201-926-6668
FAX: 201-923-6672

Trenton

Sleep Disorders Center
Capital Health System at
  Mercer
446 Bellevue Avenue
P.O. Box 1658
Trenton, NJ 08607
Attn: Debra DeLuca, M.D.
Rita Brooks, R.EEG/EP.T,
  RPSGT, CNIM
Paula Page
609-394-4167
FAX: 609-394-4352

Snoring and Sleep Apnea
  Center
Helene Fuld Medical Center

750 Brunswick
Avenue Trenton, NJ 08638
Attn: Marcella Frank, D.O.
Rita Brooks, RPSGT
609-278-6990
FAX: 609-278-6982

Westfield

Sleep Disorders Center of New
  Jersey
2253 South Avenue, Suite 7
Westfield, NJ 07090
David S. Goldstein, M.D.
Michael Lahey, RPSGT
908-789-4244
908-789-2716

NEW MEXICO

Albuquerque

Lovelace Sleep Disorders Center
Lovelace Health Systems
2929 Coors Boulevard NW,
  Suite 106
Albuquerque, NM 87120
Attn: Lee K. Brown, M.D,
  Medical Director
Nancy L. Polnaszek, Director of
  Medical Specialties
505-839-2369

University Hospital Sleep
  Disorders Center
4775 Indian School Road
  Northeast, Suite 307
Albuquerque, NM 87110
Attn: Rose Mills Barry Krakow,
  M.D.
505-272-6101
FAX: 505-272-6112

NEW YORK

Albany

Capital Region Sleep/Wake
  Disorders Center
St. Peter's Hospital and Albany
  Medical Center
25 Hackett Boulevard
Albany, NY 12208
Attn: Aaron E. Sher, M.D.
Paul B. Glovinsky, Ph.D.
518-436-9253

Bronx

Sleep/Wake Disorders Center
Montefiore Medical Center
111 East 210th Street
Bronx, NY 10467
Attn: Michael J. Thorpy, M.D.

Cooperstown

Bassett Healthcare Sleep
  Disorders Center
One Atwell Road
Cooperstown, NY 13326
Attn: Lee C. Edmonds, M.D.
Robert C. Reese, RRT,
  RPSGT
607-547-6979

Elmira

St. Joseph's Hospital Sleep
  Disorders Center
St. Joseph's Hospital

555 East Market Street
Elmira, NY 14902
Attn: Kathleen R. Reilly, BS,
  RRT
Paula Cook, RRT 607-737-
  7008

Mineola

Sleep Disorders Center
Winthrop-University Hospital
222 Station Plaza North
Mineola, NY 11501
Attn: Michael Weinstein, M.D.,
  FCCP
Maritza Groth, M.D., FCCP
Claude Albertario, RPSGT
516-663-3907
FAX: 516-663-4788
E-MAIL: mweinstein@-
  winthrop.org

New Hyde Park

Sleep-Wake Disorders Center
Long Island Jewish Medical
  Center
270-05 76th Avenue
New Hyde Park, NY 11042
Attn: Harly Greenberg, M.D.
Gershon Ney, M.D.
Jane Luchsinger, M.S.
718-470-7058
Web site: www.LIJ.edu

New York

New York Hospital-Cornell
  Manhattan Campus
520 East 70th Street
New York, NY 10021
Attn: Daniel Wagner, M.D.
Margaret Moline, Ph.D.
914-997-5751

Sleep Disorders Institute
St. Luke's/Roosevelt Hospital
  Center
1090 Amsterdam Avenue
New York, NY 10025
Attn: Gary K. Zammit, Ph.D.
  212-523-1700
FAX: 212-523-1704

The Sleep Disorders Center
Columbia-Presbyterian Medical
  Center
161 Fort Washington Avenue
New York, NY 10032
Attn: Neil B. Kavey, M.D.
  212-305-1860 or 914-948-
  0400
FAX: 212-305-5496
E-MAIL: nbk1@
  columbia.edu

Rochester

Sleep Disorders Center of
  Rochester
2110 Clinton Avenue South
Rochester, NY 14618

Attn: Donald W. Greenblatt,
  M.D.
716-442-4141
FAX: 716-442-6259

Stony Brook

Sleep Disorders Center
State University of New York at
  Stony Brook
University Hospital, MR 120 A
Stony Brook, NY 11794-7139
Attn: Marta Maczaj, M.D.
516-444-2916

Syracuse

The Sleep Center
Community General Hospital
Broad Road Syracuse, NY
  13215
Attn: Robert E. Westlake, M.D.
Bruce D. Hall, RPSGT, RRT
315-492-5877
  FAX: 315-492-5521

The Sleep Laboratory
St. Joseph's Hospital Health
  Center
945 East Genesee Street, Suite
  300
Syracuse, NY 13210
Attn: Edward T. Downing,
  M.D.
Stephen F. Swierczek, RPSGT
315-475-3379

Utica

The Mohawk Valley Sleep
 Disorders Center
St. Elizabeth Medical Center
 2209 Genesee Street
Utica, NY 13501
Attn: Steven A. Levine, D.O.,
 FCCP
Mark Cassidy, RPSGT
315-734-3484
FAX: 315-734-3494

White Plains

Sleep-Wake Disorders Center
The New York Hospital–
 Cornell Medical Center
21 Bloomingdale Road
White Plains, NY 10605

Attn: Daniel R. Wagner, M.D.,
 Medical Director
Margaret L. Moline, Ph.D.,
 Director
914-997-5751
FAX: 914-682-6911
E-MAIL: dwagnerc/
 owestnyh@nyh.med.
 cornell.edu or
mmolinec/owestnyh@nyh.med.
 cornell.edu

The Sleep Disorders Center
White Plains Columbia-
 Presbyterian Medical Center
185 Maple Avenue
White Plains, NY 10601
Attn: Neil B. Kavey, M.D.
914-948-0595

NORTH CAROLINA

Asheville

Sleep Medicine Center of
 WNC
1091 Hendersonville Road
Asheville, NC 28803
Attn: John S. Morris, M.D.
Harriet Pruitt, RPSGT
704-277-7533
FAX: 704-277-7493

Western Carolina Sleep Center
Mission/St. Joseph's Health
 System
445 Biltmore Ave., Suite 404
Asheville, NC 28801
Attn: Jean C. Hardy, RPSGT,

704-258-6708
FAX 704-258-6702

Charlotte

Carolinas Sleep Services
University Hospital
P.O. Box 560727
8800 North Tyron Street
Charlotte, NC 28256
Attn: Mindy B. Cetel, M.D.
Paul D. Knowles, M.D.
Mary Susan Esther, M.D.
Michael Stolzenbach, RPSGT
704-548-5855
FAX: 704-548-6848

Carolinas Sleep Services
Mercy Hospital South
10628 Park Road
Charlotte, NC 28210
Attn: Mindy B. Cetel, M.D.
Michael Stolzenbach, RPSGT
704-543-2213

Greensboro

Sleep Disorders Center
The Moses H. Cone Memorial
  Hospital
1200 North Elm Street
Greensboro, NC 27401-1020
Attn: Clinton D. Young, M.D.
Reggie Whitsett, RPSGT
336-574-7406

Salisbury

Sleep Medicine Center of
  Salisbury
911 West Henderson Street,
  Suite L30
Salisbury, NC 28144

Attn: Dennis L. Hill, M.D.
Deborah Kooy, RPSGT
704-637-1533
FAX: 704-637-0470
E-MAIL: drhill@-
  salisbury.net

Sleep Disorders Center
Winston-Salem North Carolina
  Baptist Hospital
Bowman Gray School of
  Medicine Medical Center
  Boulevard
Winston-Salem, NC 27157
Attn: W. Vaughn McCall, M.D.
  Linda Quinlivan
910-716-5288

Summit Sleep Disorders Center
160 Charlois Boulevard
Winston-Salem, NC 27103
Attn: J. Baldwin Smith, III,
  M.D.
Richard Doud Bey, M.D.
910-765-9431
FAX: 910-765-4889

NORTH DAKOTA

No Accredited Member Center

OHIO

Cincinnati

Sleep Disorders Center
Bethesda Oak Hospital
619 Oak Street
Cincinnati, OH 45206
Attn: Virgil Wooten, M.D.
513-569-6320
FAX: 513-569-5495

The Tri-State Sleep Disorders
  Center
1275 East Kemper Road
Cincinnati, OH 45246
Attn: Martin B. Scharf, Ph.D.
513-671-3101

Cleveland

Pulmonary Medicine Associates'
  Cardiopulmonary Sleep
  Laboratory
Pulmonary Medicine Associates,
  Inc.
15805 Puritas Avenue
Cleveland, OH 44135
Attn: Paul C. Venizelos, M.D.,
  FCCP
Babu M. Eapen, M.D., FCCP
Belinda Gray, RPSGT
216-267-5933
FAX: 216-267-5133

Sleep Disorders Center
The Cleveland Clinic
  Foundation
9500 Euclid Avenue, Desk S-51
Cleveland, OH 44195

Attn: Dudley S. Dinner, M.D.
216-444-2165 FAX: 216-445-
  4378

University Sleep Center
University Hospitals of
  Cleveland
Department of Neurology
11100 Euclid Avenue
Cleveland, OH 44106
Attn: Carl Rosenberg, M.D.
Lucica Buzoianu
216-844-1301

Columbus

Sleep Disorders Center
The Ohio State University
  Medical Center
Rhodes Hall, S1039
410 West 10th Avenue
Columbus, OH 43210-1228
Attn: Greg Landholt, RPSGT
Charles P. Pollak, M.D.
614-293-8296
FAX: 614-293-4506

Dayton

The Center for Sleep & Wake
  Disorders
Miami Valley Hospital
One Wyoming Street, Suite
  G-200
Dayton, OH 45409
Attn: James Graham, M.D.
Kevin Huban, Psy.D.
937-208-2515

Dublin

Ohio Sleep Medicine and
  Neuroscience Institute
4975 Bradenton Avenue
Dublin, OH 43017
Attn: Helmut S. Schmidt, M.D.
Betty Hammonds 614-766-
  0773
FAX: 614-766-2599
E-MAIL: 73204.100@-
  compuserve.com

Kettering

Sleep Disorders Center
Kettering Medical Center
3535 Southern Boulevard
Kettering, OH 45429-1295
Attn: Donna Arand, Ph.D.
937-296-7805
FAX: 937-296-7821
E-MAIL: donna_arand@
  Ketthealth.com

Montrose

Ohio Sleep Disorders Centers
150 Springside Drive
Montrose, OH 44333 Attn: Jose
  Rafecas, M.D.
Frankie Roman, M.D.
330-670-1290
FAX: 330-670-1292

Toledo

Northwest Ohio Sleep
  Disorders Center
The Toledo Hospital
Harris–McIntosh Tower, Second
  Floor
2142 North Cove Boulevard
Toledo, OH 43606
Attn: Pam Lang, RPSGT
Frank O. Horton, III, M.D.
419-471-5629
FAX: 419-479-6954

Sleep Disorders Center St.
Vincent Medical Center
2213 Cherry Street Toledo,
  OH 43608-2691
Attn: Joseph I. Shaffer, Ph.D.
419-321-4980

Zanesville

Sleep Disorders Center
Genesis Health Care System
Good Samaritan Medical
  Center
800 Forest Avenue
Zanesville, OH 43701
Attn: Roger J. Balogh, M.D.
Thomas E. Rojewski, M.D.
Robert J. Thompson, M.D.
614-454-5855
FAX: 614-455-7646

OKLAHOMA

Oklahoma City

Sleep Disorders Center of
  Oklahoma
Integris Health
4401 South Western Avenue

Oklahoma City, OK 73109
Attn: Jonathan R.L. Schwartz,
  M.D.
Chris A. Veit, M.S.W., RPSGT
405-636-7700

OREGON

Eugene

Sleep Disorders Center
Sacred Heart Medical Center
1255 Hilyard Street
P.O. Box 10905
Eugene, OR 97440
Attn: Rodney Roth, RRT,
  RCP
Robert Tearse, M.D.
503-686-7224
E-MAIL: rroth@peace
  health.org

Medford

Sleep Disorders Center
Rogue Valley Medical Center
2825 East Barnett Road
Medford, OR 97504
Attn: Eric Overland, M.D.
Michael Schwartz, RPSGT
Nic Butkov, RPSGT
541-608-4320
FAX: 541-608-5890

Portland

Legacy Good Samaritan Sleep
  Disorders Center

Neurology, N-450
1015 Northwest 22nd Avenue
Portland, OR 97210
Attn: John J. Greve, M.D.,
  Medical Director
Jan White, Manager
503-413-7540
FAX: 503-413-6919

Sleep Disorders Laboratory
Providence Medical Center
4805 Northeast Glisan Street
Portland, OR 97213
Attn: Keith D. Hyde, MBA,
  RRT
Dianne Hurst, CRET
Louis Libby, M.D.
503-215-6552
FAX: 503-215-6031

Pacific NW Sleep/Wake
  Disorders Program, Suite 202
1849 NW Kearney
Portland, OR 97209
Gerald B. Rich, M.D.
Ranae Beck
503-228-4414
503-228-7293

Salem

Salem Hospital Sleep Disorders
 Center
Salem Hospital
665 Winter Street
Southeast Salem, OR 97309-
 5014
Attn: Mark T. Gabr, M.D.
Stephen J. Baughman, RRT,
 RPSGT
503-370-5170
FAX: 503-375-4722

PENNSYLVANIA

Abington

Sleep Disorders Center
Abington Memorial Hospital
1200 Old York Road
2nd Floor, Rorer Building
Abington, PA 19001
Attn: B. Franklin Diamond,
 M.D.
Albert D. Wagman, M.D.
Kevin R. Booth, M.D.
215-576-2226
Web site: www.amh.org

Allentown

Sacred Heart Sleep Disorders
 Center
Sacred Heart Hospital
421 Chew Street
Allentown, PA 18102
Attn: William R. Pistone, M.D.
Ross Futerfas, M.D.
K. Alexander Haraldsted, M.D.
David J. Brooks, RRT, RPSGT
610-776-5333
FAX: 610-776-5110

Bristol

Sleep Disorders Center

Lower Bucks Hospital
501 Bath Road
Bristol, PA 19007
Attn: Howard J. Lee, M.D.
215-785-9752
FAX: 215-785-9068

Doylestown

Penn Center for Sleep Disorders
800 West State Street
Doylestown, PA 18901
Attn: Richard J. Schwab, M.D.
Alan I. Pack, M.D., Ph.D.
Louis Metzger
215-345-5003
FAX: 215-345-5047

Lancaster

Sleep Disorders Center of
 Lancaster
Lancaster General Hospital
555 North Duke Street
Lancaster, PA 17604-3555
Attn: Harshadkumar B. Patel,
 M.D.
James M. O'Connor, RPSGT
717-290-5910
FAX: 717-290-4964

Langhorne

Saint Mary Sleep/Wake
  Disorder Center
Langhorne-Newtown Road
Langhorne, PA 19047
Attn: Howard J. Lee, M.D.,
  Medical Director
James J. Burke, Administrative
  Director
215-741-6744
FAX: 215-741-6695

Paoli

Sleep Disorders Center
Paoli Memorial Hospital
255 West Lancaster Avenue
Paoli, PA 19301
Attn: Donald D. Peterson,
  M.D.
Mark R. Pressman, Ph.D.
610-645-3400

Philadelphia

Penn Center for Sleep Disorders
University of Pennsylvania
  Medical Center
3400 Spruce Street 11 Gates
  West
Philadelphia, PA 19104
Attn: Allan I. Pack, M.D.,
  Ph.D.
Richard J. Schwab, M.D.
Louis F. Metzger
215-662-7772
FAX: 215-349-8038

Pennsylvania Hospital Sleep
  Disorders Center
Pennsylvania Hospital
8th and Spruce Streets
Philadelphia, PA 19107
Attn: Charles R. Cantor, M.D.
Ronald L. Kotler, M.D.
215-829-7079
FAX: 215-625-9187

Sleep Disorders Center
Department of Neurology MCP
Hahnemann School of
  Medicine
Allegheny University of the
  Health Sciences
3200 Henry Avenue
Philadelphia, PA 19129
Attn: June M. Fry, M.D.,
  Ph.D., Chief, Division of
  Somnology
215-842-4250
FAX: 215-848-3850

Sleep Disorders Center
Thomas Jefferson University
1025 Walnut Street, Suite 316
Philadelphia, PA 19107
Attn: Karl Doghramji, M.D.
215-955-6175
FAX: 215-923-8219
E-MAIL: karl.doghramji@mail.
  tju.edu

Temple Sleep Disorders Center
Temple University Hospital
3401 North Broad Street, 4th
  Floor Rock Pavilion
Philadelphia, PA 19140
Attn: Samuel Krachman, D.O.
Thomas Berger, BA, RPSGT
215-707-8163
FAX: 215-707-3876

Pittsburgh

Pulmonary Sleep Evaluation
  Laboratory
University of Pittsburgh
  Medical Center
Montefiore University Hospital
3459 Fifth Avenue, S639
Pittsburgh, PA 15213
Attn: Nancy Kern, CRTT,
  RPSGT
Mark H. Sanders, M.D.
Patrick J. Strollo, M.D.
412-692-2880
FAX: 412-692-2888

Sleep and Chronobiology
  Center
Western Psychiatric Institute
  and Clinic
3811 O'Hara Street
Pittsburgh, PA 15213-2593
Attn: Charles F. Reynolds III,
  M.D.
412-624-2246
FAX: 412-624-2841

Scranton

Sleep Disorders Center
Community Medical Center
1822 Mulberry Street
Scranton, PA 18510
Attn: S. Ramakrishna, M.D.,
  FCCP
717-969-8931

Upland

Sleep Disorders Center
Crozer-Chester Medical Center
One Medical Center Boulevard
Upland, PA 19013-3975
Attn: Calvin Stafford, M.D.
610-447-2689
FAX: 610-447-2918
E-MAIL: staffordc@auhs.edu

Wilkes-Barre

Sleep Disorders Center
Mercy Hospital
25 Church Street
Wilkes-Barre, PA 18765
Attn: John Della Rosa, M.D.
717-826-3410
FAX: 717-820-6658

Wynnewood

Sleep Disorders Center
The Lankenau Hospital
100 Lancaster Avenue
Wynnewood, PA 19096
Attn: Mark R. Pressman, Ph.D.
Donald D. Peterson, M.D.
610-645-3400

RHODE ISLAND

No Accredited Member
Centers

SOUTH CAROLINA

Charleston

Roper Sleep/Wake Disorders
  Center
Roper Hospital 316 Calhoun
  Street
Charleston, SC 29401-1125
Attn: William T. Dawson, Jr.,
  M.D.
Wayne C. Vial, M.D.
Graham C. Scott, M.D.
Tim Fultz, M.S., RRT,
  RPSGT
803-724-2246
Web site: www.carealliance.com

Columbia

Sleep Disorders Center of
  South Carolina
Baptist Medical Center
Taylor at Marion Streets
Columbia, SC 2922
Attn: Richard Bogan, M.D.,
  FCCP
Sharon S. Ellis, M.D.,
  Neonatologist
803-771-5847 or 800-368-1971
FAX: 803-401-3080

Easley

Southeast Regional Sleep
  Disorders Center
Easley 200 Fleetwood Drive
P.O. Box 2129
Easley, SC 29640
Attn: Freddie E. Wilson, M.D.,
  Medical Director
Katrinka Scalise
864-855-7200
FAX: 864-627-9301

Greenville

Sleep Disorders Center
Greenville Memorial Hospital
701 Grove Road
Greenville, SC 29605
Attn: Don McMahan
864-455-8916
FAX: 864-455-4670

Southeast Regional Sleep
  Disorders Center
3900 Pelham Road
Greenville, SC 29615
Attn: Freddie E. Wilson, M.D.,
  Medical Director
864-627-5337
FAX: 864-627-9301

Rock Hill

Carolinas Sleep Services
1665 Herlong Court, Suite B
Rock Hill, SC 29732
Attn: Michael A. Stolzenbach,
  RPSGT, Manager
William C. Sherrill, M.D.
  Medical Director
803-817-1915

Spartanburg

Sleep Disorders Center
Spartanburg Regional Medical
  Center
101 East Wood Street
Spartanburg, SC 29303
Attn: Shari Angel Newman,
  RPSGT
864-560-6904
FAX: 864-560-7083

SOUTH DAKOTA

Rapid City

The Sleep Center
Rapid City Regional Hospital
353 Fairmont Boulevard
P.O. Box 6000
Rapid City, SD 57709
Attn: K. Alan Kelts, M.D., Ph.D.
Terry Anderson, B.S., RRCP
605-341-8037

Sioux Falls

Sleep Disorders Center
Sioux Valley Hospital
1100 South Euclid
Sioux Falls, SD 57117-5039
Attn: Liz Grav
605-333-6302
FAX: 605-333-4402

TENNESSEE

Hermitage

Summit Center for Sleep
  Related Breathing Disorders
Columbia-Summit Medical
  Center
5655 Frist Boulevard MOB-
  Suite 401
Hermitage, TN 37076
Attn: Timothy L. Morgenthaler,
  M.D.
Lee Ann Covington, RRT,
  RPSGT

615-316-3495
FAX: 615-316-3493

Jackson

Sleep Disorders Laboratory
Regional Hospital of Jackson
367 Hospital Boulevard
Jackson, TN 38303
Attn: Thomas W. Ellis, M.D.
David M. Larsen, M.D.
Charlie Carroll, RPSGT
901-661-2148
FAX: 901-661-2441

Knoxville

Sleep Disorders Center
Ft. Sanders Regional Medical
  Center
1901 West Clinch Avenue
Knoxville, TN 37916
Attn: Thomas G. Higgins, M.D.
Bert A. Hampton, M.D.
C. Keith Hulse, Ph.D.
423-541-1375
FAX: 423-541-1837

Sleep Disorders Center
St. Mary's Medical Center
900 East Oak Hill Avenue
Knoxville, TN 37917-4556
Attn: William Finley, Ph.D.,
  Director 423-545-6746
FAX: 423-545-3115
E-MAIL: bfinley@smhs.
mercy.com

Memphis

BMH Sleep Disorders Center
Baptist Memorial Hospital
899 Madison Avenue
Memphis, TN 38146
Attn: Helio Lemmi, M.D.
901-227-5337
FAX: 901-227-5652

Sleep Disorders Center
Methodist Hospitals of Memphis
1265 Union Avenue
Memphis, TN 38104
Attn: Kristin W. Lester, Manager
Robert Neal Aguillard, M.D.,
  Medical Director
901-726-REST
FAX: 901-726-7395

Murfreesboro

Sleep Disorders Center
Middle Tennessee Medical
  Center
400 North Highland Avenue
Murfreesboro, TN 37130
Attn: Timothy J. Hoelscher, Ph.D.
William H. Noah, M.D.
615-849-4811
FAX: 615-849-4833

Nashville

Baptist Sleep Center
Baptist Hospital
2000 Church Street
Nashville, TN 37236
Attn: J. Michael Bolds, M.D.,
  Director
Stephen J. Heyman, M.D.,
  Co-Director
615-329-6306
FAX: 615-284-4781

Sleep Disorders Center
Centennial Medical Center
2300 Patterson Street
Nashville, TN 37203
Attn: David A. Jarvis, M.D.
Marcie T. Poe
615-342-1670

Sleep Disorders Center
Saint Thomas Hospital
P.O. Box 380
Nashville, TN 37202
Attn: J. Brevard Haynes, Jr.,
  M.D.
Susan L. Snyder, Ph.D.
615-222-2068

TEXAS

Amarillo

NWTH Sleep Disorders Center
Northwest Texas Hospital
P.O. Box 1110 Amarillo, TX
  79175
Attn: Michael Westmoreland,
  M.D.
John Moss, CRTT
806-354-1954
 FAX: 806-351-4293

Dallas

Sleep Medicine Institute
Presbyterian Hospital of Dallas
8200 Walnut Hill Lane
Dallas, TX 75231
Attn: Philip M. Becker, M.D.
Andrew O. Jamieson, M.D.
Wolfgang Schmidt-Nowara,
  M.D.
214-750-7776
FAX: 214-750-4621
Web site: www.sleepmed.com

Sleep Disorders Center for
  Children
Children's Medical Center of
  Dallas
1935 Motor Street
Dallas, TX 75235
Roya Tompkins

John Herman, Ph.D.
Joel Steinberg, M.D.
214-640-2793, 214-640-7671

El Paso

Sleep Disorders Center
Providence Memorial Hospital
2001 North Oregon
El Paso, TX 79902
Attn: Gonzalo Diaz, M.D.,
  FCCP
Joseph Arteaga, RPSGT
915-577-6152

Sleep Disorders Center
Columbia Medical Center East
10301 Gateway West
El Paso, TX 79925
Attn: Gonzalo Diaz, M.D.
Elizabeth Baird, RPSGT
915-595-9246

Sleep Disorders Center
Columbia Medical Center West
1801 North Oregon
El Paso, TX 79902
Attn: Gonzalo Diaz, M.D.
Jean R. Joseph-Vanderpool,
  M.D.,
Elizabeth Baird, RPSGT
915-521-1257

Fort Worth

Sleep Consultants, Inc.
1521 Cooper Street
Fort Worth, TX 76104
Attn: Edgar Lucas, Ph.D.
C. Marshall Bradshaw, M.D.
John R. Burk, M.D.
817-332-7433
FAX: 817-336-2159
E-MAIL: sleepcon@flash.net
Web site: www.flash.net/
 ˜sleepcon

Houston

Sleep Disorders Center
Columbia Spring Branch
 Medical Center
8850 Long Point Road
Houston, TX 77055
Attn: Todd J. Swick, M.D.
Kristyna M. Hartse, Ph.D.
713-973-6483
FAX: 713-722-3248
E-MAIL: hartsekm@intergate.
 com or tswick@ix.
 metcom.com

Sleep Disorders Center
Department of Psychiatry
Baylor College of Medicine and
 VA Medical Center
One Baylor Plaza
Houston, TX 77030
Attn: Constance Moore, M.D.,
 Director
Max Hirshkowitz, Ph.D.,
 Co-Director
713-798-4886 or
713-794-7563
FAX: 713-798-4099 or 713-
 794-7558
E-MAIL: maxh@bcm.tmc.edu
 or cmoore@bcm.tmc.edu

Temple

Sleep Disorders Center
Scott and White Clinic
2401 South 31st Street
Temple, TX 76508
Attn: Francisco Perez-Guerra,
 M.D.
817-724-2554

UTAH

Murray

Intermountain Sleep Disorders
  Center of Murray
Cottonwood Hospital
5770 South, 300 East
Murray, UT 84106
Attn: James M. Walker, Ph.D.
Robert J. Farney, M.D.
801-269-2015
FAX: 801-269-2948

Salt Lake

Intermountain Sleep Disorders
  Center
LDS Hospital
325 8th Avenue
Salt Lake City, UT 84143
Attn: James M. Walker, Ph.D.
Robert J. Farney, M.D.
801-321-3617
FAX: 801-321-5110
E-MAIL: ldjwalke@ihc.com

Sleep Disorders Center
University Health Sciences
  Center
50 North Medical Drive
Salt Lake City, UT 84132
Attn: Laura Czajkowski, Ph.D.
Christopher R. Jones, M.D.,
  Ph.D., Medical Director
801-581-2016
FAX: 801-585-3249

VERMONT

No Accredited Member Centers

VIRGINIA

Annandale

Fairfax Sleep Disorders Center
3289 Woodburn Road, Suite
  360
Annandale, VA 22003
Attn: Konrad W. Bakker, M.D.
Marc Raphaelson, M.D.
703-876-9870

Danville

Virginia-Carolina Sleep
  Disorders Center
159 Executive Drive, Suite D
Danville, VA 24541
Attn: Della C. Williams, M.D.,
  Medical Director
Jacalyn A. Nelson, M.D.
William Underwood, RPSGT
Nancy Craig Williams, BS,
  RPSGT
804-792-2209
FAX: 804-799-8037
E-MAIL: vanc.sleep@juno.com

Norfolk

Sleep Disorders Center for
  Adults and Children
Eastern Virginia Medical School
Sentara Norfolk General
  Hospital
600 Gresham Drive Norfolk,
  VA 23507
Attn: Reuben H. McBrayer, M.D.
J. Catesby Ware, Ph.D.
Jeffery A. Scott, M.D.
Tom Bond, Psy.D.

Nancy Fishback, M.D.
757-668-3322
FAX: 757-668-2628
E-MAIL: cware@intmed1.
  evms.edu or
rmcbrayer@intmed1.evms.edu

Richmond

Sleep Disorders Center
Medical College of Virginia
P.O. Box 980710 - MCV
Richmond, VA 23298-0710
Attn: Rakesh K. Sood, M.D.
804-828-1490
FAX: 804-828-1481

Roanoke

Sleep Disorders Center
Carilion Roanoke Community
  Hospital
P.O. Box 12946
Roanoke, VA 24029
Attn: William S. Elias, M.D.
540-985-8526
FAX: 540-985-4963

Virginia Beach

Sleep Disorders Center
Virginia Beach General Hospital
1060 First Colonial Road
Virginia Beach, VA 23454
Attn: Bruce Johnson, M.D.
Yvonne Wright-Dunn, B.A.,
  RPSGT
757-481-8168
FAX: 757-496-6337

WASHINGTON

Auburn

ARMC Sleep Apnea
  Laboratory
Auburn Regional Medical
  Center
Plaza One, 202 North Division
Auburn, WA 98001
Anne W. Casey
253-735-7520

Lakewood

St. Clare Sleep Related
  Breathing Disorders Clinic
St. Clare Hospital 11315
  Bridgeport Way Southwest
Lakewood, WA 98499
Attn: Arthur Knodel, M.D.
Erin Salsbury, RPSGT
253-581-6951

Olympia

Sleep Disorders Center for
  Southwest Washington
Providence St. Peter Hospital
413 North Lilly Road
Olympia, WA 98506
Attn: Kim A. Chase, RPSGT
John L. Brottem, M.D.
360-493-7436
FAX: 360-493-4173

Renton

Sleep Center at Valley Medical
  Center
400 South 43rd Street
Renton, WA 98055
Attn: Carla J. Hellekson, M.D.,
  FAPA
William J. DePaso, M.D.,
  FCCP
206-575-3379
E-MAIL: erin_sheldon@
  valleymed.org

Richland

Richland Sleep Laboratory
800 Swift Boulevard, Suite 260
Richland, WA 99352
Attn: A. Pat Hamner, Jr., M.D.
509-946-4632
FAX: 509-942-0118,
Web site: www.richsleep.com

Seattle

Highline Sleep Disorder Center
Highline Community Hospital
14212 Ambaum Boulevard
  Southwest, Suite 201
Seattle, WA 98166
Attn: Margaret Moen, M.D.,
  Medical Director
John Lovelace, RRT
Erin Salsbury, RPSGT
206-325-7396,
E-MAIL: cmj5@earthlink.net

Providence Sleep Disorders
Center
Jefferson Tower, Suite 203
1600 East Jefferson
Seattle, WA 98122
Attn: Ralph A. Pascualy, M.D.
206-320-2575
FAX: 206-320-3339
E-MAIL: lpascualy@aol.com

Seattle Sleep Disorders Center
Swedish Medical Center/Ballard
P.O. Box 70707
Seattle, WA 98107-1507
Attn: Gary A. DeAndrea, M.D.
Noel T. Johnson, D.O.
Richard P. Swanson, RPSGT,
CRTT
206-781-6359
FAX: 206-781-6196

Virginia Mason Medical Center
Sleep Disorders Center
Virginia Mason Hospital H10-
SDC
925 Seneca Street
Seattle, WA 98101-2742
Attn: Neely E. Pardee, M.D.
Kenneth R. Casey, M.D.
Steven H. Kirtland, M.D.
Nigel J. Ball, D. Phil.
206-625-7180
FAX: 206-341-0447
E-MAIL: sdcsdc@vmmc.org

Spokane

Sleep Disorders Center
Sacred Heart Doctors Building
105 West Eighth Avenue, Suite
418
Spokane, WA 99204
Attn: Elizabeth Hurd, RPSGT
Jeffrey C. Elmer, M.D.
509-455-4895
FAX: 509-626-4578

WEST VIRGINIA

Charleston

Sleep Disorders Center
Charleston Area Medical Center
501 Morris Street
P.O. Box 1393
Charleston, WV 25325
Attn: George Zaldivar, M.D.,
FCCP
Karen Stewart, RRT, Manager
304-348-7507
FAX: 304-348-3373

Parkersburg

PM Sleep Medicine
3803 Emerson Avenue
P.O. Box 4179
Parkersburg, WV 26104
Attn: Michael A. Morehead,
M.D.
M. Barry Louden, M.D.
304-485-5041

WISCONSIN

Appleton

Sleep Disorders Center
Appleton Medical Center
1818 North Meade Street
Appleton, WI 54911
Attn: Kevin C. Garrett, M.D.
920-738-6460
FAX: 920-831-5000

Chippewa Falls

Marshfield Clinic Sleep
  Disorders Center
Marshfield Clinic
2655 County Highway I
Chippewa Falls, WI 54729
Attn: Margaret Feiler
Kevin Ruggles, M.D.
715-726-4136
FAX: 715-726-4173

Eau Claire

Luther/Midelfort Sleep
  Disorders Center
Luther Hospital/Midelfort
  Clinic
1221 Whipple Street
P.O. Box 4105
Eau Claire, WI 54702-4105
Attn: Donn Dexter, Jr., M.D.
David Nye, M.D.
715-838-3165
FAX: 715-838-3845

Green Bay

St. Vincent Hospital Sleep
  Disorders Center
St. Vincent Hospital P.O. Box
13508 Green Bay, WI 54307-
  3508
Attn: John Stevenson, M.D.
Paula Van Ert, RPSGT
920-431-3041
FAX: 920-433-8010

Sleep Disorders Laboratory,
Bellin Hospital,
744 South Webster Avenue,
Green Bay, WI 54305,
John Stevenson, M.D.,
Lee Kvaley, RRT,
920-433-7441,
920-433-7453

La Crosse

Wisconsin Sleep Disorders
  Center
Gundersen Lutheran
1836 South Avenue La Crosse,
  WI 54601
Attn: Alan D. Pratt, M.D.
608-782-7300 x2870
FAX: 608-791-4466

Madison

Comprehensive Sleep Disorders
  Center
B6/579 Clinical Science Center
University of Wisconsin
  Hospitals and Clinics
600 Highland Avenue Madison,
  WI 53792
Attn: Steven M. Weber, Ph.D.
John C. Jones, M.D.
608-263-2387
FAX: 608-263-0412
E-MAIL: smweber@macc.
  wisc.edu or
  jones@neurology.wisc.edu

Sleep Disorders Center
St. Marys Hospital Medical
  Center
707 South Mills Street Madison,
  WI 53716
Attn: Steve Dalebroux
Kathryn L. Middleton, M.D.
608-258-5266
FAX: 608-258-6176

Marshfield

Marshfield Sleep Disorders
  Center
Marshfield Clinic
1000 North Oak Avenue
Marshfield, WI 54449
Attn: Jody Scherr, RPSGT/
  R.EEG.T.
Kevin Ruggles, M.D.
715-387-5397

Milwaukee

Milwaukee Regional Sleep
  Disorders Center
Columbia Hospital
2025 East Newport Avenue
Milwaukee, WI 53211
Attn: Marvin Wooten, M.D.
Joni Tombari, Program Director
414-961-4650
FAX: 414-961-8712

St. Luke's Sleep Disorders
  Center
St. Luke's Medical Center 2801
  West
Kinnickinnic River Parkway,
  Suite 445
Milwaukee, WI 53215
Attn: David Arnold
Michael N. Katzoff, M.D.
414-649-5288
FAX: 414-649-5875

WYOMING

No Accredited Member Centers

Appendix B

Sleep Disorders

The following are brief descriptions of the 78 recognized sleep disorders described in the *International Classification of Sleep Disorders, Diagnostic and Coding Manual,* which is published by the American Sleep Disorders Association.

Dyssomnias

The dyssomnias are disorders that cause either difficulty initiating or maintaining sleep, or cause excessive sleepiness. They are divided into three types: *intrinsic sleep disorders, extrinsic sleep disorders,* and *circadian rhythm disorders.*

Intrinsic sleep disorders

These are disorders that originate or develop within the body.

1. *Psychophysiological insomnia*
People with psychophysiological insomnia react to situations that are psychologically stressful with bodily tension or other physical complaints (upset stomach, headache), and they learn to associate certain things (i.e., going to bed) with emotions that prevent sleep (fear of going to sleep). People with this disorder typically have a focused absorption on their sleep problems, which itself interferes with sleep.

2. *Sleep state misperception*

This disorder involves an honest complaint of insomnia or excessive sleepiness when there is no objective evidence that sleep is disturbed or lacking. People in middle or late adulthood can develop this disorder because they are not able to sleep as long or as well as they could in former years.

3. *Idiopathic insomnia*

Idiopathic insomnia is a lifelong inability to get adequate sleep that has no observable cause. We assume that this difficulty is due to an abnormality of sleep-wake control systems in the brain. It may be due to a problem in the sleep-inducing and -maintaining systems, or hyperactivity in the arousal systems.

4. *Narcolepsy*

Narcolepsy is a disorder characterized by excessive sleepiness, abnormal REM sleep, cataplexy (sudden muscle weakness), hypnagogic hallucinations, and problems sleeping at night. The cause of narcolepsy is not known, but we are now closing in on a gene that contributes to the disorder. This is the only sleep disorder that we know is due to a flaw in the primary sleep systems in the brain.

5. *Recurrent hypersomnia*

People with this disorder have recurrent episodes of extreme sleepiness and huge sleep needs. Episodes of hypersomnia usually last several days to several weeks, and occur twice a year, on average (although they can occur as many as 12 times a year). Patients sleep as much as 18 to 20 hours a day during these episodes, waking only to eat and go to the bathroom. The best described cause of this is Klein-Levin syndrome, which mostly afflicts teenage boys. Patients with this syndrome have not only hypersomnia but also binge eating and hypersexuality.

6. *Idiopathic hypersomnia*

Idiopathic hypersomnia is a disorder in which the patient complains of excessive sleepiness and prolonged sleep at night. The sign that sets people with this disorder apart from normal long sleepers and narcoleptics is that there are numerous episodes of non-REM sleep that last for up to two hours. For this reason, this disorder is sometimes called non-REM narcolepsy. Since extreme sleepiness and large sleep need can be a symptom of many other sleep disorders, like narcolepsy and sleep apnea, it's important to rule out these before making this diagnosis.

7. Posttraumatic hypersomnia

This is excessive sleepiness that develops as the result of physical injury or disease in the central nervous system. It can be caused by brain injury, neurosurgery, infection, or spinal cord injury. The hypersomnia usually goes away over weeks or months.

8. Obstructive sleep apnea syndrome

In obstructive sleep apnea, breathing is blocked during sleep when the airway pulls shut. This causes sleep disruption, dropping oxygen levels in the blood, and cardiovascular problems. This disorder and the problems it leads to are fully described in Chapter 7.

9. Central sleep apnea syndrome

This is a rare type of apnea that occurs not when the throat is blocked but when the patient can't make the effort necessary to pull air into the lungs. It is usually the result of problems in the neurological control of breathing, or with the muscles associated with breathing.

10. Central alveolar hypoventilation syndrome

During sleep, everyone naturally takes less air into the lungs than when awake. If there are problems with gas exchange in the lungs (for instance, caused by emphysema), there may be problems getting enough oxygen during the night, and sleep is disturbed. Because we naturally take in a larger volume of oxygen during the day, there may not be similar problems during the day.

11. Periodic limb-movement disorder

PLM disorder occurs when the sleeper periodically moves a limb (usually a leg) in exactly the same way over the course of the night. A typical movement would be a kick or flex of the leg every 10 seconds. These movements disrupt sleep and lead to insomnia and daytime sleepiness.

12. *Restless legs syndrome*

This syndrome is characterized by uncomfortable feelings (tingling, itching, crawling, pulling, or aching, for example) in the legs right before falling asleep. These feelings are relieved by moving the legs but return when movement stops. This obviously interferes with falling asleep and can cause severe insomnia. Usually patients accumulate large sleep debts after many nights of restless legs, until the resulting powerful sleepiness overcomes the unpleasant feelings and the patient sleeps. Once enough sleep debt is worked off, however, the feelings once again interfere with sleep.

Extrinsic sleep disorders

These disorders are those that originate outside the body. These can be caused by environmental or behavioral factors.

1. *Inadequate sleep hygiene*

People with this disorder have habits that aren't compatible with good sleep or maximum daytime alertness. Caffeine or other drugs near bedtime, or stressful activities before bed, are common problems of sleep hygiene.

2. *Environmental sleep disorder*

This is a complaint of insomnia due to heat, cold, noise, light, or some other condition in the sleep environment. The patient's own sensitivity to the stimulus is usually more important than the level of the stimulus itself. Sensitivity usually increases toward morning, when sleep debt is low.

3. *Altitude insomnia*

This problem occurs when people sleep at high altitudes and are not accustomed to low air pressure and lower than normal oxygen levels. It is usually accompanied by fatigue, headache, and loss of appetite.

4. *Adjustment sleep disorder*

This is a transient insomnia caused by a temporary stressful event. To be diagnosed with this disorder, the insomnia must appear at the same time as an unusual stressful event, and must go away after the event is over.

5. Insufficient sleep syndrome

This is the name given to the experience of someone who persistently fails to get enough sleep to stay normally alert when awake.

6. Limit-setting sleep disorder

Usually found in children, limit-setting sleep disorder occurs when someone stalls or refuses to go to bed. When an absolute bedtime is set and met, then the child falls asleep quickly. When limits (bedtimes) are not set and enforced, or enforced only sporadically, a child's sleep will be delayed, and total sleep may not be enough to meet his sleep needs.

7. Sleep-onset association disorder

This is another disorder usually associated with childhood. In this disorder, the individual is unable to sleep unless certain conditions are met: the light is on, the window is open, the presence of a favorite blanket. When the conditions are met, the child can sleep easily. This rigidity may not normally be a problem, except when the sleep conditions can't be met (a different room, power outage, blanket is in the wash).

8. Food allergy insomnia

Although the name of this disorder is food allergy insomnia, it is usually a food intolerance, such as a lack of enzymes to easily digest milk, that leads to discomfort and difficulty sleeping.

9. Nocturnal eating (drinking) syndrome

This syndrome is characterized by repeated awakenings, with an inability to return to sleep without eating or drinking. This is usually a disorder of childhood, but adults can also become conditioned to eating or drinking at certain times of the night. Once learned, this conditioning leads to repeated awakenings and reinforcement of the pattern.

10. Hypnotic dependent sleep disorder

This inability to sleep is caused by tolerance to or withdrawal from a drug used as a sleep inducer. Such medications commonly include members of the benzodiazepine group.

11. *Stimulant dependent sleep disorder*

Insomnia resulting from dependence on or withdrawal from stimulant drugs such as amphetamines, cocaine, caffeine, or athsma medications.

12. *Alcohol-dependent sleep disorder*

As the name suggests, people with this problem depend on alcohol to get to sleep at night. This usually leads to tolerance—people need more and more alcohol to get to sleep. They also tend to wake up in the middle of the night as the alcohol wears off. For this disorder to be diagnosed, the patient must have used alcohol to help them get to sleep for at least 30 days.

13. *Toxin induced sleep disorder*

A sleep problem caused by the ingestion of poisonous toxins or heavy metals. This is usually found in people who work around these substances, or in children who ingest lead paint or other toxic compounds around the house.

Circadian rhythm sleep disorders

These disorders are grouped together because they share a common theme of disrupting the way sleep occurs over a 24-hour period.

1. *Time zone change (jet lag) syndrome*

This common disorder is the result of rapidly changing time zones, usually as the result of jet flight. The disagreement between the body's internal clock and local time causes trouble getting to sleep at night, daytime sleepiness, and physical problems like stomach upset.

2. *Shift-work sleep disorder*

Transient insomnia or excessive sleepiness that results when work schedules change or are incompatible with nonwork sleep-wake cycles.

3. *Irregular sleep-wake pattern*

This is a disorder in which individuals have not set times for sleeping and for waking up, with the result that they can have trouble sleeping or waking when they try to do either. People who are restricted to bed, or who are in an environment without a regular daily routine can be at risk for developing this disorder.

4. *Delayed-sleep-phase syndrome*
This is a disorder in which nightly sleep is delayed until long after the desired sleep time. This results in sleep-onset association disorder and trouble waking at the desired time.

5. *Advanced-sleep-phase syndrome*
This is a disorder in which nightly sleep and irresistible sleepiness come before the desired time, and the patient wakes up earlier than desired in the morning.

6. *24-hour sleep-wake syndrome*
People with this syndrome have the kind of sleep pattern usually seen in experiments where people are isolated from time cues. They sleep as if they have a free-running biological clock, and have a daily sleep delay of 1 to 2 hours after the previous night's sleep time.

Parasomnias

These disorders are not primarily disorders of sleep and wake states per se—rather, they are disorders of partial arousal or disorders that interfere with sleep stage transitions.

Arousal disorders
1. *Confusional arousals*
Also called sleep drunkenness or excessive sleep inertia, this disorder is an extreme example of the slowness most people feel upon awakening. People with confusional arousals respond poorly to commands or questions, and they have major memory impairment of things that have just happened or happened a short time before. Behaviors are often strange, such as picking up a lamp and talking because the person believes it is a phone. These typically occur when someone is aroused from a deep sleep in the first part of the night.

2. *Sleepwalking*
Sleepwalkers engage in behaviors not usually associated with sleep, such as sitting up in bed, walking about, or even frantic attempts to "escape." These actions are apparently initiated during slow wave sleep. Sleepwalking may end by itself when the sleepwalker returns to bed and goes back to sleep, but if the sleepwalker wakes, he is often extremely confused.

3. *Night terrors*

This disorder is characterized by a sudden arousal from slow wave sleep with a piercing scream or cry and signs of intense fear. The individual usually sits up in bed with eyes open, but is unresponsive to other people or stimuli. If awakened, the patient is confused and disoriented. People usually can't remember the event or have vague, dreamlike images of it. This is usually a disorder of childhood.

Sleep-wake transition disorders

1. *Rhythmic movement disorder*

This a group of repeated movements (usually in the head and neck) that typically occur immediately before sleep. This disorder is usually found in children age one or younger. The child may lie prone and repeatedly lift the head or entire upper body, and then forcibly bang the head back on the pillow. Or the child may sit against the wall or headboard and repeatedly bang the back of his head against it. Because of this, the disorder is sometimes called "head banging," but it can involve other movements, such as a body rolling or rocking on hands and knees.

2. *Sleep starts*

These are sudden, brief contraction of muscles in the legs, arms, or head, which occur just as people are falling asleep. These hypnagogic jerks are felt by most people at some time, but when they are very strong or frequent they can lead to insomnia.

3. *Sleep talking*

This problem can be precipitated by emotional stress, fever, or sleep disorders such as night terrors or even sleep apnea. Sleep talk is usually benign, although it may bother bed partners or family members. The talk is usually brief and devoid of emotional content, but it can be a long speech or infused with anger and hostility. Sleep talking can be spontaneous or induced by conversation with the sleeper.

4. *Nocturnal leg cramps*

As the name suggests, these are leg cramps (usually in the calf) that occur spontaneously during sleep. They may last for only a few seconds or as long as 30 minutes. The cramps cause arousal and disturb sleep. Their cause is not well understood.

Parasomnias usually associated with REM sleep

1. *Nightmares*
Frightening dreams that usually awakened the sleeper from REM sleep.

2. *Sleep paralysis*
Sleep paralysis is a common part of REM sleep itself but is a disorder when it strikes outside REM sleep. Usually, people with sleep paralysis are unable to perform voluntary movements either right before they go to sleep or upon waking in the morning. Sleep paralysis most often lasts for several minutes and then disappears.

3. *Impaired sleep-related penile erections*
In men, erections are a natural part of REM sleep. When REM-related erections are not present, it indicates a physical cause of impotence. Diagnosis of this disorder can be a useful way of differentiating between psychological and physiological impotence.

4. *Sleep-related painful erections*
Sometimes the erections associated with REM sleep can be so intense as to be painful. This may cause nighttime awakenings during REM sleep, and subsequent sleep loss.

5. *REM sleep-related sinus arrest*
This is a rare disorder in which the heart will periodically stop beating during REM sleep. Heart stoppages can last up to nine seconds before starting again. The cause of this disorder is unknown, and is different from cardiac arrest caused by sleep apnea.

6. *REM sleep behavior disorder*
In this disorder, the usual REM-associated muscle paralysis is absent, so that people act out the dreams they are having. Punching, kicking, leaping, and running from the bed are common.

Other parasomnias

1. *Sleep bruxism*
Grinding or clenching teeth during sleep. The sound of grinding teeth can be unpleasant to others who hear it, and can cause excessive tooth

wear in the individual. It can also lead to jaw pain and headaches while awake.

2. Sleep enuresis (bedwetting)

Urination at night is found in every infant, but as children are toilet trained, they become more able to control their bladder at night. Usually, though, regular bedwetting disappears after the age of five. It is estimated that regular bedwetting occurs in 40 percent of 4-year-olds, 10 percent of 6-year-olds, 5 percent of 10-year-olds and 3 percent of 12-year-olds. When there are no other neurological, psychiatric, or urological problems that may cause bedwetting, it is called "primary enuresis." There is evidence that primary enuresis is hereditary. A single recessive gene is thought to be responsible, and there is a high prevalence of primary enuresis among blood relatives of a child with this disorder. If both parents were late bedwetters as children, their child has a 77 percent chance of being a bedwetter. If one parent was a late bedwetter, then the child has a 44 percent chance of having frequent bedwettings after the age of five.

3. Sleep-related abnormal swallowing syndrome

People with this disorder have inadequate swallowing of their saliva while sleeping. Saliva builds up in the mouth, then flows down the throat and is breathed into the lungs. This causes choking and coughing, and wakes up the sleeper.

4. Sudden unexplained nocturnal death syndrome

As the named suggests, this syndrome is typified by sudden death in healthy young adults while they sleep. Neither clinical history nor autopsy provides an explanation for death. The first signs are labored breathing, gasping, and choking, but the disorder is not sleep apnea. Fibrillation (spasm) of the heart muscle has sometimes been detected. Southeast Asian men between 25 and 44 years of age are most often the victims of this disorder, and there are descriptive terms in many Asian languages that suggest sudden unexplained nocturnal death syndrome has long been popularly recognized.

5. Primary snoring

Primary snoring is simply loud upper airway breathing sounds without signs of sleep apnea or diminished breathing.

6. *Infant sleep apnea*

Central or obstructive apneas during sleep in infants. Premature infants are more at risk for this disorder than infants born at term. Infants born before 31 weeks of gestation have about a 50 to 80 percent chance of developing apnea, whereas 7 percent of infants born at term have apnea.

7. *Congenital central hypventilation syndrome*

This is a failure of the automatic control of breathing, so that not enough air is pulled into the lungs. It is usually worse during sleep than during wakefulness. It usually gets better over 6 to 12 months, although children may have to be hospitalized when they get colds or flus until they are four or five years old.

8. *Sudden infant death syndrome*

This is an unexplained sudden death during sleep for which there is no adequate explanation. The cause is still a mystery, although risk factors include laying an infant on his stomach, respiratory infections, being one of a multiple birth, or being born to a substance abusing mother.

9. *Benign neonatal sleep myoclonus*

This is a jerking of the limbs and trunk, or repetitive stretching. The disorder is rare but harmless. The cause is not known.

Medical and psychiatric sleep disorders

Sleep disorders associated with medical disorders

1. *Alcoholism*

Alcohol abuse and dependency commonly disturb sleep. After 30 minutes of alcohol consumption, subjective sleepiness increases and stays high for four hours. After that, sleep become fragmented as the lowered alcohol level increases arousals. When alcoholics abstain from alcohol, sleep can be severely disrupted, and the short episodes of sleep they do get are often plagued by nightmares and other anxiety dreams.

2. *Sleeping sickness*

Also called African sleeping sickness or Gambina trypanosomiasis, this is a chronic protozoan brain infection that produces excessive sleepiness.

3. *Nocturnal cardiac ischemia*
Chest pains due to atherosclerotic heart disease that keep the sleeper awake at night.

4. *Chronic obstructive pulmonary disease*
Lung or bronchial problems that inhibit lung function (like emphysema) can cause severe insomnia.

5. *Asthma*
Asthma attacks during sleep usually awaken the sleeper.

6. *Sleep-related gastroesophageal reflux*
Some people wake from sleep with a sour taste in their mouth or with heartburn. This is because some of the stomach contents have been regurgitated into the esophagus during the night.

7. *Peptic Ulcer*
The pain of ulcers can waken the sleeper frequently during the night.

8. *Fibrositis syndrome*
Also called fibromyositis or fibromalgia. This syndrome is characterized by diffuse muscle and bone pain, chronic fatigue during the day, and unrefreshing sleep at night.

Sleep problems associated with neurological disorders

1. *Degenerative brain disorders*
The many cerebral degenerative disorders can disrupt sleep at night. These include Huntington's disease, Alzheimer's disease, Pick's disease, Parkinson's disease, ALS, and others. Fatal familial insomnia is a rare, inherited degenerative disorder that begins with sleep troubles and progresses within a few months to a total lack of sleep, and then death.

2. *Sleep-related epilepsy*
Epileptic seizures can be found in either wakefulness or sleep, and there are some types that are found mostly in sleep. These seizures disrupt sleep.

3. *Sleep-related headaches*
Headaches can also strike during sleep, and in some people sleep-related headache is more common than waking headaches.

Sleep disorders associated with psychiatric disorders

1. *Psychoses*
Psychoses like schizophrenia and those that are drug-induced are characterized by delusions, hallucinations, incoherence, catatonic behavior, or inappropriate emotions. Insomnia or excessive sleepiness is also common in individuals suffering from such psychoses.

2. *Mood disorders*
Mood disorders include depression, mania, and hypomania. Insomnia is usually the result, but excessive sleepiness can occur too.

3. *Anxiety disorders*
Anxiety disorders are characterized by unusually great anxiety and avoidance of whatever seems to cause it. Anxiety disorders can create sleep-onset association disorders or sleep-maintainance insomnia.

4. *Panic disorder*
Panic disorders are commonly called phobias: claustrophobia (fear of enclosed spaces), agoraphobia (fear of open spaces), and the like. Extreme fear and anxiety can occur unexpectedly, and panic episodes can waken people from their sleep.

Proposed sleep disorders
These are sleep problems for which there is not enough information available to firmly establish them as discrete disorders.

1. *Short sleeper*
A short sleeper is someone who regularly takes less than 75 percent of the sleep time usually required in his or her age group, and feels no negative effects from this shortened sleep. Psychologically, short sleepers are basically normal, with a tendency to hypomanic behavior. They are usually smooth, efficient people who are distinct "nonworriers."

2. *Long sleepers*

Long sleepers need substantially more sleep than most people. This usually means sleeping 10 hours or more for adults. The timing and structure of sleep is normal in true long sleepers—when making this diagnosis it is important to rule out other problems that might lead to long hours in bed. Long sleep is usually acquired in childhood, firmly established by adolescence, and remains a lifelong pattern. Psychologically, long sleepers tend to be more introverted than others, and often appear mildly depressed or anxious when interviewed by researchers. They are often described as worriers.

3. *Subwakefulness syndrome*

Some people complain about a lack of daytime alertness, but they have no nighttime sleep disruption and seem to be getting adequate sleep. There is no objective evidence of severe, excessive sleepiness, but a display of daytime drowsiness can occur. This syndrome may be a less severe version of idiopathic hypersomnia, or may be caused by some other, unrecognized medical or psychiatric disorder.

4. *Fragmentary myoclonus*

Myoclonus is manifest by brief, involuntary jerks or twitches. Some people get this during non-REM sleep throughout the night. The proposed disorder is very rare and harmless.

5. *Sleep hyperhydrosis*

Also known as night sweats, which commonly afflict people when they have a fever. There are some people, however, who sweat heavily at night without any signs of fever or other disorders. Some people sweat excessively during sleep all their lives. The worst problem is sleep disruption, and people often have to get up to change pajamas or sheets.

6. *Menstrual-associated sleep disorder*

There are three forms of menstrual-associated sleep disorders: premenstrual insomnia, premenstrual hypersomnia, and menopausal insomnia. As these three names suggest, menstrual-associated sleep disorder can lead to either less sleep or more sleep than normal.

7. *Pregnancy-associated sleep disorder*
Pregnancy can also lead to either insomnia or excessive sleep and sleepiness. Pregnant women usually start the pregnancy feeling excessive need for sleep, and end pregnancy with insomnia due to physical discomfort. In rare cases, pregnancy and the postpartum period may be associated with nightmares, night terrors, or postpartum psychosis.

8. *Terrifying hypnagogic hallucinations*
When people fall asleep normally, closed eyes and a state of drowsiness give way to reverie, and vague thoughts and images flow through the mind just as sleep is descending. Rarely, these common, unthreatening hypnagogic images can turn threatening, and seem real, partly as a result of how quickly they follow wakefulness. These hallucinations are common in people with narcolepsy, who regularly go into REM sleep right after falling asleep.

9. *Sleep-related laryngospasm*
Very rarely, some people have a spasm of the throat that closes off the airway and halts breathing during sleep. The result is similar to a single episode of apnea, but these patients do not have apnea. Typically, the patient will wake up choking and jump out of bed, clutching the throat. Episodes last anywhere from a few seconds to five minutes. People who get these laryngospams typically experience them only two or three times per year. Drinking water usually speeds the relaxation of throat muscles.

10. *Sleep choking syndrome*
This sleep disorder is also rare, but its victims have episodes of choking almost nightly, and sometimes more than once a night. The patient wakes with feelings of fear, anxiety, and impending death. Fear is always associated with the choking, but patients don't suffer from nightmares, night terrors, or other forms of nocturnal anxiety attacks. They also don't suffer from obstructive sleep apnea. The cause is unknown.

Appendix C

Sleep Web Sites

The Internet has become a very useful network and clearinghouse for information about sleep and sleep disorders. Here's a concise list of some of the most useful sites:

SleepNet
Everything you wanted to know about sleep disorders but were too tired to ask. SleepNet links to over 200 sites.
www.sleepnet.com

American Sleep Disorders Association
A professional medical association representing practitioners of sleep medicine and sleep research.
www.asda.org

National Sleep Foundation
Dedicated to prevention of catastrophic accidents caused by sleep deprivation and excessive sleepiness and to enhanced quality of life for millions who suffer from sleep disorders.
www.sleepfoundation.org

Sleep Medicine Home
This home page lists resources regarding all aspects of sleep, including

the physiology of sleep, clinical sleep medicine, sleep research, federal and state information, patient information, and business-related groups.
www.users.cloud9.net/~thorpy/

The Sleep Well

A reservoir of information on sleep, sleep disorders, and sleep-related events.
www.stanford.edu/~dement/

Children and Sleep Disorders

Children's sleep-disorders symptoms are often different from the symptoms of an adult.
www-leland.stanford.edu/dement/children.html

Restless Legs Syndrome Support Page

Restless Legs Syndrome (RLS) is a movement disorder characterized by unusual sensations that occur typically deep within the legs, occasionally in the arms, and infrequently in other body parts. These sensations compel the sufferer to move the affected extremity to achieve relief. Because RLS is worse during the evening and at night, it can lead to severe insomnia and excessive daytime sleepiness.
www.rls.org

A.P.N.E.A. NET

Dedicated to providing news and education to sleep apnea patients and their family members, and to increasing public awareness of sleep apnea through patient activism.
www.apneanet.org

Sleep & The Traveler

Good information and helpful hints about traveling through different time zones.
www.healthtouch.com/level1/leaflets/sleep/sleep032.htm

American Fibromyalgia Syndrome Association

AFSA is a non-profit organization dedicated to research, education, and patient advocacy for fibromyalgia. The Web page includes information about AFSA, some research projects and grant applications, and resources.
www.AFSAfund.org.